Helix–Loop–Helix Transcription Factors

THIRD EDITION

Trevor D. Littlewood and Gerard I. Evan

Biochemistry of the Cell Nucleus Laboratory,
Imperial Cancer Research Fund, London

OXFORD   NEW YORK   TOKYO
OXFORD UNIVERSITY PRESS
1998

Oxford University Press, Great Clarendon Street, Oxford OX2 6DP

Oxford New York
Athens Auckland Bangkok Bogota Bombay
Buenos Aires Calcutta Cape Town Dar es Salaam
Delhi Florence Hong Kong Istanbul Karachi
Kuala Lumpur Madras Madrid Melbourne
Mexico City Nairobi Paris Singapore
Taipei Tokyo Toronto Warsaw
and associated companies in
Berlin Ibadan

Oxford is a trade mark of Oxford University Press

Published in the United States
by Oxford University Press, Inc., New York

A catalogue record for this book is available from the British Library

Library of Congress Cataloging in Publication Data
Littlewood, Trevor D.
Helix–loop–helix transcription factors / Trevor D. Littlewood and
Gerard I. Evan. – 3rd ed.
(Protein profile)
1. Helix–loop–helix motifs. I. Evan, Gerard I. II. Title.
III. Series.
QP552.T68L58 1997   572.8′65–dc21   97-39870
ISBN 0 19 850248 6 (Pbk)

Typeset and printed by Alden Group, Oxford

Helix–Loop–Helix Transcription Factors

THIRD EDITION

Series preface

The Protein Profile *series has been developed from a recognition that individuals find it increasingly difficult to access readily the enormous amount of information accumulated by the international research community; information which is crucial for the efficiency and quality of their activities.*

The *Protein Profile* series aims to provide a practical, comprehensive and accessible information source on all major families of proteins. Each volume of *Protein Profile* is focused on a single family or sub-family of proteins, and contains tables and figures presenting as comprehensive an accumulation of structural, kinetic and biochemical information available on that particular protein group, coupled to an extensive bibliography. Every volume will be refined and updated to provide users with a practical up-to-date single source of information by the publication of new editions approximately every two years.

Content

The text provides a brief overview of the biological context of the function of the protein group followed by an overview of available information on:

- function
- kinetic and biochemical properties
- sequences, sequence relationships and sequence features
- domain structure
- mutations
- 3-D structure
- binding sites of protein
- ligand binding sites and interactions with drugs
- derivatization sites
- proteolytic cleavage sites

Each volume follows the same format but with different emphases depending on the protein family. The text is extensively supported by tables and figures listing key information gathered from the literature with comprehensive reference to primary sources.

Available protein sequences, or where there are very large numbers, representatives from each sub-group, are aligned in an appendix at the back of each issue.

Available references pertinent to the properties, structure and function of the proteins are listed in a full bibliography. References are numbered for access in the text, but are also arranged alphabetically under headings to allow browsing. Reviews are listed at the beginning and key papers are identified.

An **online version** of the Protein Profile series will be available during 1998. For the latest information about the series, see our web page at
`http://www.oup.co.uk/protein_profile`

Protein Profile

online

Protein Profile is the most comprehensive resource available for information on protein families. **Protein Profile** is available as a series of books, but will also be published online from the middle of 1998 – a new service which will provide a focal point for information in the field of protein science.

A subscription to **Protein Profile Online** will give you:

> ➣ online access to all the **Protein Profile** volumes published by Oxford University Press

> ➣ frequent updates of the data

> ➣ links to abstracts or, if you subscribe to online journals, to complete papers

> ➣ links back to the original sequence and structural data

There is no better way of getting quickly to the information you need.

Protein Profile Online will be introduced during 1998 and there will be a free trial period for you to explore and provide us with feedback on the content and presentation. If you would like to be informed by e-mail or post of the latest news of **Protein Profile Online** please complete the online information request form which you can find at:

http://www.oup.co.uk/protein_profile/?b97

Alternatively, you can write to: Journals Marketing Department, Oxford University Press, Great Clarendon Street, Oxford OX2 6DP, UK. *Tel: +44 (0)1865 267907 Fax: +44 (0)1865 267835 E-mail: jnl.orders@oup.co.uk*

Contents

Bibliography 49

Appendix: Protein sequence alignments 139

List of Figures

List of Tables

Abbreviations

ADD1, adipocyte determination- and differentiation-dependent factor 1
Ah, aryl hydrocarbon
AP4, activator protein 4
Arnt, Ah receptor nuclear translocation protein
AS-C, Achaete-Scute complex (*Drosophila*)
BETA, β cell E box transactivator
bZIP, basic-leucine zipper
CBF1, centromere binding factor 1 (yeast)
CD, circular dichroism
CDEI, conserved DNA element I
cdk, cyclin-dependent kinase
CKII, casein kinase II
class A, class of ubiquitously expressed HLH proteins
class B, class of HLH proteins exhibiting temporally or spatially restricted expression
CNS, central nervous system
Da, Daughterless protein (*Drosophila*)
Del, Delila protein (*Antirrhinum*)
Dpn, Deadpan protein (*Drosophila*)
E box, Ephrussi box, consensus sequence CANNTG
EBV, Epstein–Barr virus
EGF, epidermal growth factor
Emc, Extramacrochaetae protein (*Drosophila*)
ERK1, extracellular-regulated kinase (MAPK)
ES, embryonic stem
E(spl), Enhancer of split protein (*Drosophila*)
FIP, Fos-interacting protein
Ga14, galactose control protein 4
GCN4, general control protein 4 (yeast)
GSKIII, glycogen synthetase kinase III
HEB, HeLa E box binding factor
Hen, helix–loop–helix encoded in neuroblastoma protein
Hes, Hairy- and Enhancer of split-related mammalian proteins
HLF, hepatic leukaemia factor
hnRNP, heterogeneous ribonucleoprotein particle
HPLC, high-performance liquid chromatography
hsp90, heat shock protein 90
ICRE, inositol/cholrine response element
Id, inhibitor of differentiation protein
IFN, interferon
Ig, immunoglobulin
IgE, immunoglobulin E
IgH, immunoglobulin heavy chain
IgM, immunoglobulin M
ITF, immunoglobulin transcription factor
L-Sc, Lethal of Scute protein (*Drosophila*)

LTR, long terminal repeat
Lyl, lymphoid leukaemia protein
Mad, Max-associated dimer protein
MADS, MCM1, agamous deficiens, serum response factor
Mash, mammalian Achaete-Scute homologue protein
Max, Myc-associated x protein
MCK, muscle creatine kinase
MEF2, myocyte specific enhancer-binding factor 2
Mi, microphthalmia protein
MLP, major late promoter of adenovirus
MRF4, muscle regulatory factor 1
Mxil, Max interactor 1 protein
MycER, c-Myc-oestrogen receptor
Myf, myogenic factor
MyoD, myogenic determination factor
N box, consensus sequence CACNAG
NGF, nerve growth factor
NSCL, neurological stem cell leukaemia protein
ODC, ornithine decarboxylase
p107, 107 kDa protein related to Rb
PAS, Per, Arnt-AhR, Sim domain
PCR, polymerase chain reaction
PDGF, platelet-derived growth factor
PKA, cAMP-dependent kinase
PKC, protein kinase C
PNS, peripheral nervous system
Rb, retinoblastoma protein
REF, rat embryo fibroblast
Scl, stem cell leukaemia protein
SDS-PAGE, sodium dodecyl sulphate-poly-acrylamide gel electrophoresis
SH2, Src homology domain 3
SRE-1, sterol regulatory element-1
SREBP, sterol regulatory element binding protein
Tal, T cell acute leukaemia protein
SV40, Simian virus 40
T-ALL, T cell acute lymphoblastic leukaemia
TBP, TATA-binding protein
TCR, T cell receptor
TFII-I, transcription factor II-I
TFE3, transcription factor E3 binding
TFEB, transcription factor enhancer binding
TFEC, transcription factor C
TGF-β, transforming growth factor β
USF, upstream stimulatory factor
WRPW, four amino acid sequence conserved in some HLH proteins
YY1, Yin-Yang-1 protein

Introduction

What are HLH proteins?

The transcription of genes within eukaryotic cells is controlled by complex interactions between transcription factors and specific DNA recognition sequences in target genes. These DNA-binding transcription factors fall into a number of groups, each defined by shared sequence and, presumably structural, motifs. One such motif is the helix–loop–helix (HLH), first identified in an immunoglobulin enhancer-binding polypeptide as well as several other proteins known, or suspected, to be transcription factors [741]. The HLH region has also sometimes been referred to as the 'Myc homology domain', doubtless in deference to the notoriety and perceived importance of Myc proteins in carcinogenesis. However, the HLH motif is present in many proteins of diverse biological function and unified only by their common involvement in transcriptional regulation (reviewed in [3, 4, 32, 34, 43, 51, 62, 64, 69, 1312]). The HLH domain is a dimerization domain that mediates homo- and/or hetero-dimerization with other HLH proteins. The HLH domain is usually adjacent to a short region of basic residues that constitutes the sequence-specific DNA interaction interface; hence such proteins are often referred to as bHLH proteins. A second group of bHLH proteins contains an additional dimerization domain, the leucine zipper [1148], immediately C-terminal to the HLH. These proteins are commonly referred to as bHLHZ proteins. Members of a third group of HLH proteins lack a functional DNA-binding domain and act as negative regulators of bHLH proteins. Proteins containing HLH domains are found throughout evolution (Table 1) and, in many cases, have been isolated more than once from different species, giving rise to a somewhat confusing nomenclature (see Table 2 for a

TABLE 1 Cloned HLH proteins

Group	Family	Proteins	MW (kDa)	Source	References
bHLHZ proteins	Myc	c-Myc	60/64	Mammalian	156, 252, 393, 830, 1071
		N-Myc	62/68	Mammalian	505, 580, 706, 955, 971, 1268
		L-Myc	*68–70	Mammalian	306, 557
		v-Myc	various *gag–myc* fusion proteins	Retroviral transduction of chicken c-*myc*	87, 847
		B-Myc	(19.5)	Mammalian	111
		S-Myc	(47)	Mammalian	979
	Max	Max	*21/22	Mammalian	168
	Mad	Mad1	35	Mammalian	1214
		Mxi1	35	Mammalian	1257
		Mad3	29	Mammalian	1624
		Mad4	32	Mammalian	1624
	AP4	AP4	48	Mammalian	1234, 1772
	USF	USF1	43	Mammalian	426
		USF2	44	Mammalian	950, 1202, 1218, 1716

TABLE 1 Continued

Group	Family	Proteins	MW (kDa)	Source	References
	Ig enhancer binding	TFE3	59	Mammalian	134
		TFEB	(60)	Mammalian	214
		TFEC	(45)	Mammalian	1123
	Mi	Mi	(55)	Mammalian	482, 496
	SREBP	SREBP1a	68 (precursor 125)	Mammalian	1061, 1062, 1109, 1015
		SREBP2	59–68 (precursor ~120)	Mammalian	495
bHLH proteins	Ubiquitous (class A)	E12/E47	*56–70	Mammalian	547, 741,
		ITF-1	(60)	Mammalian	470, 471
		ITF-2	70	Mammalian	470, 472
		HEB	(70)	Mammalian	494
		Daughterless (Da)	82	*Drosophila*	221, 269
	Neurogenic	Single-minded (Sim)	(75)	*Drosophila*	265, 748
		NeuroD	60	Mammalian	1705, 1804
		MATH1	(38)	Mammalian	1324
		MATH2	(39)	Mammalian	1374, 1933
	Achaete–Scute family	Lethal of Scute (L-sc) (T3)	(29)	*Drosophila*	89
		Scute (T4)	(38)	*Drosophila*	1039
		Achaete (T5)	(23)	*Drosophila*	1039
		Asense (T8)	(54)	*Drosophila*	89, 418
		Atonal	34	*Drosophila*	1645
		Mash1	34	Mammalian	532
		Mash2	(28)	Mammalian	532
	Myogenic	MyoD	42	Mammalian	184, 786
		Myogenin	33	Mammalian	184, 185, 894
		Myf5	(29)	Mammalian	187
		MRF4	35	Mammalian	186
	Haemato-poeitic	Lyl1	29	Mammalian	601, 1040
		Lyl2	(30)	Mammalian	1040
		Tal1	37/42, 22/24	Mammalian	96, 98, 135, 231, 232, 412, 1389, 1514
		Tal2	(12)	Mammalian	1098
		Hen1	20	Mammalian	136, 199, 650
		Hen2	15.6	Mammalian	199, 407, 650
		Vav	95	Mammalian	554, 555
	Others	Arnt1	87	Mammalian	485, 860
		Arnt2	85	Mammalian	1603
		Ah receptor	95	Mammalian	206, 346
		Twist	(55)	*Drosophila*	1005
		Delilah	40	*Drosophila*	102
		bHLH–EC2	(25)	Mammalian	824, 1395, 1418
		Scleraxis	~30	Mammalian	1469
		GbHLH1.4	(55)	Mammalian	1589
		Trachealess (Trh)	150	*Drosophila*	2048

TABLE 1 Continued

Group	Family	Proteins	MW (kDa)	Source	References
		BETA3	50	Mammalian	1855
		Thing1	(24)	Mammalian	1468, 1470, 1608, 1958
		Thing2	(24)	Mammalian	1468, 1470, 1608, 1958
	Yeast bHLH proteins	Cbf1	39.4	*Saccharomyces cerevisiae*	121, 209, 702
		Pho4	(34)	*S. cerevisiae*	153, 634, 769, 1111
		Ino2p	(34)	*S. cerevisiae*	1814
		Ino4p	(18)	*S. cerevisiae*	1616
		Rtg1p	(20)	*S.cerevisiae*	1896
		Esc1	(52)	*Schizosaccharomyces pombe*	151
	Plant bHLH proteins	R-Lc	(67)	Maize	662
		R-S	(67)	Maize	795
		Sn	(68)	Maize	1459
		B-Peru	(64)	Maize	832
		Delila (Del)	(70)	*Antirrhinum*	420
HLH proteins lacking a functional DNA-binding domain	Enhancer of split (E(spl))	M4	(17)	*Drosophila*	574
		M5	(20)	*Drosophila*	574
		M7	(21)	*Drosophila*	574
		M8	(20)	*Drosophila*	574
	Mammalian homologues of E(spl)	Hes1	(30)	Mammalian	898
		Hes2	(22)	Mammalian	515
		Hes3	(25)	Mammalian	898, 1903
		Hes5	18.5	Mammalian	79
		Hairy	(37)	*Drosophila*	888
		Deadpan (Dpn)	(43)	*Drosophila*	161
		Extramacro-chaetae (Emc)	(22)	*Drosophila*	344, 391
		Id1	14	Mammalian	143, 1481
		Id2	(15)	Mammalian	1204
		Id3	15	Mammalian	241
		Id4	(15)	Mammalian	866, 1832

Identified HLH proteins are grouped into related families and broad functional groups and the source of the clone and relevant references indicated. For each protein the apparent molecular weight determined from SDS–PAGE is shown. A range of molecular weights (*) indicates known splice variants and/or post-translational modifications. Molecular weights estimated from the protein sequence are indicated in parentheses. P indicates that a partial sequence only is available.

summary). A comparison of the proteins listed in Table 1 is presented in the Appendix.

Not all proteins that possess helix–loop–helix motifs are transcription factors. For example, certain HLH proteins are components of the calcium signalling pathway [16, 48]. However, in this review we will only consider further those HLH proteins that appear to have some role in transcriptional regulation. In this regard, recent elucidation of the three-dimensional structure of isolated bHLH–DNA and bHLHZ–DNA complexes has provided new insights into the way in which these proteins form dimers and interact with their specific DNA recognition sites.

TABLE 2 Proteins with more than one name

Name	Alternative name(s)	Source	References
Max	Myn	Mouse	1244
USF	MLTF1		215
	UEF		715
	NF-λ2	Mouse	228
	CPBF	Rat	1475
USF2	FIP		1218
SREBP	ADD1	Rat	1015
	HLH106	*Drosophila*	1989
E12	BCF1	Human	1043
	Pan2	Rat	753
	XE3	*Xenopus*	1927
	ZFE12	Zebrafish	2062
E47	ALF2	Mouse	1193
	Pan1	Rat	753
	A1	Mouse	1056
HEB	HTF4	Human	1120
	ALF1A/ALF1B	Mouse	1193
	SCBPα/SCBPγ	Rat	648
	REBα/REBβ	Rat	575
	BETA1	Hamster	2112
ITF2	ME1	Mouse	758
	GE1	Chicken	758
	TFE	Dog	527
	XEL1 and XE2	*Xenopus*	1927
	MITF2A and MITF2B	Mouse	1945
MyoD	Myf-3	Human	184
	CMD1	Chicken	649
	Xlmf1	*Xenopus*	907
	Dmyd	*Drosophila*	784
	Nautilus	*Drosophila*	705
	CeMyoD/hlh1	*Caenorhabditis elegans*	588, 1308
	Sum1	Sea urchin	1035
	Amdr1	*Halocynthia roretzi*	1338
Myf5	Bmyf	Cattle	129, 243
Myogenin	Myf-4	Human	184
		Mouse	330, 331
MRF4	Myf-6	Human	186, 861
	Herculin	Mouse	712
Tal1	Scl	Human, mouse	96, 135, 137
	Tcl-5	Human	373
Hen1	NSCL-1	Mouse	136, 650
	Nhlh1	Mouse	1795
Hen2	NSCL-2	Mouse	407, 650
	Nhlh2	Mouse	407

TABLE 2 Continued

Name	Alternative name(s)	Source	References
Scute	Sisterless-b	*Drosophila*	349, 781
Mash1	hASH1	Human	122
	XASH1	*Xenopus*	370
MATH2	NEX1	Rat	1374
NeuroD	BETA2	Hamster	1804
Thing1	Hxt	Mouse	1468
	eHAND	Mouse	1470
Thing2	Hed	Mouse	1468
	dHAND	Mouse	1958
HLH-EC2	Meso1	Hamster	1395
	Paraxis	Mouse	1418
Hes1	Rhl	Rat	366
Id-3	HLH462	Mouse	241
	HLHIR21	Human	302
	Heir-1	Human	345
Cbf1	Cpf1	*S. cerevisiae*	702
	Cp1	*S. cerevisiae*	121
	GF11	*S. cerevisiae*	1495

Clones encoding HLH proteins which have been isolated several times and given different names are shown above. For clarity, the name in the left-hand column is used in this review.

The functions of bHLH proteins

Most known bHLH proteins are transcriptional regulators. That is, they are proteins that are able to alter the genetic programme of cells by repressing or activating specific genes, often genes involved in control of growth and differentiation. Not surprisingly, therefore, inappropriate expression of genes encoding both bHLH and bHLHZ proteins is frequently associated with tumorigenesis and/or developmental dysfunctions.

bHLH proteins can be divided into two broad functional groups by their patterns of expression. In the first group, expression is restricted to cells of a particular lineage. These are sometimes referred to as 'class B' bHLH proteins and examples are the myogenic factors MyoD, Myf5, MRF4 and myogenin. The second group ('class A' bHLH proteins) are expressed fairly ubiquitously. These proteins, for example the E12 transcription factor, typically form heterodimers with the lineage-specific bHLH proteins. A similar classification holds for the bHLHZ proteins. One group comprises members whose expression is either tissue-specific (e.g. the restricted expression of N-Myc [524, 732, 733]) or else correlated with a specific cellular state, for example c-Myc in proliferation, apoptosis and, in some cell types, the potential to differentiate (reviewed in [3, 25, 31, 39, 47, 49]). In order to function, members of this first group must dimerize with members of the second group of bHLHZ proteins which are ubiquitously expressed (e.g. the obligate interaction between the Myc proteins and the ubiquitous bHLHZ protein Max (reviewed in [3])). The functions of both classes of bHLH and bHLHZ proteins are reviewed in this section.

bHLH proteins involved in myogenesis

Several bHLH proteins are involved in the determination of myocytes. The archetypal bHLH family member MyoD1 was originally isolated by screening a monocyte library with a myoblast-specific subtracted probe [293]. Its bHLH domain was first noted because of its limited homology with the bHLH domain of the c-Myc oncoprotein and was even occasionally referred to as 'a Myc homology domain' [741]. Subsequently, however, three further members of the MyoD family were isolated, Myf5 [187], MRF4 [186, 712, 861] and myogenin [184, 185, 330, 331, 1094]. Myogenic bHLH regulatory proteins have been identified in mammals, birds, frogs, fish, sea urchins, insects and nematodes. This remarkable conservation is exemplified by the fact that myogenic bHLH factors from sea urchins and nematodes can induce mammalian myogenesis [588, 589, 1035, 1308]. All four proteins, MyoD1, Myf5, MRF4 and myogenin, share considerable sequence homology which extends beyond the bHLH region, and may have been derived by duplication from a single ancestral gene [1357]. All have the property, when constitutively expressed, of converting a range of different mesenchymal cell types into muscle (reviewed in [7, 8, 21, 22, 23, 43, 50, 52, 63, 67–69, 1298, 1300]). Genetic analysis indicates that MyoD and Myf5 share overlapping functions in generating and/or maintaining muscle cell identity of different skeletal muscle cell lineages [1408] and in localizing myoblasts to muscle compartments, whereas myogenin appears to be required for full differentiation into myotubes [188, 881, 882, 1409, 1768, 1872]. The functions of MRF4 and myogenin appear to be only partially overlapping since mice with targeted mutations in the *myogenin* gene display severe skeletal muscle deficiencies and die perinatally [461, 744] (reviewed in [22, 23, 67, 1314] whereas animals with mutant MRF4 display defective axial myogenesis and rib pattern formation, possibly due to down-regulation of Myf5 [1410, 1528], and die at birth [1842] (reviewed in [1822]). None the less, each of the myogenic proteins probably exerts unique functions in certain situations. Whereas initial experiments demonstrated that Myf5, specifically, is required for normal rib cage development [188, 1560], other experiments show that insertion of the *myogenin* gene into the *myf5* locus (simultaneously disrupting Myf5 function) gives rise to mice with a normal rib cage [2035]. This suggests that the ability of myogenic proteins to compensate for each other's functions may depend, at least partly, on their temporal expression. All four myogenic bHLH proteins bind the same DNA sequence with comparable affinities and their ability to activate specific genes may reside in non-conserved amino acids outside the bHLH domain [670, 1166].

The myogenic bHLH proteins are involved in a complex network of autoregulation and cross-regulation (reviewed in [41, 67]) which involves interaction with non-bHLH intermediate regulators such as members of the MEF2 family [200, 642, 1393, 1557, 1663, 1786, 1880, 2054] (reviewed in [41, 52, 1823]) and other unidentified factors [301, 1550]. For example, MyoD, Myf5 and myogenin all up-regulate their own expression, MyoD and/or Myf5 are required for expression of myogenin, and Myf5 can induce MyoD. In contrast, the universal expression of MyoD in myocyte populations derived from *myf5* homozygous mutant embryonic stem (ES) cells and its premature expression during differentiation of these cells *in vitro* suggests that Myf5 may down-regulate MyoD during early myogenesis, possibly via E box motifs in the *myoD* enhancer [556, 1410]. Similarly complex cross-activation is also known to occur in bHLH proteins involved in *Drosophila* neurogenesis (Fig. 1).

Although members of the MyoD family can each form homodimers, the active myogenic species are thought to be heterodimers between a MyoD family member and a member of the *E2A*-encoded family of ubiquitously expressed bHLH proteins (E12, E47 and ITF1) [1178, 2133]. Commitment to myogenesis is further regulated by three other processes. First, the promoter context of the target gene plays an important role in transcriptional activation by MyoD. Many of the MyoD target genes possess two MyoD binding sites to which MyoD binds cooperatively [144, 1128, 1195, 1663]. Although binding of MyoD

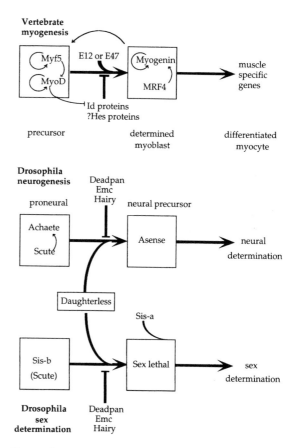

Figure 1
Comparison of HLH protein networks involved in vertebrate myogenesis and *Drosophila* neurogenesis and sex determination. The diagrams illustrate common features of developmental processes involving HLH proteins; they do not include all the factors or cross-regulations. With the exceptions of Sex lethal and Sis-a, all the factors shown are HLH proteins. Thin arrows indicate cross-regulation and autoregulation. (Redrawn from [32].)

is necessary, it is not sufficient for transcriptional activation and may be influenced by neighbouring DNA-binding proteins or the requirement for co-activators or repressors [2100]. Second, MyoD can repress potential inhibitors of its own activity. For example, MyoD represses expression of both the c-*fos* [1018] and fibroblast growth factor receptor (both of which antagonize MyoD) and post-translationally inactivates Id, an HLH protein lacking a basic domain which heterodimerizes with bHLH proteins to form non-DNA binding (and hence non-functional) heterodimers. Third, the cell cycle arrest concomitant with differentiation [1335] requires the Rb protein whose activity is negatively regulated by cyclin-dependent kinases (cdks) through phosphorylation. MyoD can activate expression of the cdk inhibitor p21 during differentiation of murine monocytes and in non-myogenic cells [1571, 1573]. The increase in p21 correlates with diminished levels of cdk2 protein and activity thus relieving the negative regulation of Rb.

bHLH proteins involved in neurogenesis

There are many general similarities between mechanisms underlying vertebrate myogenesis and those regulating *Drosophila* neurogenesis (Fig. 1; reviewed in [26, 32]). Whereas MyoD and related bHLH proteins specify muscles in vertebrates, Achaete, Scute and other bHLH proteins specify the initial steps in neural development in *Drosophila* [1315].

Achaete and *scute* are proneural genes expressed in a temporally regulated fashion in the wing imaginal disc and they are required for the formation of thoracic macrochaetae (reviewed in [9]). Reminiscent of the situation in vertebrate myogenesis, Achaete and Scute exhibit cross-regulation and some degree of functional overlap. For example, the *achaete* gene promoter contains several E box elements that are targets for transactivation by Scute [686]. In addition, the *achaete–scute* gene complex encodes two other bHLH proteins, Asense and Lethal of Scute [89]. *Asense* is expressed after neural precursor formation and *lethal of scute* acts as a proneural gene in the central nervous system during embryonic development [312, 475, 1407, 1644], and may be involved in the segregation of muscle progenitors [1424]. Although genetic analysis of these four bHLH proteins using loss-of-function mutants indicates that each has distinct functions, ectopic expression of any one of them induces micro- and macro-chaetae, suggesting that they are sufficiently similar to complement one another functionally [9, 32, 475, 884]. Achaete, Scute and Lethal of Scute are all involved in neuroectodermal transcription of the *enhancer of split* (E(spl)) gene family which encodes seven partially redundant bHLH proteins [304, 587].

As with the myogenic factors, members of the Achaete–Scute complex function as transcriptional regulators by forming DNA-binding heterodimers with the ubiquitously expressed *Drosophila* bHLH protein Daughterless [1221]. The importance of such dimerization is illustrated by the requirement of these proteins for the bHLH region, as shown by mutagenesis studies. Indeed, the bHLH of the Lethal of Scute protein is not only necessary but, by itself, sufficient to mediate its proneural function and to activate proneural genes [475]. The evolutionary conservation of *achaete–scute* genes is exemplified by the ability of the product of the single *achaete–scute* gene of *Hydra vulgaris* (CnASH) to dimerize with the *Drosophila* Da protein and functionally complement an *achaete* and *scute* double mutant in flies [1564]. A gene encoding a further proneural bHLH protein has been isolated from *Drosophila* by PCR using degenerate primers based on the sequence of the *acaete–scute* genes [1645]. This protein, Atonal, binds to the E box as a heterodimer with Daughterless and is involved in the formation of chordotonal organs (internal stretch receptors) and the first photoreceptor to appear in the eye imaginal disc (R8) of the compound eye [1645, 1646]. *Atonal* is expressed in the proneural clusters and sense organs that give rise to the embryonic and adult chordotonal, but not external, sense organs. A further *Drosophila* bHLH protein, Singleminded, appears to act as a master regulator of CNS midline development [748]. Sim also possesses a PAS protein interaction domain, and its activity may be regulated by the release of bound hsp90 following interaction with Per (a PAS-containing protein that lacks an HLH), Arnt (see below) or with further unidentified members of the bHLH–PAS family [1953, 2140]. The *Drosophila tracheless* gene (*trh*) encodes a bHLH–PAS protein which shows the highest homology to the Sim protein [2048]. *Trh* is expressed in the nuclei of the tracheal cells throughout development and is required for tracheal development and in the salivary gland ducts [1633, 2048]. Ectopic expression of *trh* generates extra tracheal pits and leads to the expression of tracheal markers [2048]. It is likely that Trh dimerizes with other bHLH–PAS proteins such as Sim or Arnt.

Activity of the Achaete–Scute bHLH proteins is inhibited by the product of the *extramacrochaetae* gene, an HLH protein which lacks a basic domain and functions as a 'dominant negative' in a manner analogous to the role of Id in myogenesis [344, 391, 1027]. Two other related genes, *hairy* and *deadpan*, also encode bHLH proteins that act as negative regulators of Achaete–Scute proteins in the formation of neuronal precursors in the PNS [161, 888]. Point mutations in the HLH and basic region of Hairy both abolish its activity, demonstrating the requirement for dimerization and DNA binding for its activity *in vivo* [1052]. It has been suggested that transcriptional repression by the Hairy/E(spl) family of proteins involves two mechanisms: (1) repression of transcriptional activators such as the Achaete–scute proteins through the HLH and a further conserved region C-terminal to the HLH and (2) repression by recruitment of co-repressors such as the Groucho protein via interaction with the C terminal WRPW motif [1052, 1477, 1526, 1838].

In vertebrates, several groups of bHLH proteins are known to be involved in neurogenesis (reviewed in [1307]). First, mammalian homologues of the *Drosophila* genes *achaete–scute* have been identified by the PCR using oligonucleotide primers based on the conserved amino acid sequence of *achaete–scute* genes [532]. Two genes so isolated, *mash1* and *mash2*, both show greater homology in the bHLH region with the *achaete–scute* genes than with any other known mammalian HLH protein. *mash1* is briefly expressed in the midgestational embryonic rodent nervous system and a null mutation in the *mash1* gene eliminates sympathetic and parasympathetic neurons and enteric neurons of the foregut [383, 434, 654, 1730]. It is also transiently induced during retinoic acid-induced differentiation of P19 murine embryonal carcinoma cells into neurons [533]. Interestingly, MEF2A is also induced in differentiating P19 cells and in the nervous system [2138]. Functional and physical interaction between Mash1 and MEF2A indicates that MEF2 transcription factors may cooperate with neural specific bHLH regulators such as Mash1 in a manner similar to the interaction between MEF2 and MyoD in myogenesis ([2138], and see above). *mash2* transcripts are much less abundant than *mash1* but

are also restricted to neuronal precursors *in vivo* [532]. Mouse embryos homozygous for a targeted disruption of the *mash2* gene die from placental failure at 10 days postcoitum. Rescue of the placental phenotype of *mash2*$^{-/-}$ embryos with wild-type extraembryonic tissue demonstrates that Mash2 is not required for embryonic development but is needed at post-implantation for the generation of differentiated trophoblast cell types [1568]. In contrast to *mash1*, *mash2* mRNA is expressed in undifferentiated P19 cells and disappears following retinoic acid-induced differentiation, implying a different role to *mash1* [533]. Expression of *mash* genes has not been detected in non-neural tissues or cell lines. *mash1* expression precedes overt neuronal differentiation, as judged by the appearance of neuron-specific markers such as neurofilament, by 12–24 hours. Like its *Drosophila* counterparts (the Achaete–Scute proteins), Mash1 is expressed in precursors of both central and peripheral neurons. Moreover, in the brain, Mash1 is observed in subsets of neuroepithelial cells and, in the PNS, exclusively in precursors of the sympathoadrenal/enteric serotonergic lineage [526, 654, 1396]. Thus, the temporal and spatial restriction of Mash1 expression is very similar to that observed for *Drosophila* Achaete–Scute proteins, suggesting that Mash1 plays an analogous role in neural determination in vertebrates [435]. However, whereas the myogenic factors are sufficient to induce myogenesis, enforced Mash1 expression in undifferentiated P19 cells is not sufficient to induce a phenotypic change associated with neurogenesis [533]. In summary, the sequence conservation of a family of *Drosophila*, *Xenopus* [370, 1022], *Hydra* [1564] and mammalian HLH proteins and their parallel patterns of expression during neurogenesis indicates remarkable evolutionary conservation of neurogenic development in a wide variety of animals.

A second group of mammalian bHLH proteins involved in neurogenesis has also been cloned by virtue of their *Drosophila* homologues. However, not all of these mammalian homologues show analogous patterns of expression to their *Drosophila* cousins. For example, the rat hairy-like gene (*rhl* [366], also known as *hes1*; [898]), which encodes the rat homologue of the *Drosophila* protein Hairy, is involved in negative regulation of neuronal precursor formation

[514]. Unlike the *Drosophila* gene, expression of which is restricted to subsets of ectodermal cells, *hes1* expression is widespread during mammalian embryogenesis and in the adult [898]. *Hes1* expression is induced by NGF stimulation of PC12 cells with kinetics characteristic of immediate-early genes, suggesting a role in the transduction of external signals [366]. The Hes1 protein represses transcription by binding a sequence called the N box (CACNAG), the recognition site of the *Drosophila* counterpart of Hes1 (Enhancer of split) [992, 1011], and decreases the transcription of E box genes resulting from the activity of other bHLH proteins such as E47 [898]. Furthermore, *Hes1* inhibits the function of MyoD and Mash1 to promote the myogenic conversion of C3H10T1/2 cells [898] and neuronal differentiation of PC12 cells in response to NGF [366]. Mice homozygous for a targeted disruption of the *hes1* gene exhibit severe neurulation defects and die during gestation or immediately postnatal [1634]. In the developing brain of such mice expression of the neural differentiation factor Mash1 is up-regulated and postmitotic neurons appear prematurely, suggesting that Hes1 controls the timing of neurogenesis and regulates neural tube morphogenesis. Three further mammalian genes with homology to the *Drosophila* genes *hairy* and *enhancer of split* have been isolated, *hes2* [515], *hes3* [898] and *hes5* [79]. The Hes2 protein, like Hes1, shows widespread expression in a variety of embryonic and adult tissues and appears to be a negative regulator of promoters containing both E box and N box motifs [515]. In contrast, Hes3 appears only to be expressed in the cerebellar Purkinje cells, and Hes5 expression is specific to the developing nervous system [79, 898, 1977]. Although all the Hes factors analysed thus far act as negative regulators of neuronal precursor formation, their mechanisms of action differ. For example, whereas Hes1 and Hes2 bind to both E box and N box motifs [898], Hes2, at least, exerts no inhibitory effects on E47, MyoD or Mash1 [515]. Secondly, Hes5 binds to the N box motif and significantly reduces transcription from promoters with this sequence, but is unable to bind the E box. None the less, Hes5 does partially inhibit E47-induced transcription from promoters bearing E boxes, possibly by forming non-DNA-binding heterodimers [898] with

E box proteins. Finally, Hes3 binds neither E nor N boxes. Like Hes5, however, Hes3 suppresses E box-dependent transcription, probably by sequestering E47 into inactive non-DNA-binding heterodimers [515, 898] in an analogous way to the Id proteins (see below).

Hes1 also antagonizes the activity of MATH1, a mammalian bHLH protein structurally related to the *Drosophila* Atonal protein (~70% identity in the bHLH region [1324]). Transcripts of both *MATH1* and a related gene *MATH2* ([1933], previously cloned and named NEX1 [1374]) are detected in the developing central nervous system and not in non-neural tissues, suggesting that these proteins play a role in the differentiation of neural cells [1324, 1933].

Screening of a chick brain library by PCR using degenerate primers based on the *Drosophila daughterless* gene identified a further gene encoding a bHLH protein, GbHLH1.4 [1589]. Although GbHLH1.4 exhibits considerable homology with the ubiquitously expressed class A proteins HEB and E12, and is widely expressed at early stages of development, its expression becomes progressively restricted as embryogenesis proceeds. At later stages, transcripts are restricted to the developing nervous system, heart, limbs and craniofacial primordia [1589], suggesting that it is involved in the differentiation of these tissues.

A third group of genes involved in mammalian neurogenesis is exemplified by two genes independently isolated by two groups by their homology with the haematopoietic bHLH factor, Tal1 [231, 232] (also known as Scl [96, 97, 135] see below). These genes, known as *NSCL-1* [136] or *hen1* [199] and *NSCL-2* [407] or *hen2* [199], encode proteins of 133 and 135 amino acids, respectively, in which the *C*-terminal 75 amino acids of each contains a highly homologous bHLH region. The *N*-terminal portions of these proteins diverge markedly, although the significance of this has not been established. Similarity in genomic structure between the *hen1* and *hen2* genes [650] suggests a close evolutionary relationship. *hen1* and *hen2* are coexpressed in the developing central and peripheral nervous systems of 11–13-day-old mouse embryos, suggesting a role in neurogenesis, reminiscent of that mediated by *achaete–scute* genes in *Drosophila*. Both *hen1* and *hen2* are expressed in cell lines derived from tumours of neural or neuro-endocrine origin and *hen1* transcription is activated during NGF-induced neural differentiation of PC12 cells [1165]. Little is known about the specific targets of either Hen1 or Hen2 bHLH proteins and, thus far, only Hen1 has been shown to form active dimers: it homodimerizes and forms heterodimers with E12 or E47 that bind a specific DNA sequence [1165]. None the less, both Hen1 and Hen2 possess all the credentials of bona fide transcriptional regulators.

Recently, Lee [1705] isolated a further bHLH protein involved in neurogenesis by virtue of its inter-action with the *Drosophila* Daughterless protein in a yeast two-hybrid system [2126]. This protein, NeuroD, has also been isolated from pancreatic islet cells ([1804] and see below). It is transiently expressed in embryonic tissues that contain terminally differentiating neurons. Ectopic expression of NeuroD in *Xenopus* is able to convert both non-neural ectodermal and neural crest cells into neurons [1705]. Conversion of the non-neural component of neural crest cells, which give rise to the connective tissue and cranial skeleton, into neural lineage is accompanied by loss of expression of Xtwi (the *Xenopus* homologue of the *Drosophila* bHLH protein Twist). Moreover, ectopic expression of Xtwi decreases NeuroD expression. Thus, two members of the bHLH protein family, NeuroD and Twist, may compete to determine the fate of different cell types derived from the neural crest.

bHLH proteins in sex determination

Many of the HLH proteins involved in the initial steps of *Drosophila* neurogenesis are also involved in sex determination (Fig. 1) (reviewed in [26, 32, 53]). *Drosophila* sex is determined by the ratio of X chromosomes to autosomes (X : A). The dosage of *scute* – also known as *sisterless-b* [349, 781, 782] – and *sisterless-a*, which encodes a bZIP protein [350], both of which are located on the X chromosome, act as positive transcriptional activators of the female-specific gene sex-lethal which promotes female development. In addition, the Daughterless protein acts as a common

bHLH dimerization partner in both neurogenesis and sex determination, and Extramacrochaetae, Hairy and Deadpan are each able to inhibit both pathways [32, 781, 782].

bHLH proteins involved in haematopoiesis

Several HLH proteins have been identified as encoded by genes at genetic loci involved in translocations and are thus implicated in the malignant development of T cells. The *scl* locus was originally defined by the position of breakpoints within a kilobase region of chromosome 1 from patients with T cell acute leukaemia (T-ALL) [135, 231, 232]. The *scl* gene, also known as *tal1* [231, 232] or *tcl-5* [373], encodes an HLH protein with homology to *lyl1*, a gene on chromosome 19 also implicated in T cell leukaemogenesis [135, 231, 232]. Although translocation of the *tal1* gene is observed in only 3% of T-ALL cases, an additional 25% of patients harbour deletions of the *tal1* gene not detectable by karyotype analysis [157, 198, 535]. Thus, both t(1;14) translocations and deletions disrupt the *tal1* gene, bringing its coding sequences under the control of regulatory elements in either the TCRδ gene or the *sil* gene [97], both of which are normally expressed in T cells [190, 198, 231]. Although Tal1 can cooperate with v-Abl to enhance T cell tumourigenesis in mice [1513], enforced expression of Tal1 in murine bone marrow is insufficient to generate leukaemia [1512]. Analyses of the normal *tal1* gene demonstrate a pattern of expression restricted to cells of early haematopoietic lineages, notably erythroid, mast and early myeloid cells [135, 424, 542, 731, 1932]. Enforced over-expression of Tal1 can block monocytic differentiation of M1 murine myeloid cells and, interestingly, the differentiation of C2C12 muscle precursor cells [1555]. This suggests that Tal1 and MyoD can compete for a common partner (e.g. E12/E47). Utilization of different 5′ untranslated exons of *tal1* occurs in differing haematopoietic cell lineages [96, 2103], giving rise to two protein products: a full-length polypeptide of ~42 kDa (residues 1–331 [96]) and a truncated form of 24 kDa (residues 176–331 [895]). Both forms contain the bHLH (residues 188–239) and are, therefore, capable of DNA binding and dimerization, but differ in the presence of a transactivation domain. However, it is not known whether these two proteins have distinct functions. Tal1 protein is most abundant in erythroid cell lines and in foetal and adult haematopoietic populations rich in erythroid precursors [424, 1797]. Consistent with this, tal1-deficient embryos lack nucleated red blood cells as a result of the failure to produce primitive erythroid cells [1935], and die between E8.5 and E10.5. However, the effect of Tal1 loss on early erythropoiesis does not exclude a potential role for Tal1 during later erythroid maturation [98]. There is also evidence to support a role for Tal1 in growth and differentiation of neural [28] and endothelial cells [503] and in inhibiting apoptosis of the Jurkat T cell line in reduced serum concentrations [1713]. Tal1 is unable to bind DNA by itself, presumably due to its inability to form homodimers [492, 1181]. Instead, like other tissue-specific bHLH proteins (such as myogenic and neurogenic factors), Tal1 interacts with the ubiquitously expressed E2A gene products and the resulting heterodimers bind an E box motif [492, 1180, 1181, 1233, 1255]. Recent data suggest that sequences outside of the Tal1 bHLH are important for DNA binding. Deletion of the C-terminal 53 amino acids (which leaves the bHLH intact) reduces protein binding to the Tal1 DNA site [1713]. Moreover, the truncated Tal1 protein (amino acids 1–279) appears to act as a dominant negative, perhaps by sequestering the class A heterodimeric partner E12 or E47 [1713].

The tal2 gene is related to tal1 and was identified on the basis of sequence homology [1098]. The tal2 gene is also located at the site of translocations found in some cases of T-ALL. The t(7;9)(q34;q32) translocation places the tal2 gene from chromosome 9 adjacent to the TCR β chain on chromosome 7, resulting in deregulation of tal2 expression. The Tal2 protein contains a bHLH domain with a high degree of homology to both Tal1 and Lyl1 [1098] and binds a specific DNA sequence as a heterodimer with E12 or E47 [1293]. Both Tal1 and Tal2 and the related Lyl1 protein (see below) also associate with RBTN1 and RBTN2, related polypeptides that possess two tandem LIM domains (a cysteine-rich sequence that

coordinates zinc atoms) [2149, 2151]. This interaction requires the bHLH domain, and the fact that RBTN1 and 2 associate with Tal1/E47 heterodimers suggests that residues on the exposed surface of the heterodimer mediate RBTN interaction [2151].

The lyl1 gene shares several features with tal1. It was identified through its involvement in t(7;19) translocations in T-ALL [1040]. The translocation occurs between the TCR β locus and the first intron of lyl1 resulting in a truncated lyl1 transcript. However, since the predominant initiation codon of lyl1 is situated in exon 2, the main effect of the translocation is to bring expression of lyl1 under the control of promoter elements in the TCR β gene. The lyl1 and tal1 genes share a similar structure and their protein products display 84% homology in the bHLH domain, suggesting recent evolution from a common ancestral gene [96]. Lyl1 and Tal1 both heterodimerize with products of the E2A gene (E12, E47 and ITF1) and bind closely related DNA sequences containing an identical CAGATG core [1181, 1233, 1255, 1780]. Like tal1, differential splicing of the lyl1 5′ untranslated region correlates with expression of two alternative sizes of transcripts in different haematopoietic cell types, the smaller class (∼1.5 kb) being typical of erythroid lineage and the larger class (∼2.3 kb) present in B lymphocytes [1040]. In addition, differential splicing within the coding region of the mouse lyl gene generates two polypeptides, Lyl1 and Lyl2 [1040]. Finally, there is considerable overlap with Tal1 expression, particularly in erythroid and monocyte lineages, but Lyl1 is also expressed in B lymphocytes [424, 601, 1040]. In T cells there is normally little, if any, expression of lyl1, and it is likely that the deregulated expression of lyl1 that results from translocation contributes to the neoplastic phenotype.

In summary Tal1, Tal2 and Lyl1 comprise a discrete subset of bHLH proteins whose deregulated expression can contribute, via recognition of a common set of target genes, to the development of T cell leukaemias.

When first isolated, several features of the Vav protein were inferred from the nucleotide sequences of the human and murine genes [554, 555, 1264, 1281, 1461]. In particular, the N-terminal region disrupted by oncogenic mutation [554, 1461] is rich in leucine residues, and it was proposed to comprise an HLH and leucine zipper. However, subsequent analysis [1402] and amendment of the published sequence [1320] along with characterization of the protein indicates that Vav is not a member of the HLH family of proteins.

A cDNA encoding a putative bHLH protein has been isolated from stimulated blood mononuclear cells [1938, 2059]. However, the predicted basic region of GOS8 has little homology with the basic region of other bHLH proteins, and the presence of a helix-destabilizing proline residue in the predicted helix 1 casts some doubt on whether GOS8 is a bona fide member of the bHLH class of proteins.

Other tissue-specific bHLH proteins

Several other bHLH proteins appear to have roles in the regulation of particular cell lineages in different species. For example, the bHLH protein Twist is expressed during the earliest stages of differentiation of the *Drosophila* mesoderm. It is responsible, in conjunction with the maternal transcription factor Dorsal, for activating and maintaining expression of early mesoderm-specific genes including Snail (a zinc finger transcription factor) [636, 859]. Snail, in turn, is a transcriptional repressor that is expressed throughout the prospective mesoderm but that forms a sharp posterior boundary which helps establish the boundary between mesoderm and neuroectoderm [513]. The spatial distribution of Snail appears to be established by a combination of overlapping gradients of the Dorsal and Twist proteins. Thus, the bHLH protein Twist is involved in determining the temporal and spatial differentiation of mesoderm. In addition to a role in specifying early mesoderm, the relative amounts of Twist participates in the choice between alternative mesodermal fates. Thus, high levels of Twi are required for somatic myogenesis and block the formation of other mesodermal fates [1376]. In vertebrates, subdivision of mesoderm may also depend on Twist homologues such as mTwi (mouse [1087]), XTwi (*Xenopus* [1611]), Meso-1 [1395] and bHLH-EC2 [824]. In the mouse, mTwi is initially

found throughout the somatic mesoderm, and down-regulation in the myotome is concomitant with up-regulation of myogenic bHLH proteins and members of the MEF2 protein family [1957]. This reciprocal expression pattern suggests that mTwi may influence mesoderm cell fate by inhibiting somatic myogenesis. In fact, ectopic expression of mTwi (and, interestingly, *Drosophila* Twist) can inhibit muscle differentiation of murine cells *in vitro* by inhibiting transactivation by MEF2 and sequestering the heterodimeric partners of myogenic bHLH proteins (E12 and E47) [1957]. The Daughterless, Achaete and Scute proteins that are involved in neurogenesis and sex determination in *Drosophila* may also play a role in the formation of embryonic mesoderm [417].

The paraxial mesoderm in vertebrates gives rise to a variety of cell types in the embryo, including the musculature, the axial skeleton and dermis. The sequential and overlapping expression patterns of three bHLH proteins, bHLH–EC2 ([824] known as Paraxis in the mouse [1418] and Meso1 in the hamster [1395]), Scleraxis [1469] and the mammalian homologue of Twist (mTwi [1087]) in the paraxial mesoderm and developing somites suggests that they are involved in specifying somite-derived cell lineages. A third Twist-related bHLH protein, Dermo-1, is expressed in a subset of mesenchymal cell lineages including developing dermis. It binds an E box consensus in the presence of E12 but fails to activate transcription [1720]. Like mTwist, Dermo-1 represses the transcriptional activity of myogenic bHLH proteins, possibly by sequestering E12 [1587, 1720].

Two genes encoding bHLH proteins involved in implantation have recently been cloned by three independent groups. The first, called Thing1 [1608] or Hxt [1468] or eHAND [1470], is expressed in early trophoblast and in differentiated giant cells. Trophoblasts are among the first cell lineages to be established in the mammalian embryo that contribute to the extraembryonic structures that form the placenta. Overexpression of Hxt induces trophoblast cell differentiation *in vitro*, suggesting that it has a role in trophoblast cell commitment and differentiation [1468]. The second gene encodes a closely related protein (87% identical in the bHLH domain), called Thing2 [1608] or Hed [1468] or dHAND [1470], and is expressed in maternal deciduum surrounding the implantation site. Interestingly, of the sequence mismatches in the bHLH domains of these two proteins, an asparagine in the Thing2 basic domain, which is highly conserved in the basic regions of other bHLH proteins (Fig. 2), is replaced by a proline residue in Thing1. This feature is reminiscent of the Hairy, Deadpan and E(spl) proteins of *Drosophila*, and it is possible that, like E(spl) proteins, Thing1 may bind an N box element.

The *Drosophila* bHLH protein, Delilah, is expressed exclusively in epidermal cells that function as attachment sites for the somatic muscles [102]. Expression of Delilah persists in embryos which lack mesoderm (*snail* mutants) indicating that expression is not induced by the attachment of underlying muscles and that Delilah plays a part in epidermal cell proliferation. The cDNA encoding Delilah was isolated from an expression library by screening with the mammalian E12 bHLH protein (see below). Since Delilah cannot homodimerize or bind DNA alone it may interact with the ubiquitously expressed Daughterless protein *in vivo*.

Many mammalian genes with E boxes in their control elements show cell type-specific expression and are probably regulated by HLH proteins. For example, pancreatic cell-specific transcription of the mammalian insulin gene is mediated, at least in part, by binding of bHLH proteins – both the ubiquitously expressed E12, E47 and HEB are components of the regulatory factor that binds to the E box consensus sequence *cis*-acting DNA element, GCCATCTG in the insulin promoter [261, 942, 1056, 2016, 2112]. Recently, a tissue-specific 'class B' bHLH partner that acts with E47 in the control of insulin expression has been isolated from a hamster insulin tumour [1804]. This protein, BETA2, is a component (along with E47) of the native insulin E box complex and, consistent with this, Northern analysis demonstrates that *BETA2* mRNA is expressed in pancreatic α and β cell lines. BETA2 expression is also observed in the brain and intestine, and Lee *et al.* [1705] have isolated an identical protein (named NeuroD) that is transiently expressed in differentiating neurons during mouse embryonic development. Interestingly, there is evidence that islet cells are derived from the ectoderm via neural crest cells, and insulin transcripts have been detected in mouse brain [1484] at about the same time as NeuroD RNA is first detected [1705]. Insulin expression may also be controlled through the action of dominant negative inhibitors of bHLH protein function: exogenous expression of Id, a negative regulator of bHLH proteins (see below), suppresses E box-mediated transcription of the insulin gene [261]. Second, BETA3, a bHLH protein related to BETA2/NeuroD (53.4% amino acid identity) and mTwi (48.3% identity), represses the transactivation of an insulin E box reporter by BETA2/E47 [1855]. BETA3, like BETA2/NeuroD, is a 'classB' bHLH protein, with highest levels of expression in kidney, brain and lung cells. Although BETA3 interacts with E47, the dimer is unable to bind the insulin E box, and repression of BETA2/E47 activity appears to be due to the ability of BETA3 to reduce the amount of BETA2/E47 heterodimer or E47 homodimer bound to DNA. Similarly, BETA3 also inhibits the MyoD/E47 induction of the muscle creatine kinase promoter, suggesting that, like Dermo-1, BETA3 may act to sequester E47 [1855]. Expression of BETA3 in the brain indicates that it may also play a role in the regulation of neurogenesis by BETA2/NeuroD.

Ubiquitously expressed (class A) bHLH proteins

The widely accepted view of tissue-specific regulation by the bHLH family of DNA-binding transcriptional regulators is that dimerization of a bHLH protein of tissue-restricted expression (class B) with a ubiquitously expressed member (class A) is generally required for functionality. Given that the number of class A proteins appears to be small, it is likely that each single class A protein dimerizes with many different bHLH proteins and thereby exerts profound effects on the genesis and maintenance of many different cell lineages. Some examples of this are now considered.

Early experiments with mutations of the widely expressed Daughterless bHLH protein demonstrated that it was involved in multiple, seemingly unrelated, aspects of development in *Drosophila* [10, 221, 249,

266, 267, 269, 276, 1024]. The first mutant allele, da^1, resulted in death only of the daughters of homozygous mutant mothers. The fact that daughters die even if they are genetically wild-type at this locus (i.e. da^+/da^+) indicates a requirement for maternal expression, and recent data suggest that maternally derived transcripts are transferred to the zygotes and translated early in embryogenesis [268]. Intriguingly, at higher temperatures, nearly all of the sons die as well, irrespective of their da genotype, indicating that the requirement for da^+ expression in their mothers is not sex-specific and may be involved in oogenesis. Unexpectedly, a search for genes required for development of the nervous system in embryos revealed that dead embryos lacking zygotic da^+ expression completely lack a PNS and parts of the CNS [220]. Thus, the daughterless gene is involved in the regulation of at least three developmental pathways in *Drosophila* – sex determination, oogenesis and neurogenesis. Daughterless is widely distributed throughout most tissues during development [268] and there is accumulating evidence that its pleiotropic effects are mediated through its interaction with other bHLH proteins whose expression is temporally or spatially restricted (see above).

Genes encoding a series of closely related bHLH proteins, E12/E47/ITF1 [470, 471, 741, 1121], ITF2 [470, 472, 527] and HTF4/HEB [494, 1120], have been isolated from mammalian cDNA expression libraries by screening for binding of labelled E box sequences. Whilst all these genes are expressed fairly ubiquitously, they none the less direct tissue-specific transcription programmes through their heterodimeric interactions with lineage-restricted bHLH proteins. For example, in muscle cells, E12-like proteins heterodimerize with muscle-specific factors of the MyoD family and mediate expression of muscle-specific genes (see above).

The human $E2A$ gene encodes several related polypeptides, E12, E47/HE47 and ITF1, all produced through alternative splicing [984]. Products of the $E2A$ gene are involved in many cell lineages, including regulation of expression of the immunoglobulin heavy and light chain genes in B lymphocytes [521]. Although homozygous E2A mutant mice develop to full term apparently normally, they subsequently display a high rate of postnatal death, and the surviving mice exhibit retarded growth [1366, 2080]. These animals contain no B cells, whilst other haematopoeitic lineages including T cell, granulocyte, macrophage and erythroid are intact. B cell differentiation is blocked at an early step (prior to Ig gene DJ rearrangement). Interestingly, heterozygous embryos produce, on average, about half as many mature B cells as wild-type embryos, suggesting the importance of a threshold of E2A activity in the pre-B cell [2079], which may be further modulated by expression of Id proteins [1968]. The fact that cell lineages other than B cells are intact indicates that E2A is not essential for determination of many cell types. In these cells, loss of E2A may be compensated for by other class A bHLH proteins such as HEB and ITF2 (see below). Why HEB and/or ITF2 cannot compensate for E2A in B cell lineages is unclear.

The $E2A$ gene maps to chromosome region 19p13, a site associated with translocations (t(1;19)(q23;p13)) in acute lymphoblastic lymphoma [700]. In a subset of B cell precursor acute lymphoblastic leukaemic cells (those that have cytoplasmic IgM heavy chains), translocations involving the $E2A$ gene frequently result in the synthesis of transcripts resulting from a fusion between $E2A$ and the homeobox gene PBX1 on chromosome 1q23 [820]. This generates a fusion protein that retains the transcriptional activator domain of the $E2A$ protein but whose bHLH is replaced by the homeobox domain of Pbx1. Expression of this protein is oncogenic when expressed in NIH3T3 cells, suggesting that the hybrid gene product(s) contribute to leukaemogenesis [545, 546, 626]. The $E2A$–Pbx1 hybrid protein acts as a constitutive transcriptional activator of genes regulated by members of the Pbx family [626, 660]. Similarly, the t(17;19) (q21–22;p13.3) translocation in ALL results in a hybrid transcription factor comprising the transcriptional activation domain of the $E2A$ product and the bZIP domain of the hepatic leukaemia factor (Hlf) [501]. The hybrid $E2A$–Hlf protein is presumed to exhibit different transcriptional activity on Hlf target genes compared to the wild-type Hlf protein.

The human $E2$–2 gene encodes the bHLH protein ITF2 [472]. Like ITF1 (identical to E47 except for its first coding exon [471]), ITF2 is expressed in a variety of cell types and binds to the $\mu E5/\kappa 2$ motif present in both heavy and κ light chain enhancers [470]. ITF1 and ITF2 homo- and hetero-dimerize via their HLH domains and each possesses a distinct additional domain that acts as a transcriptional activator [470]. A canine counterpart of ITF2 (TFE) has been isolated from a thyroid cDNA expression library with the thyroglobulin gene promoter [527]. Two alternatively spliced forms of mouse ITF-2, termed MITF-2A and -2B, differ in their N termini [1945]. Whereas MITF-2A transactivates the cardiac α-actin promoter (which contains an E box) when co-expressed with MyoD, MITF-2B inhibits MyoD transactivation of the promoter, probably by forming inactive heterodimers [1945]. The inhibitory activity requires the N-terminal 83 amino acids which are absent from MITF-2A.

Another ubiquitous bHLH factor is HEB (also known as HTF4), which binds specifically to the E box motifs in the $\kappa E2$ immunoglobulin enhancer [494, 1120], the simian virus AP4 site [1120], the CD4 enhancer [899], the LTR of HIV-1 [1122] and, in murine fibroblasts, to the LTR of several murine type C retroviruses [2110]. HEB is closely related to E12/E47/ITF1 and ITF2, and, like them, is expressed in many tissues [494]. In addition to forming homo-dimers, HEB also heterodimerizes with E12 and ITF2, and with myogenin, indicating a role in myo-genesis [494]. The murine homologue of HEB is ALF1A [1193]. A second protein, ALF1B, generated by alternative splicing of the ALF1 gene, differs by the insertion of 24 amino acids [1193]. Alternative splicing of the rat homologue also produces two proteins, REBα and REBβ, that differ by the insertion of 24 amino acids [575]. Although ALF1 and REB expression is widespread, alternative RNA splicing results in tissue-specific ratios of ALF1A/ALF1B and REBα/REBβ [575]. The 24 amino acid insert specific to REBβ mediates an inhibitory effect on DNA binding [575]. Like the alternatively spliced domain of E2A products that prevents homodimerization of E12 [2147], a similar inhibitory domain present in REBβ restricts homodimerization [575]. In contrast, no differences in the transactivation of a reporter gene by ALF1A and ALF1B was observed [1193] and the significance of differential expression of ALF1A and ALF1B remains unclear [1193].

Several further potential transcriptional modulators have been described that contain a putative HLH domain, such as Fli-1 [843], Mel-18 [516] and Erg-3 [869]. However, none of these proteins has been shown to interact directly with E box sequences, and they will not be considered further.

Yeast bHLH proteins

Several HLH proteins have been described in the budding yeast *Saccharomyces cerevisiae*. Elucidation of the roles of these proteins has been greatly facilitated by the availability of *null* mutants and some of these studies are described below.

The centromere-binding protein CBF1 [209], encoded by the yeast *CEP1* gene (also known as *CP1* and *CPF1* [121, 702]), is a member of the bHLH family of proteins. It is required for two distinct processes: optimal chromosome segregation and methionine prototrophy [209]. Its role in chromo-some segregation is mediated through its binding to conserved DNA element I (CDEI) in the centromeres. The degenerate CDEI sequence (RTCACRTG, where $R = $ purine) contains the E box consensus sequence CANNTG. Consensus CDEI sites are also present in the promoter regions of most methionine bio-synthetic genes (*MET*), suggesting that the vital role of CBF1 in methionine metabolism is mediated through its transcriptional modulation of *MET* genes. However, CBF1 lacks a functional transactiva-tion domain, and may have no direct role in the transcription of *MET* genes [1666, 2108]. Rather, it has been proposed that binding of CBF1 at *MET* promoters acts to facilitate the binding of MET4, a bZIP factor that appears to be the direct trans-activator of *MET* gene transcription [1006]. Although the exact mechanism of CBF1 function is unknown, it has been suggested that binding of CBF1 alters the chromatin structure of CDEI-contain-ing promoters, perhaps by interacting with other chromatin proteins, thus allowing access to transcrip-tion factors [690, 702]. Indeed, the *C*-terminal 87 amino acids of Cbf1 contains a potential amphipathic helix which may modulate protein–protein inter-actions [1497].

Transcription of the acid phosphatase gene *PHO5* requires two positively acting factors, Pho2 and Pho4, and is inhibited by Pho80 [1112]. A detailed analysis of deletion and insertion mutants of the Pho4 protein has demonstrated that a bHLH motif at its *C* terminus is required for its activity and that Pho4 binds *PHO5* DNA as a dimer [769]. The Pho80 polypeptide blocks Pho4 function by direct interaction (squelching) with sites on the Pho4 protein not involving the bHLH domain [528]. Two other regions of the Pho4 protein are also important for its ability to stimulate transcription of the *PHO5* gene. The first, situated in the *N*-terminal 109 amino acids, contains a tripartite transcriptional activation domain rich in acidic residues [769] and may play a role in chromatin disruption during promoter activation [1969, 1970, 2116]. Deletion of a second region (amino acids 172–227) also abolishes Pho4 activity, and available data suggest that this may comprise the Pho80 interaction domain [528]. Moreover, Pho80 has homology to yeast cyclins and a complex with Pho85 (a $p34^{cdc2/CDC28}$ related protein kinase) phosphorylates Pho4 which correlates with negative regulation of the *PHO5* gene [1273, 1299]. Nuc-1, a homologue of Pho4 which regulates transcription of genes encoding phosphorous acquisition enzymes in the fungus *Neurospora crassa* [549], also contains a domain required for interaction with negative regulatory factors [548]. As expected, the bHLH region of Nuc-1 is essential for its function. In addition, an atypical zipper domain containing a heptad repeat of alanine and methionine residues adjacent to helix 2 is also required for dimerization and function of Nuc-1 [1849].

Rtg1p is a bHLH protein of *S. cerevisiae* that is required for basal and regulated expression of *CIT2*, the gene encoding a peroxisomal isoform of citrate synthase [1896]. Although Rtg1p binds to a 76 bp region in the 5′ flanking region of the *CIT2* gene, this sequence does not contain an E box or an N box, both of which are canonical DNA binding sites recognized by most bHLH proteins [1896].

In *S. cerevisiae*, activation of the fatty acid synthase genes via the inositol/choline response element (ICRE) is governed by the activity of two bHLH proteins, Ino2p [1813] and Ino4p [1616], which form a heterodimer [1917, 1920]. The consensus binding site for Ino2p/Ino4p in the ICRE has been defined as 5′-WYTTCAYRTGS-3′ (where W = A or T, Y = C or T, R = A or G and S = C or G) [1917]. Heterodimer formation and DNA-binding specificity is dictated by the respective bHLH domains. However, transcriptional activation of target promoters requires a functional Ino2p protein. Consistent with this, deletion studies have identified two separate transcriptional activation domains in the *N*-terminal part of Ino2p [1920].

The yeast Sin3 protein (also known as SD11, UME4, RPD1 and GAM2) is a transcriptional repressor of a number of diverse yeast genes [1037, 1059, 1060]. The *SIN3* gene encodes a protein with four paired amphipathic helix motifs resembling an HLH domain [1059]. Evidence suggests that the Sin3 protein regulates transcription through direct protein–protein interactions with other transcription factors rather than by binding DNA. For example, expression of the *HO* gene (which encodes an endonuclease responsible for initiating mating-type switching) is controlled by Sin3. *HO* gene expression is suppressed by the SDP1 protein, and this suppression is antagonized by a further protein, I-SDP1. Sin3 interacts with I-SDP1, so allowing the SDP1 repressor to bind and suppress *HO* expression. The mammalian homologue of Sin3 interacts with the Mad family of bHLHZ proteins and acts as a co-repressor of transcriptional activity (see below). Consistent with this mode of action, the Sin3 protein lacks a DNA-binding domain adjacent to any of the paired amphipathic helix motifs.

The recently described Esc1 bHLH protein of *Schizosaccharomyces pombe* promotes sexual differentiation by modulating responses to decreases in cyclic AMP as a result of nitrogen starvation [151]. Immediately following the bHLH is a putative leucine zipper possibly making Esc1 the first yeast bHLHZ protein to be identified (see below) [151]. Although the bHLHZ region is required for activity the individual contribution of the leucine zipper has not been determined. The discovery of an HLH protein in *S. pombe* that is involved in differentiation demonstrates the importance of HLH proteins in differentiation processes of diverse species.

Plant bHLH proteins

Mutants within the maize anthocyanin biosynthetic pathway responsible for the development of the red and purple coloration display a diverse pattern of different pigmented phenotypes. In recent years many of these mutants have been localized to members of the R and B gene families [663, 832]. The R gene product Lc, was the first plant protein shown to possess an HLH motif [662]. R and B genes encode HLH proteins that control the temporal and spatial distribution of anthocyanin in maize. Pigmentation is also controlled by the C/P family of genes that encodes polypeptides which, whilst not bHLH proteins, appear to act in concert with products of the R and B genes.

R and B proteins share a considerable degree of amino acid homology, particularly between their HLH domains, and all are bona fide transcription factors. R regulates the expression of three enzymes involved in anthocyanin biosynthesis [662, 663]. Transient transfection of R and B genes demonstrates that they are functionally equivalent [410, 663], and phenotypic variation arises through temporal and spatial differences in R/B gene expression rather than from functional differences. Notably, the 5′ untranslated region of the R and B genes is extremely heterogeneous compared to the coding sequences and elements within the 5′ regions of the B genes Peru and I are responsible for their tissue-specific expression [831]. The 5′ region of B genes is also involved in paramutation, an allele-specific interaction that leads to a heritable change in one allele at a high frequency [1844, 1845]. Whereas the complex regulation of R/B genes is beginning to be unravelled, the potential combination of dimerization partners and their effect on plant pigmentation and development has not been elucidated.

In *Antirrhinum*, anthocyanin pigmentation is controlled by the product of the *delila* gene, which encodes a bHLH protein with extensive homology to products of the R genes in maize [420, 1760]. Thus, despite the many differences in morphology and colouration between maize and *Antirrhinum*, the control of anthocyanin pigmentation in both is mediated by conserved bHLH regulators. It is a

reasonable assumption that, as in vertebrates, plant bHLH proteins may be involved in the control of a number of differentiation pathways.

Other bHLH proteins

DNA-binding proteins with homology to the bHLH family are also implicated in diverse signal transduction pathways. For example, the dioxin receptor mediates signal transduction by the potent extracellular toxin 2,3,7,8-tetrachlorodibenzo-*p*-dioxin (dioxin) and indolocarbazole derivatives [1676]. It binds, as a dimer of two bHLH proteins, the ligand-binding aryl hydrocarbon receptor (AhR) [206, 346] and the auxillary factor Arnt (AhR nuclear translocation [485, 860]) to target sequences of the xenobiotic metabolizing enzymes, XRE [692, 1304]. The specific temporal and spatial expression of AhR indicates that it may be important in normal embryonic development [1318]. In the absence of ligand, a latent, non-DNA-binding form of the receptor is found in the cytoplasm associated with hsp90. Treatment with dioxin releases hsp90, allowing dimerization with Arnt, translocation to the nucleus and DNA-binding [1077, 1078, 1493, 2154]. In contrast to other bHLH and bHLHZ proteins, which recognize the symmetrical consensus DNA-binding site CANNTG, the Ah receptor–Arnt complex binds to the asymmetrical consensus XRE (A/T)NGCGTG [2093, 2106], consistent with the variation in the AhR basic region compared with other bHLH proteins including Arnt (Table 2). Interestingly, the Arnt homodimer binds specifically to, and can activate, the Adenovirus major late promoter, which contains a CACGTG E box consensus [1336, 1953, 2114]. Since the XRE contains an E box half-site (GTG) it is possible that this sequence is recognized by Arnt [2093] and the other half of the XRE interacts with AhR. In fact, the basic region of AhR (amino acids 27–39) deviates from the usual bHLH consensus (see Fig. 2), and an additional basic region (amino acids 9–20) is required for XRE binding [1363, 1539, 2099].

Functional domains within AhR and Arnt have been identified by deletion analysis. The PAS domains of AhR are required for ligand binding and association with hsp90 [1337, 1465, 1540], and act synergistically with the HLH to mediate interaction with the other bHLH–PAS proteins, Arnt and Sim [1953, 2134]. Screening of a mouse cDNA library (from 11.5-day-old embryos) with cDNAs encoding the bHLH/PAS regions of Arnt and AhR revealed the existence of a cDNA encoding a second Arnt protein [1603]. This protein, Arnt2, is very similar to Arnt with 81% identity in the N-terminal region (57% overall identity), and the bHLH regions of 55 amino acids are identical except for three changes. Arnt2 shares many biochemical properties with Arnt, but their patterns of expression are different. Whereas Arnt2 mRNA is specifically expressed only in the brain and kidney of adult mice, Arnt is expressed ubiquitously [1603]. Wang *et al.* [2024–2026] have characterized a further bHLH–PAS factor in cultured mammmalian cells under reduced O_2 conditions. Hypoxia-inducible factor (HIF-1) is necessary for transcriptional activation mediated by the erythropoietin gene enhancer in hypoxic cells. It consists of two bHLH–PAS subunits: HIF-1β, which is identical to Arnt, and HIF-1α, which is related to, but distinct from, Sim. Thus, Arnt proteins appear to be a common subunits used by AhR, Sim and HIF-1α and possibly others [1319, 1426, 1430, 1506, 2131] and may play physiological roles in the regulation of E box-containing genes. Further studies indicate that DNA binding by HIF-1 is modulated by phosphorylation, although the phosphorylation sites have not been identified [2025, 2026]. Whereas the HLH-PAS and basic domains are required, respectively, for dimerization and XRE binding [1540, 1876], the C-terminal halves of AhR and Arnt mediate transcriptional activation [1641, 1719, 1740, 2045] and the AhR C-terminus appears to be the predominant transactivator [1540, 1677, 1952].

Comparison of the sequence of the Epstein–Barr virus (EBV) nuclear antigen-1 (EBNA-1) with known bHLH proteins suggests that it, too, contains a bHLH domain [1632, 2086]. Deletions which remove part of the predicted helices 1 or 2 abolish binding to oriP, a fragment of EBV DNA required for episomal replication. Although oriP contains the CANNTG consensus, the requirement of this site has not been demonstrated.

bHLHZ proteins

One large group of HLH proteins is characterized by the possession of a second dimerization motif, the leucine zipper: these are the bHLHZ proteins. The α-helical leucine zipper was first identified as a domain that mediates dimerization between members of the bZIP family of transcription factors (reviewed in [30]). In bHLHZ proteins the leucine zipper is invariably positioned immediately C-terminal to the HLH, in effect generating an extended helix 2, and this may serve to restrict promiscuous interactions with other HLH and bZIP proteins (see below). With the exception of the AhR/Arnt dimer and SREBP proteins (see below), all known bHLHZ proteins bind to E box (CANNTG) DNA elements. The varied functions of these bHLHZ proteins are outlined below.

The Myc, Max, Mad, and Mxi1 proteins

The *myc* genes comprise a family of structurally and functionally related genes [305, 306] that encode bHLHZ proteins. The archetypal member, c-*myc*, was first isolated as the chicken cellular homologue of the viral v-*myc* gene [871]. The c-*myc* gene is highly conserved throughout chordate evolution [1356] and has been observed in such diverse organisms as man [156, 252, 280], mice [156], birds [1066, 1067], amphibians [570, 1000], fish [1026, 1836, 2076], sea stars [1055] and Drosophila [1545a, 1916a]. To date, *myc* homologues have not been identified in *S. cerevisiae*.

The human c-*myc* gene encodes two phosphoproteins of 439 and 453 amino acids [20, 24] generated by alternative translational start sites [447]. Although there is some evidence that the two c-Myc polypeptides exhibit distinct functions [1578], this has not been found by others [1394]. Two other well-characterized *myc* genes, N-*myc* and L-*myc*, share extensive homology with c-*myc* in their coding regions and encode similar-sized nuclear proteins [307, 355, 580, 955, 971, 1356]. Multiple c-Myc and N-Myc polypeptides are produced as a result of alternative translation initiation sites [447, 673]; multiple L-Myc polypeptides are derived by alternative splicing of the mRNA [295, 557]. Two B-*myc* genes have been identified; they are conserved in the mouse, rat and human genome and have homology to intron one, exon two and non-coding sequences in exon three [111, 1355, 1631]. B-*myc* RNA is expressed in many tissues, notably the brain [1631], and the longest open reading frame predicts a protein of 178 amino acids [111, 1355]. The predicted truncated protein product lacks *C*-terminal amino acids essential for biological activity of the c-Myc protein [974]. Nonetheless, homology with the transactivation domain of c-Myc and ability to inhibit transformation and transcriptional activation by c-Myc has led to the suggestion that B-*myc* regulates c-Myc activity by interacting with an adapter protein(s) required for contacting the transcriptional machinery [856, 1355].

S-*myc* was isolated from a rat genomic library and comprises a single exon with homology to both the second and third c-*myc* exons [979]. Although, expression of the s-*myc* gene has not been reliably detected in rat tissues or cell lines, transfection of the gene (in the absence of an artificial promoter) into the RT4-AC rat tumour cell line produced significant amounts of RNA, suggesting that it may not be a transcriptionally inert pseudogene [979]. Moreover, transfection of s-*myc* into glioma cells suppressed their tumourigenicity in nude mice [629, 979, 1350, 1351], possibly by inducing apoptosis in the recipient cells [109]. Myc proteins are also modified by phosphorylation (see Table 5 below). All are implicated in promoting cell cycle progression (reviewed in [25, 1302]), transcriptional modulation (reviewed in [3, 49, 64]), differentiation [258, 311, 821, 1310, 1788] and induction of apoptosis [29, 39, 109, 146, 356, 933, 937, 1042, 1097, 1302, 1305, 1551, 1679, 1831]. Extensive deletion analysis has been carried out in order to identify functional domains within the Myc protein. The *C*-terminal region of Myc proteins comprises the basic (DNA-binding) region including a nuclear localization signal and the HLHZ dimerization domain, whilst the *N*-terminal portion contains a transcriptional activation domain (see below). Generally, deletion or disruption of any one of these domains abolishes the ability of Myc to promote cell proliferation [25, 338, 356] and apoptosis [29, 356], autosuppress [794], inhibit differentiation [384, 1811] and co-transform rat embryo fibroblasts

[974]. There are, however, exceptions. For example, a naturally occurring mutant of feline c-*myc* transduced by feline leukaemia virus (T17 v-*myc*) in a spontaneous T cell lymphosarcoma lacks part of the *N* terminus (amino acids 49–124 of feline c-Myc) which forms part of the transactivation domain [1541]. It also has a 3 bp insertion in the basic domain, although this seems to have no effect on DNA binding. The T17 mutant retains oncogenic potential in T cells. In contrast to wild-type feline c-*myc*, the T17 mutant gene is unable to induce transformation or apoptosis in chicken embryo fibroblasts, suggesting that these functions are uncoupled from the leukaemogenic potential in this mutant. Although members of the Myc family of oncoproteins have highly related structures and properties, suggesting that they have similar functions (albeit with some exceptions [1788]), redundancy in Myc protein function is minimized by complex spatial and temporal differences in expression of c-, N- and L-*myc* genes. At the onset of gastrulation, N-*myc* is abundantly expressed in embryonic cells while c-*myc* transcripts predominate in extraembryonic tissues [315]. Throughout midgestation the distribution of N-*myc* transcripts is restricted to particular organs such as the brain and kidney while the expression of c-*myc* is broader [315, 732, 911]. L-*myc* is expressed in the developing kidney, lung and central nervous system, with the highest levels in the neuroectoderm of the brain and neural tube [1584]. In contrast to homozygous null c-*myc* and N-*myc* mice which die at embryonic days 10 and 12, respectively [229, 290, 905, 969], homozygous null L-*myc* mice are healthy, reproductively competent and represented in expected frequencies from heterozygous matings [1584]. Although overlapping expression patterns of *myc* family members may complement the deficiency in L-*myc* expression, compensatory changes in the level of c- or N-*myc* were not detected in homozygous null L-*myc* animals [1584]. Given the role of Myc proteins in proliferation and differentiation it is, perhaps, not surprising that members of the *myc* family of proto-oncogenes are frequently activated during oncogenesis by a variety of mechanisms that lead, primarily, to deregulated expression (reviewed in [19, 47, 61, 95]).

Although Myc is unable to transform rat embryo fibroblasts (REFs) by itself, it can cooperate with a number of other gene products including oncogenically activated *ras* alleles fully to transform REFs [614]. Since deregulated expression of *myc* is a potent inducer of apoptosis under certain conditions, it is not surprising that cooperation with proteins that promote cell survival is a common finding. For example, Bcl-2 cooperates with Myc to promote cell survival *in vitro* [166, 363, 1051] and tumourigenesis in transgenic mice [975, 1295], probably by inhibiting apoptosis of cells with deregulated *myc* expression. Although the requirement for the tumour suppressor p53 in Myc-mediated apoptosis is controversial [1594, 1618, 1710, 1904, 2019], it is possible that loss of p53 function (the most common mutation in human tumours) may contribute to Myc-mediated tumourigenesis [1397, 1511].

Given that progress through the cell cycle is governed by cdks and their regulatory subunits, the cyclins (reviewed in [1311]), the transcriptional activation of these genes might provide one mechanism by which Myc exerts its mitogenic effect. Although cotransfection of primary fibroblasts with *cyclin D1* (the regulatory subunit of certain cdks active during the G_1 phase of the cell cycle) and *myc* does not lead to a transformed phenotype [1735], they cooperate to generate B cell neoplasia. Whereas $E\mu$–*cyclin D1* transgenic mice exhibit only subtle changes in the cycling of B cells and only rarely develop tumours, B cell lymphomagenesis is much more rapid in mice that co-express both *cyclin D1* and *myc* transgenes than in mice expressing either transgene alone [1400, 1734]. Furthermore, the spontaneous lymphomas of *myc* transgenic animals often ectopically express the endogenous *cyclin D1* gene [1400], suggesting that Myc and cyclin D1 can cooperate in oncogenesis. It is not, however, clear whether Myc directly promotes *cyclin D1* expression [525, 1473, 1955]; indeed, the evidence indicates that overexpression of Myc in fibroblasts represses *cyclin D1* expression [525, 805, 1755], possibly by interacting with an initiator element in the *cyclin D1* promoter [805]. Conversely, transfection of cyclin A or D1 into HeLa or Saos-2 cells stimulates transcription of reporter constructs containing the Myc P2 promoter [1826]. Of the genes encoding cyclins D2 and E and cdks 2 and 4, only cyclin E is moderately up-regulated by Myc [452, 525]. However, activation of Myc in quiescent rat fibroblasts can facilitate activation of both cyclin E- and cyclin D1-dependent kinases without significant changes in the amount of these complexes [1960]. Partial activation of the cyclin E–cdk2 complex by Myc correlates with the release of inhibitory components (including the kinase inhibitor p27) from the complex; full activation requires additional signals supplied by growth factors [1960]. Ectopic activation of Myc leads to induction of cyclin A mRNA in both proliferating cells and cells undergoing apoptosis [481, 525, 1371]. Thus, Myc may exert its mitogenic effects by affecting the expression or activity of cell cycle regulatory components.

A GST–c-Myc fusion polypeptide that contains only the c-Myc bHLHZ region specifically binds to the core DNA sequence CACGTG *in vitro* [1163]. This bacterially expressed Myc fragment is presumed to form a homodimer. However, full-length Myc proteins do not homodimerize *in vitro* or in cell extracts and fail to bind DNA [1186, 1225]. Rather, Myc proteins dimerize with the heterologous bHLHZ protein Max [90, 168, 169, 735, 1186, 1217, 1256, 2153], and the Myc/Max heterodimers bind specifically to the core DNA sequence CACGTG [168, 169, 1186, 1213, 1244]. Max contains a bHLHZ DNA-binding motif similar to that of Myc [168, 1244]. Consistent with this, the ability of Myc to prevent growth arrest and induce apoptosis requires heterodimerization with Max [91, 2121]. Given that dimerization with Max is required for most of the biological functions of Myc it is likely that Max is present in the same range of species as Myc proteins. Interestingly, phylogenetic analyses indicate that Max exhibits significantly less sequence variation than Myc proteins, and it is suggested that this reduced variability reflects evolutionary pressures acting to preserve the dimerization capability with Myc and related proteins ([1356], see below).

Max is ubiquitously expressed. Two predominant Max proteins have been described, and they differ by the presence or absence of a nine amino acid insertion N-terminal to the basic domain [168, 1244]. Both Max proteins are extremely stable and they are coexpressed in a variety of cell types [3, 154]. In addition to the alternatively spliced exon in the N terminus, several naturally occurring forms of alternatively spliced *max* mRNAs have been reported [672, 1014, 1346]. A variant protein, termed dMax, has a deletion spanning the basic domain, helix 1 and loop region, presumably as a result of alternative splicing [1346]. Although dMax associates with Myc, the dimer fails to bind a consensus CACGTG site, suggesting that dMax may function as a dominant negative regulator of Myc function [1346].

It is clear that Max is essential for most, if not all, of the functions of Myc. DNA binding, transcriptional activation, co-transformation, induction of cell proliferation and apoptosis are all dependent on the association with Max [90, 91, 272, 2121]. The only exceptions to this are the effect of Myc on the expression of cyclin D1, which appears to be independent of dimerization with Max [805], and the apparent lack of a functional Max protein in the rat pheochromocytoma cell line, PC12 [1610]. In addition to forming heterodimers with Myc, the Max protein also forms homodimers that recognize the same DNA sequence as Myc [154, 552, 1186, 1213, 1260], and experimental overexpression of Max attenuates Myc-induced transcription, co-transformation, cell proliferation and tumourigenesis [90, 431, 592, 672, 846, 1726]. However, in the presence of the Myc protein, the Myc/Max heterodimer is preferentially formed and stabilized [1213].

Recently, four related proteins have been described that specifically associate with Max but not with Myc proteins [1214, 1257, 1624]. These proteins, Mad1 [1214], Mad3 [1624], Mad4 [1624] and Mxi1 [1257], form heterodimers with Max that efficiently bind the Myc/Max consensus binding site. Like Myc, Mxi1 and Mad proteins are unable to bind DNA by themselves. Mad/Max and Mxi1/Max heterodimers repress transcription through the same binding sites activated by Myc/Max heterodimers, and ectopic expression of Mad or Mxi1 antagonizes transcriptional activation by Myc [1214, 1257, 1624, 2061]. Moreover, Mad and Mxi proteins inhibit co-transformation by Myc and Ras [610, 1624, 1681, 2146], suggesting that they antagonize Myc *in vivo*. The mechanism of repression by Mad and Mxi1 involves the recruiting of mammalian homologues of the yeast transcriptional co-repressor, Sin3, to the Mad/Max or Mxi1/Max heterodimer [1361, 1624, 1870, 2146]. Mutants of

Mad in which the N-terminal domain required for interaction with mSin3 is deleted fail to inhibit transactivation and co-transformation by Myc [1681].

Analysis of the expression patterns of Myc and Mad family members in mammalian cells that can be induced to differentiate *in vitro* indicates that loss of *myc* expression and an increase in *mad* expression correlates with growth arrest and differentiation [116, 620, 1483, 1623, 1624] (reviewed in [1306]). Ectopic expression of Mad1 inhibits the proliferative response of NIH3T3 cells to signalling through the colony-stimulating factor-1 receptor and requires an intact mSin3 interaction domain suggesting that the ability of Mad1 to inhibit proliferation involves transcriptional repression [1897]. Studies *in vivo* demonstrate that, in normal epidermis, colonic mucosa and the developing CNS, *myc* expression is restricted to proliferating cells while expression of *mad1*, *mad3* and *mad4* is restricted to differentiating cells [315, 732, 1054, 1448, 1623, 2010]. In the testis, *mad1* expression is associated with the completion of meiosis and early development of haploid cells [2010]. In contrast, *mxi1* is expressed in both proliferating and differentiating myeloid leukaemia cell lines [620, 1257] and in the developing spinal cord and epidermis [1624]. Nonetheless, the downregulation of *myc* during differentiation suggests that Mxi1/Max heterodimers will predominate. Thus, the ability of Mad proteins to suppress the biological functions of Myc and the inverse relationship in their patterns of expression constitutes a switch in heterocomplexes (Myc/Max versus Mad/Max), which may be reflected in activation or repression of common target genes mediating cell proliferation and differentiation.

The correlation of *mad* expression with reduced proliferation (concomitant with differentiation) and the ability of Mad1 and Mxi1 to suppress Myc-dependent transformation are consistent with a potential function of Mad family proteins as tumour suppressors. Indeed, ectopic expression of *mad* inhibits proliferation and tumourigenicity of human astrocytoma cells [1439], and allelic loss and mutation at the *mxi1* locus has been detected in prostate cancers [1501].

Several studies have sought to identify Myc-regulated target genes. Such a search is complicated by the fact that expression of Myc correlates with the entry of cells into the cell cycle, a process during which many genes are subject to regulation that is only indirectly affected by c-Myc. Only a few of the genes so far isolated that appear to be modulated by c-Myc contain the Myc consensus binding site in their control elements and are thus candidates for direct c-Myc regulation. They include genes for *p53*, ornithine decarboxylase (*ODC*), *α-prothymosin* and an embryonically expressed gene, *ECA39*. The *p53* CACGTG consensus binding site is bound by c-Myc and USF [851, 852, 1200]. This CACGTG element is conserved between the mouse and human promoter and is located downstream from the transcription initiation site [851, 852]. High levels of c-Myc protein activate, and high levels of Max repress, the human p53 promoter, and there is a correlation between the levels of c-Myc protein and p53 mRNA in Burkitt's lymphoma and other B cell lines [1898]. Moreover, antisense *c-myc* RNA leads to a reduction in the levels of c-Myc protein and p53 RNA, suggesting a direct role for c-Myc in the transcriptional regulation of p53 [1898]. ODC, a rate-limiting enzyme of polyamine biosynthesis essential for progression from the G_1 phase to the S phase, is constitutively expressed in FDC-P1 myeloid cells that constitutively express *c-myc* [297] and may be transactivated by c-Myc through a CACGTG motif found in *ODC* intron 1 [140, 141, 792, 1050, 1851, 1993]. Moreover, overexpression of ODC has been implicated in cell transformation [114] and apoptosis [778, 1830]. *ECA39* is expressed in certain embryonic and adult tissues and in several tumours with elevated levels of c-Myc. The *ECA39* gene contains a functional Myc-binding site located downstream from its transcription initiation site [152]. Transfection of *c-myc* prevents the normal down-regulation of this gene which occurs in embryonic stem cells undergoing differentiation. By ectopic activation of a conditional mutant of c-Myc in rat fibroblasts, the c-Myc–oestrogen receptor (MycER) chimera [338], in which activity of MycER is dependent on the presence of exogenous β-oestradiol, the growth-regulated *prothymosin-α* gene has been identified as a c-Myc target [339]. Although both the rat and human *prothymosin-α* genes contain Myc-binding sites [392, 1784], other

data fail to support a role for Myc in activating transcription of the human *prothymosin-α* gene [1785]. It is intriguing that all known c-Myc-regulated genes possess their c-Myc recognition DNA element downstream of the transcription start site, and this may account for some of the reported differences in the transactivation of synthetic reporters and intact promoter/enhancer regions of supposed Myc target genes (see [1414, 1486, 1829]). In addition, the rat *prothymosin-α* gene possesses a mechanism of discriminating Myc/Max complexes and closely related bHLHZ proteins that bind the same sequence such as USF and TFE3 [1486]. Whereas Myc/Max is capable of activating from a distal element (relative to the transcription start site), USF is not (although USF does bind this site). Consistent with this, most USF binding sites are proximal to the transcription start site. A second E box element discriminates against transactivation of *prothymosin-α* by TFE3 [1486], probably by binding a repressor protein reminiscent of the way in which transactivation of the IgH gene by MyoD and TFE3 is inhibited in non-B cells [395, 2118].

In summary, there is considerable evidence that Myc proteins regulate transcription of a number of genes. As yet the effects of Mad/Max and Mxi1/Max heterodimers on the transcriptional activities of these Myc target genes have not been determined. Although other experiments have suggested a role for Myc proteins in DNA replication [245, 246, 506, 507, 977], many of these experiments have not been successfully duplicated by others [441, 442].

USF

Upstream stimulatory factor (USF, also known as MLTF1 or UEF) was first described as an activity in HeLa cell nuclei which bound to, and activated, an E box sequence upstream of the adenovirus major late promoter [215, 715, 901]. Extensive purification of USF activity yielded two polypeptides of 43 and 44 kDa, respectively [900, 902]. Subsequent cloning of the gene for the smaller polypeptide (commonly referred to as USF[43] or just plain USF) showed it to be a member of the bHLHZ family of proteins. Like other bHLHZ proteins, USF binds to its target

DNA as a dimer [426, 1143, 1202]. The USF leucine zipper is required for stable dimerization and DNA binding by the intact USF protein. However, a truncated USF bHLH mutant lacking a leucine zipper is still able to bind DNA in a sequence-specific manner, suggesting that the zipper is partially dispensable [426, 1202]. Recent data suggest that zipper interactions within USF dimers are not important for DNA binding but, rather, the leucine zipper alters the kinetics of DNA association [2104, 2113]. In this regard, it is interesting that the sea urchin USF protein, which is required for activation of the sea urchin U6 small nuclear RNA by RNA polymerase III [645], lacks a *C*-terminal leucine zipper [586]. However, with the exception of the bHLH domain, sea urchin USF exhibits little homology with the human and *Xenopus* USF proteins (which share some 80% identity at the amino acid level [556, 1012]), and it is thus only distantly related to vertebrate USF.

USF is expressed ubiquitously in many cell types and activates transcription through binding to the E box sequence CACGTG present in the regulatory regions of a number of genes, including metallothionein I [216], γ-fibrinogen [238, 1782], the murine Hox2.3 gene [1132], histone H5 [322], immunoglobulin λ2 chain [228], class I alcohol dehydrogenase [1196], β-globin [192], human insulin [845], L-pyruvate kinase [1491, 2012], cardiac ventricular myosin light chain 2 [1803], the pancreatic islet homeobox factor STF-1 [1928], fatty acid synthase [2022], cyclin B1 [1454], CD2 [1827], mouse cAMP-dependent protein kinase regulatory subunit type IIβ [1943], and the tumour suppressor *p53* [852, 1572]. *In vitro* DNA-binding studies suggest that USF is also involved in the TGF-β1-stimulated transcription of plasminogen activator inhibitor type I [862] and the interferon-regulated expression of the *HLA-B* gene [405]. Other studies demonstrate that USF cooperates with Varicella–Zoster virus IE62 protein to activate a bidirectional viral promoter [698, 1769]. One clue as to the molecular function of USF comes from studies of its stimulation of the adenovirus major late [1874, 2081, 2115] and HIV-1 [1490] promoters. This is mediated via pyrimidine-rich initiator elements in conjunction with a novel initiator-binding factor, TFII-I [401, 1171, 1246], suggesting a role in basal

transcription. *In vitro* studies suggest that USF may also play an important role in establishing the transcriptional potential of cellular genes during chromatin assembly [1091]. A second protein with a highly related bHLHZ region to USF has recently been isolated [1202]. This protein, dubbed USF2, also binds to CACGTG and may be identical to the 44 kDa polypeptide originally copurified with USF[43] (USF1) from HeLa cell nuclei [900, 902, 950]. USF1 and USF2 (USF[44]) can each homodimerize and heterodimerize with each other, and USF2 has also been isolated via its association with the Fos protein (FIP, see below [1218]). USF1 and -2 are ubiquitously expressed, although their relative abundance varies. For example, USF2 homodimers are not detected in HeLa cells due to the abundance of USF1 [950]. Whereas no difference in preferred DNA-binding sites or activation potential has been detected *in vitro*, the divergence of the *N*-terminal regions of USF1 and -2 suggest that they may have different activities *in vivo* [950, 1737]. Recent data demonstrate that, while both USF1 and -2 inhibit the transformation of rat embryo fibroblasts by *myc* and *ras*, USF2 (but not USF1) can inhibit E1A-mediated transformation [1738], suggesting that members of the USF family may act as negative regulators of cell proliferation. Another protein with related properties to USF has been described that activates the C4 promoter of the rodent complement system [390]. Whether this represents the rat homologue of USF2 has not been determined.

Immunoglobulin enhancer-binding bHLHZ proteins

The immunoglobulin heavy chain (IgH) enhancer is important for the transcriptional activation of rearranged heavy chain genes and contains a number of E box protein-binding sites. One of these sites, μE3 (CATGTG), is recognized by several bHLHZ factors. TFE3 is a ubiquitous activator of the IgH enhancer that binds the μE3 site [134] as well as regulatory elements important in lymphoid-specific, muscle-specific and some ubiquitously expressed genes [874]. TFE3 exists *in vivo* as two alternatively spliced isoforms with different transactivation potentials [874, 1888].

TFE3S, which lacks an exon encoding an *N*-terminal acidic activation domain, can act as a dominant negative of the larger form, TFE3L [1348]. A proline-rich domain present in the *C* terminus of both TFE3S and TFE3L acts synergistically with the acidic domain of TFE3L to activate μE3 reporter constructs [1348]. A 38 amino acid region at the *C* terminus of TFE3 shares 45% identity (including three conserved proline residues) with the related proteins TFEB and Mi, suggesting that this domain may contribute to transactivation in a number of HLHZ proteins. TFEB was isolated by screening a human B cell line expression library with an E box sequence from the adenovirus major late promoter (MLP) that is also known to bind USF (CACGTG [214]). Not surprisingly, TFEB also binds to E boxes in the IgH enhancer. TFEB specifically binds DNA both as a homodimer and as a heterodimer with TFE3 [314], and TFEB and TFE3 homo- and hetero-dimers all exhibit a greater affinity for the MLP site than for the μE3 site *in vitro* [377]. A third bHLHZ protein that binds the IgH μE3 enhancer has been isolated by the PCR from rat chondrosarcoma cDNA using oligonucleotide primers derived from the bHLH coding region of TFE3 [1123]. Predictably, this protein, TFEC, is closely related to TFE3 and TFEB: its basic domain is identical and its HLH shows 88 and 85% identity with the same domains in TFE3 and TFEB, respectively. TFEC forms heterodimers with TFE3 [1123] but, in contrast to TFE3, TFEC does not contain an acidic domain and is unable to transactivate a reporter gene containing four tandem repeats of the μE3 enhancer element. Moreover, TFEC also inhibits the transactivation of the reporter by TFE3 when cDNAs of these proteins are cotransfected [1123]. This suggests that TFEC may regulate the activity of TFE3 (and possibly TFEB) by competing either for its dimerization partners or, as a homodimer, for its DNA-binding sites. While TFEC mRNA is found in many tissues in adult rats, the relative abundances of TFEC and TFE3 RNAs vary considerably [1123]. Elucidation of the precise biological roles of the TFEB/TFE3/TFEC group of bHLHZ proteins awaits further data regarding their intracellular interactions and identification of their target genes.

AP4

The enhancer-binding protein AP4 is a transcription factor that activates both viral and cellular genes by binding to the E box sequence CAGCTG [1234]. AP4-binding sites have been identified in the SV40 late promoter [1772], amylase 2A [1529] and in the LTRs of the feline immunodeficiency virus [716] and Maedi–Visna virus [760].

Other bHLHZ proteins

The mouse microphthalmia phenotype is characterized by the presence of one or more defects, such as lack of pigmentation, small eyes, a reduction in the number of mast cells, early onset deafness and bone abnormalities (reviewed in [1309]). Additionally, the human homologue, microphthalmia-associated transcription factor (MITF), has recently been shown to be mutated in two families with Waardenburg's syndrome type II, characterized by partial deafness and patch pigmentation of the hair, skin and eyes [1962]. All these pathologies result from a defect in a single gene, reminiscent of the diverse effects of mutations in the *Drosophila* gene *daughterless*. This implies that the gene responsible for microphthalmia has a role in many diverse cell types. Recently, a mutant line of mice with microphthalmia was found to have an insertion in a gene (*mi*) encoding a bHLHZ protein [482, 496]. The insertional mutant results in deletion of some of the *mi* coding region and transcriptional failure. Other spontaneously arising *mi* alleles contain deletions at other positions in the *mi* gene, strongly suggesting that mutation of this single gene is responsible for the mutant phenotype (reviewed in (1309)). For example, the original *mi* allele has a small in-frame deletion that deletes a single arginine residue from the putative basic domain [482]. The mutant Mi protein may, therefore, be a non-DNA-binding mutant which, in the same way as Id and Extramacrochaetae (see below), can form non-functional heterodimers with partners. Moreover, the *mi* gene is transcribed in a number of mouse tissues, consistent with multiple defects in different tissues characteristic of microphthalmia [496]. The Mi protein is most closely related to murine TFE3 with more than 70% identity at the amino acid level [496], and can form stable dimers with TFE3, TFEB or TFEC but not with Myc, Max, USF or E47 [1309, 2129]. Dimers containing Mi can activate transcription through both an E box (CACGTG) and through recognition of the conserved pigmentation promoter M box element (CATGTG), and an alternatively spliced exon located outside the bHLHZ modulates DNA recognition by the basic domain.

Screening of a rat adipocyte λgt11 expression library with an oligonucleotide containing an E box led to the isolation of the ADD1 bHLHZ protein [1015]. ADD1 activates transcription through a binding site in the 5′ flanking region of the fatty acid synthetase gene which is expressed in differentiating adipose cells, suggesting that it plays a role in the determination of adipocytes [1015, 1671].

Two closely related proteins, designated SREBP1 and 2, were isolated from nuclear extracts of HeLa cells by DNA affinity chromatography with the sterol regulatory element (*SRE-1*) [495, 1061, 1109]. Sequence comparison indicates that SREBP1a is the human homologue of ADD1 with over 70% identity throughout the whole protein and only one conservative change in the bHLH region. SREBP1 activates transcription through a binding site in the 5′ flanking region of the fatty acid synthetase gene which is expressed in differentiating adipose cells, suggesting that it plays a role in the determination of adipocytes [1015, 1671]. SREBP proteins also activate transcription of the low-density lipoprotein receptor through interaction with the sterol response element-1 (SRE-1), and may be involved in regulating plasma cholesterol levels [1109, 1905, 1965, 2070, 2096]. Unlike other bHLHZ proteins, SREBP1 exhibits a dual DNA-binding specificity [2102]. It is able to bind both an E box (CACGTG) present in the carbohydrate response element (which, in response to carbo-

hydrate, regulates genes involved in fatty acid and triglyceride metabolism) and a non-E box sequence shown to be important in cholesterol metabolism [1905, 2070, 2096], the sterol regulatory element-1 (SRE-1; ATCACCCCAC) [1062, 1109]. The SREBP proteins share with Max three amino acids in the basic domain that contact the sequence CACGTG [1109, 1144], and it is likely that one subunit of the dimer contacts the E box half-site TCAC while the other binds the GGGT half of the SRE-1. The dual binding of SREBP to GGGT or CAC depends on a critical tyrosine residue in the SREBP basic domain (Y335 in Fig. 2) [2102], which is conserved in the *Drosophila* homologue HLH106 [1989]. Mutation of this tyrosine to arginine abolishes binding to SRE-1 without affecting E box binding. The equivalent arginine in other bHLH proteins is conserved (Fig. 2) and is important for DNA binding specificity [1142–1144, 1149]. Conversely, substitution of a tyrosine for the equivalent arginine in USF allows USF to acquire dual DNA-binding specificity similar to that of SREBP [2102]. Recently, Wang *et al.* [1062] have shown that SREBP1 is synthesized as a precursor that is attached to the nuclear envelope and endoplasmic reticulum. In sterol-depleted cells this membrane-bound precursor is cleaved to release the bHLHZ-encoding *N* terminus which then translocates to the nucleus [1062, 1104, 1911, 2087]. Cleavage of SREBP is carried out by members of the cysteine protease family, such as CPP32 [2032] and Mch3 [1833], which are implicated in apoptosis in animal cells. While it is assumed that the HLHZ region mediates dimerization, it is of note that the presumed leucine zipper is shorter than that in other bHLHZ proteins, and it is possible that SREBP proteins are examples of a diverged group of bHLHZ proteins. Preliminary evidence suggests that SREBP1 forms homo-oligomers [495].

Structure/function relationships of HLH proteins

The bHLH proteins bind DNA as dimers and usually recognize short palindromic sequences (CANNTG) such that each protein monomer binds one half-site. Immediately N-terminal to the HLH or HLHZ dimerization domain is a region of basic amino acids (b) presumed to mediate DNA binding. Sequence specificity is assumed to reside in the combination of the two basic domains in the dimer. Exceptions to this linear arrangement of basic domain and dimerization domain are a number of proteins with no recognizable basic domain such as Extramacrochaetae and Id (Fig. 2). These proteins, which are unable to bind DNA, inhibit the activity of bHLH proteins by dimerizing with them to form inactive, non-DNA-binding, heterodimers.

In structure, the bHLH domain comprises a short stretch of hydrophilic (often basic) residues (b) followed by a set of mainly hydrophobic residues located in two short segments (helix 1 and helix 2) and separated by a non-conserved sequence of variable length (the loop). The distribution of conserved residues within the HLH is consistent with the formation of two helices separated by a stretch of amino acids unfavourable for helix formation. Several groups have investigated the identities of amino acids at the beginning and end of such helices [1134, 1138, 1153, 1155] (reviewed in [1154]). These studies indicate that, apart from proline and glycine, there are certain amino acids that are more likely to be found at the boundaries of helices (referred to as the N cap and C cap residues). The N cap preferences, asparagine, serine and threonine, are often conserved at the beginning of the helices of HLH proteins. Recently the co-crystal structures of isolated homodimers of the E47, MyoD and USF bHLH and the Max bHLHZ each complexed with its specific recognition site have been reported [1142, 1143, 1144, 1149] (reviewed in [1137, 1141, 1152, 2049]) (Fig. 3).

These structures, described in detail below, confirm the previously held belief that the conserved HLH and

leucine zipper (Z) domains mediate dimerization and that each basic domain contacts bases in the CANNTG half-site.

```
                --BASIC DOMAIN--          .
      Max   17  RFQSAAD KRA HHNALERKRR DHIKDSFHSL  46
    c-Myc  348  SDTEENV KRR THNVLERQRR NELKRSFFAL 377
      Mad   50  SKKNNSSS RS THNEMEKNRR AHLRLCLEKL  79
     Mxi1   25  TSNTSTAN RS THNELEKNRR AHLRLCLERL  54
      AP4   25  RDQERRI RRE IANSNERRRM QSINAGFQSL  54
      USF  193  RTTRDEK RRA QHNEVERRRR DKINNWIVQL 222
     TFE3  134  ALLKERQ KKD NHNLIERRRR FNINDRIKEL 163
      FIP  137  RTPRDER RRA QHNEVERRRR DKINNWIVQL 166
       Mi  198  ALAKERQ KKD NHNLIERRRR FNINDRIKEL 227
  SREBP1a  317  SAQSRGE KRT AHNAIEKRYR SSINDKIIEL 346
      E12  543  KAEREKE RRV ANNARERLRV RDINEAFKEL 572
       Da  548  KAIREKE RRQ ANNARERIRI RDINEALKEL 577
    Twist  347  ETDEFSNQ RV MANVRERQRT QSLNDAFKSL 376
      Sim    1          MKE KSKNAARTRR EKENTEFCEL  23
    Scute   93  YNVDQSQSVQ RRNARERNRV KQVNNSFARL 122
    Mash1  109  LPQQQPAAVA RRNERERNRV KLVNLGFATL 138
     MyoD  103  RKTTNAD RRK AATMRERRRL SKVNEAFETL 132
     Lyl1  143  HQPQKVA RRV FTNSRERWRQ QHVNGAFAEL 172
     Tal1  181  GPHTKVV RRI FTNSRERWRQ QNVNGAFAEL 210
     Tal2    1      MTRKI FTNTRERWRQ QNVNSAFAKL  25
     Hen1   69  RRRATAKY RT AHATRERIRV EAFNLAFAEL  98
     Arnt   83  SADKERLA RE NHSEIERRRR NKMTAYITEL 112
      AhR   20  KTVKPIPAEG IKSNPSKRHR DRLNTELDRL  49
     Cbf1  216  TDEWKKQ RKD SHKEVERRRR ENINTAINVL 245
     Pho4  244  GALVDDD KRE SHKHAEQARR NRLAVPLHEL 273
       Lc  406  AQEMSGTGTK NHVMSERKRR EKLNEMFLVL 435
     Peru  375  TVTAQENGAK NHVMSERKRR EKLNEMFLVL 404

     Hes1   28  PKTASEH RKS SKPIMEKRRR ARINESLSQL  57
     Hes5   10  MLSPKEKN RL RKPVVEKMRR DRINSSIEQL  39
  E(spl)M7   7  MSKTYQY RKV MKPLLERKRR ARINKCLDEL  36
    Hairy   25  ETPLKSD RRS NKPIMEKRRR ARINNCLNEL  54
      Dpn   34  GLSKAEL RKT NKPIMEKRRR ARINHCLNEL  63

      Emc   20  ASGRIQRHPT HRGDGENAEM KMYLSKLKDL  49
      Id1   71  GTRLPALLDE QQVNVLLYDM NGCYSKLKEL 100
      Id2   72  LGISRSKTPV DDPMSLLYNM NDCYSKLKEL 101
      Id3   25  ARGRGKSPST EEPLSLLDDM NHCYSRLREL  54
      Id4   49  RCKAAEAAAD EPALCLQCDM NDCYSRLRRL  78
```

Figure 2

The basic region of HLH proteins. The basic (DNA-binding) domains of representative HLH proteins are aligned to emphasize the conserved residues (shown in bold type). Notably, these residues are missing from HLH proteins which are unable to bind DNA (bottom group) or interrupted by a proline residue in proteins which exhibit a preference for the N box DNA sequence (middle group). For each protein the region shown is indicated by the amino acid numbers adjacent to the sequence. The first conserved hydrophobic residue of helix 1 is indicated by ●. The complete amino acid sequences of these proteins and the alignment of basic and HLH domains are shown in the Appendix.

Dimerization of HLH proteins

The Max homodimer forms a parallel, left-handed, four-helix bundle with a stable hydrophobic core. All of the conserved hydrophobic amino acids from helices 1 and 2 are buried within this core. Helix 1 packs against helix 2 in the same molecule and also against helix 2' of the apposing subunit. Extensive van der Waals contacts and limited electrostatic interactions stabilize the HLH four-helix bundle (Fig. 3). Studies by Davis and Halazonetis [291] on mutant Myc/Max heterodimers demonstrate the requirement of all of the conserved hydrophobic amino acids in bH1 and H2 for stable interaction with DNA and suggest that the parallel, four-helix bundle is, indeed, the structure responsible for DNA binding. Although probably sharing the same overall structure, bHLH and bHLHZ proteins vary in the sequence, amino acid composition and length of the interhelical loop. Analysis of the three-dimensional structures of E47, USF, MyoD and Max suggests that the minimum length of the loop is at least four or five amino acids. Consistent with this, all known members of the bHLH and bHLHZ families exhibit loop lengths of between 5 and 24 amino acids. Moreover, shortening of the eight amino acid loop of MyoD to only four amino acids abolishes DNA-binding activity [1156]. In addition to base and phosphate contacts between the basic region and the DNA recognition element, residues in the loop regions of USF and Max also interact with the phosphodiester backbone of DNA.

Modelling of Max on the known structure of GCN4 indicates that the Max zipper is a *C*-terminal extension of helix 2 that forms a parallel, two-stranded coiled-coil comparable in length to the zipper domains of many bZIP proteins [30] (Fig. 4(a)). End on, the helical leucine zipper can be represented as a helical wheel in which the seven amino acids of each repeat are referred to by the letters **a**–**g** and the residues of the opposing helix as **a'**–**g'** (Fig. 4(b)). The leucine residues of the zipper are aligned at position **d**. Hydrophobic residues are also common at position **a**, giving the 4,3 repeat of hydrophobic residues characteristic of coiled-coil structures. Examination of the helical wheel diagram shown in Fig. 4(b)

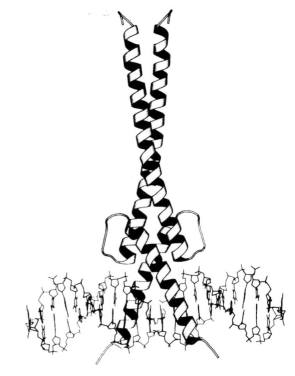

Figure 3

Three-dimensional structure of the Max–DNA complex. Cartoon representation of the Max bHLHZ (amino acids 22–113) homodimer–DNA complex. Helix 2 and the leucine zipper of each monomer are shown extending upwards from the DNA. The helical regions comprising helix 1 of the HLH and the basic domain diverge allowing the basic region (at the *N* terminus) to contact the major groove of the DNA. (Figure courtesy of A. R. Ferré-D'Amaré and S. K. Burley. Reprinted with permission from *Nature* [1144], copyright (1993) Macmillan Magazines Limited.)

shows that these hydrophobic residues lie along the apposing contact surface of the two helices. There are, however, several differences between the structure of the leucine zippers of Max and those of classical bZIP proteins. First, polar amino acids are more common at positions **a** and **d** of the bHLH leucine zipper helix than in the bZIP leucine zipper. Second, charged residues occupy more of the flanking **e** and **g** positions in bHLH zippers than in the zippers of bZIP proteins. Electrostatic interactions between these residues in the Myc/Max heterodimer are important for dimerization; reversed phase HPLC and

(a)

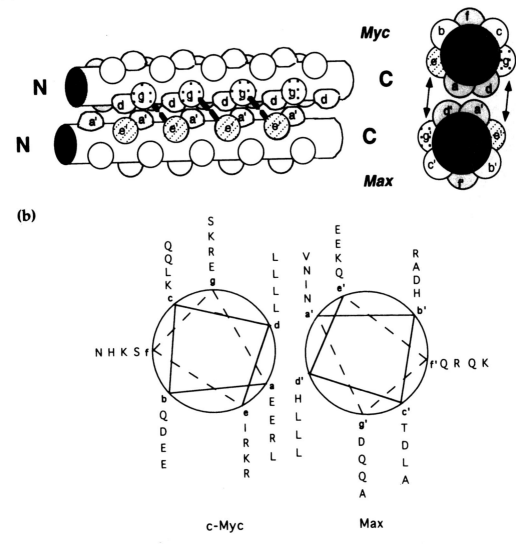

Figure 4
Interactions between the Myc and Max leucine zippers. (a) A model representing the parallel alignment of leucine zipper domains. The transverse view (right) clearly shows the proximity of the hydrophobic **a** and **d** residues of the two helices, and the arrows indicate electrostatic interactions that occur between charged residues at positions **e** and **g**. (b) The amino acid sequence of the human c-Myc and Max leucine zippers are displayed as helical wheels in order to emphasize the character of adjacent residues.

circular dichroism (CD) spectroscopy of synthetic peptides corresponding to the leucine zippers of Max and Myc suggest that the major interaction involves a histidine side-chain in the Max zipper (H81) and two glutamic acid side-chains in the Myc zipper (E410 and E417) at the heterodimeric interface [2089]. However, few of these potential electrostatic interactions appear to form interhelical salt bridges in the structure of the Max homodimer [1144], and this may account for the decreased stability of the Max homodimer compared to the Myc/Max heterodimer [90, 1213]. Third, the Max bHLHZ dimer exhibits considerably more buried surface than the GCN4 leucine zipper, resulting in extensive van der Waals contacts between the two helices. Additional CD data [1136] indicate that, in the absence of DNA, the bHLHZ of USF exists as a tetramer whereas the bHLH alone exhibits a mass consistent with dimers, suggesting a role for the leucine zipper in stabilizing higher-order oligomers. Using gel filtration chromatography, velocity sedimentation and chemical cross-linking, others have shown that USF exists as a dimer in solution in the presence or absence of DNA and that the leucine zipper is necessary for stabilizing the dimer [2122].

The functions of many bHLH and bHLHZ proteins depend on hetero-dimerization with other HLH family members (see below). Residues within the zipper segment of bHLHZ proteins greatly influence and, in some cases determine, their dimerization specificity [2139]. In the main, bHLHZ proteins are unable to associate with HLH proteins lacking a leucine zipper, although exceptions have been noted [1202]. Despite the similar structure of the HLH domain of both classes of protein, the instability of dimers of bHLH proteins lacking a leucine zipper indicates that other contacts in the structure of bHLH proteins are involved in the formation of stable dimers. For example, the E47 homodimer may be stabilized by two features [1142]. First, an additional turn in helix 1 increases the buried surface of the HLH four-helix bundle providing for an extra salt bridge between subunits. Second, glutamine residues at positions 364 (helix 1), 373 (loop) and 381 (helix 2) form hydrogen bonds. This triad of glutamines is a unique feature of E proteins (E12, E47, ITF1, ITF2 and HEB) and may contribute to the marked stability of their homodimers compared with other bHLH proteins such as MyoD. Further data suggest that residues in the loop and helix 2 can affect the rate with which E47 forms homodimers or heterodimers [1231].

The E12 and E47 proteins are distinguished by alternative splicing of the E2A gene, giving rise to an additional sequence in E12 (known as the 'A domain'), immediately N-terminal of the basic domain, that inhibits E12 activity [984]. DNA-binding studies suggested that this inhibitory domain prevents the E12 basic domain from contacting DNA [984]. However, more recent data indicate that the inhibitory domain blocks homodimerization of E12 and not DNA binding [2147]. Moreover, specific amino acids in MyoD helix 2 (Glu139 and Glu149) have been identified that are required to overcome the E12 inhibitory domain during the formation of MyoD/E12 heterodimers [2147]. These residues are not required for MyoD to heterodimerize with E12 containing mutants in the inhibitory domain nor E47 which lacks this domain altogether. Interestingly, all of the other myogenic bHLH proteins that dimerize with E12 have glutamic acid residues in the same position of helix 2 as MyoD. Since E12 dimerizes with a number of tissue-specific factors and negative regulators such as Id proteins, the regulation of dimerization specificity dictated by the inhibitory domain may contribute to the differentiation of several cell lineages.

DNA binding by HLH proteins

Most bHLH proteins bind as dimers to the consensus DNA hexamer CANNTG (also known as an 'E box') where N represents any base, most commonly either CG or GC (see Table 3 and references therein). Analysis of the DNA-binding ability of various bHLH and bHLHZ mutant proteins has established the importance of the basic domain for sequence-specific DNA-binding. Circular dichroism studies of isolated bHLH and bHLHZ domains [1133, 1143, 1149, 1173] suggest that DNA induces a transition to an α-helical structure in the basic DNA-binding domain [2088, 2091]. Recently, the three-dimensional structures of the Max bHLHZ and USF, E47 and MyoD bHLH domains complexed with their cognate DNA sites have been determined [1142, 1143, 1144, 1149] (reviewed in [1137, 1141, 1152]). The basic region of the Max bHLH domain is a helical extension of helix 1 (H1) that is orientated parallel to the major groove of the binding site (Fig. 3). The C-terminal helix comprises helix 2 and the leucine zipper as one continuous extended α helix. In the homodimer, two H1 regions pack against each other and against the two H2 regions to form a left-handed, parallel, four-helix bundle. The two leucine zippers that form

Table 3 Preferred DNA-binding sites

Protein	DNA sequence	Reference
Max/Max	RAN*CACGTG*NTY	168, 1175, 1179, 1203, 1244
c-Myc/Max	RAC*CACGTG*GTY	1162, 1163, 1175, 1183, 1197, 1203
Mad/Max	CACGTG	1214
Mxi1/Max	CACGTG	1257
AP4	CAGCTG	1234
USF	CACGTG	426, 900, 1160
	YYAYTCYY (R = pyrimidine)	1171
USF2	CACGTG (MLP)	1218
TFE3	MLP (CACGTG) >μE3 (CATGTG)	134
TFEB	MLP (CACGTG) >μE3 (CATGTG)	214
TFEC	μE3 (CATGTG)	1123
Mi	CACGTG, CATGTG	2129
SREBP1a, SREBP2	T*CACCCCAC*	495, 1109
	CACGTG	
E47	μE5κE2 CAGGTG	741
	CACCTG	1164
E12/MRF4	CAGCTG	1237
E12/ myogenin	CAGCTG	1237
E12/MyoD	CACCTG	1164, 1169
E12/Mash1	CACCTG	1182
E12/Mash2		
E47/Thing1	CATCTG	1608
E12/Tal1	μE2, CAGCTG	1180, 1181
E47/Tal1	μE5, CACCTG AA*CAGATG*GT	
E12/Tal2	CAGATG	1293
ITF1/Lyl1	AACAGATG(T/g)T	1780
E12/Hen1	CAGCTG	1165
ITF2	μE5κE2 (CAGGTG)	470
HEB	μE2	494, 1122
	AAG*CAGCTG*CTT	
MyoD	A*CAGCTG*T	1164
Mash1, Mash2	CACCTG	1182
Hen1	CAGCTG	1165
Arnt/Ah receptor	T-GCGTG (XRE-1)	1096, 2093, 2106
Hes1	N box > E box	898
Hes2	N and E boxes	515
Hes5	N box > E box	79
E(spl) proteins	N box, CACNAG	1011
Pho4	CACGTG	1177

This table lists the preferred binding site for each HLH protein dimer *in vitro*. Where only one protein is indicated it is presumed to bind as a homodimer. Further details of the binding sites can be found in the references.

part of the second α-helical region form a parallel, left-handed coiled-coil similar to the structure of bZIP proteins such as GCN4 [1150].

In common with other bHLH proteins, Max homodimers and Myc/Max heterodimers bend DNA towards the minor groove [1173, 1210]. The Max homodimer makes several contacts with conserved nucleotides in its binding site (Fig. 5). Foremost amongst these are hydrogen bonds from the cytosine and adenine of the *CANNTG* to a key glutamic acid. This glutamate residue (position 32 of the Max protein) is conserved in all bHLH and bHLHZ proteins with known DNA-binding activity (see Fig. 2 and the sequence

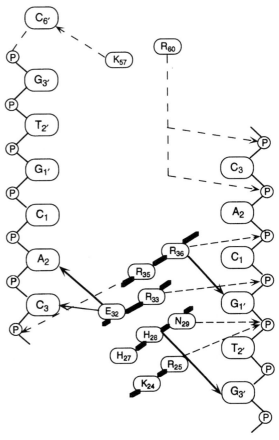

Figure 5
Summary of contacts between Max homodimer and DNA. A schematic summary of the contacts made by Max bHLHZ (amino acids 22–113). For simplicity, only contacts made by one monomer of Max are shown. Amino acid side-chain nucleotide contacts are indicated by solid arrows and contacts with the DNA phosphate back-bone by broken arrows.

alignment in the Appendix). Substitutions of this glutamate residue generally destroy DNA binding [1176]. Spaced approximately one helical turn N-terminal to the conserved glutamic acid is a histidine residue (position 28) that is conserved in Max proteins from all species [168, 1014, 1244] and is also present in the basic domains of the bHLHZ proteins Myc, TFE3, TFEB and USF. Bromouracil-mediated photo-cross-linking studies indicate that the analogous histidine in the human c-Myc protein (at position 336 in the basic region) contacts, or is close to, the thymidine of the CANNTG, suggesting that the Myc/Max heterodimer binds DNA in a similar way to the Max homodimer [1139, 1157]. In Max, H28 donates a hydrogen bond to the $3'$ guanidine of the consensus CACGTG sequence and appears to displace the arginine side-chain at position 25 such that it swings out of the major groove and makes a phosphate contact (Fig. 5). In contrast, the equivalent arginine of MyoD (R111) is buried in the DNA major groove and contacts the $3'$ guanidine of the consensus CAGCTG [1149]. The conformation of the arginine residue at this position seems to be important in transcriptional activity of target genes rather than DNA binding. The conformation of R111 is influenced by the nature of the residues at positions 114 (which lies in an analogous position to H28 of Max) and 115 (alanine and threonine, respectively). Consistent with this, introduction of A114, T115 and K124 (amino acid positions refer to human MyoD), which are conserved in the myogenic proteins, into equivalent positions of E12 (551, 552 and 564, respectively) confers myogenic activity on E12 [1170], suggesting that the cis-acting negative sequences in the MCK enhancer seem to be directed at the bHLH region of E12 [2118]. Thus, the conformation of the conserved arginine (position 111 of MyoD) may be important for transcriptional activation of muscle-specific genes [2137].

Specificity for nucleotides at the central two positions of the consensus CANNTG element (usually CG or GC) depends upon the identity of amino acids close to the conserved glutamic acid. The amino acid residue one helical turn to the C-terminus of the conserved glutamic acid (i.e. residue 36 of Max) is an important determinant of this specificity (see Table 3 and Fig. 2). Dimers of bHLH proteins that

possess an arginine at this equivalent position prefer CG as the two central bases (e.g. USF, Max, Myc, Mad, TFE3, and the yeast transcription factors Pho4 and CBF1). In contrast, proteins with smaller, non-polar residues at this position favour GC (e.g. AP4, MyoD and E12). Indeed, the preference for CAGCTG exhibited by MyoD and AP4 can be altered to CACGTG simply by substituting, respectively, the leucine or methionine at this position with arginine [1162]. In the Max homodimer, the arginine at position 36 hydrogen bonds with the central guanidine of the appropriate half-site. The identity of the amino acid at position 31, immediately N-terminal to the conserved glutamic acid at position 32 also influences the preferred site. In proteins that bind CAGCTG this residue is arginine, and in proteins recognizing CACGTG it is a non-polar amino acid (see Table 3 and Fig. 2). In general, the basic region makes a large number of additional contacts with phosphate moieties throughout the entire DNA recognition element. Lastly, in Max, a lysine in the loop region between Helices 1 and 2 stabilizes the loop by making direct contact with the phosphodiester backbone. It has been suggested that this latter contact may play a part in selection of bases flanking the CANNTG core [1144] that has been described for Myc and Max [1160, 1162, 1203].

At present our knowledge of the interactions of HLH proteins with each other and with DNA is limited and based largely on crystal structures of Max, USF, E47 and MyoD complexed to their cognate DNA sites. These four stuctures have, however, demonstrated the overall conservation of the bHLH fold, and it is likely that other bHLH and bHLHZ proteins behave in the same way. For example, amino acids required for base contacts in the Max homodimer are also essential for the DNA-binding activities of TFEB and Myc, suggesting similar protein–DNA interactions. Moreover, HLH proteins that do not bind DNA and act as negative regulators of bHLH proteins either do not possess any region with homology to the DNA-binding α-helical basic region (e.g. Id and Emc) or contain a helix-destabilizing proline residue (e.g. Hairy and Hes proteins). In contrast, residues determining the hydrophobic core essential for the formation of the four-helix bundle (see above) are well conserved in Id and Emc, consistent with the fact that they are still able to form stable dimers with appropriate bHLH partners.

Nuclear localization of HLH proteins

As DNA-binding transcription factors, bHLH and bHLHZ proteins must localize to the nucleus. In general, sequences within the basic domain of bHLH and bHLHZ proteins appear sufficient to direct the protein to the nucleus. In other bHLH and bHLHZ proteins, however, additional sequences have also been identified that direct nuclear localization. Some examples are discussed below.

With the exception of *Xenopus* maternal Myc [440, 1000, 1708], all Myc proteins localize to the nucleus [88, 342, 354, 445, 799]. Nuclear localization of c-Myc is mediated by a region encoded in the third exon and has been defined as amino acids 320–328 (PAAKRVKLD) [282, 283, 974]. This sequence is evolutionarily conserved amongst known c-*myc* genes, and a similar sequence (PPQKKIKSE) occurs in N-Myc [283]. Related sequences have also been identified in Max [552] and ALF1 [1193]. Absence of any analogous nuclear localization sequence in murine and human L-Myc proteins [633] may be compensated for by a second peptide sequence conserved between c-, N- and L-Myc proteins and which functions both as a surrogate nuclear localization signal [282] and comprises part of the basic domain responsible for sequence-specific DNA-binding (see above). Indeed, the existence of two nuclear localization signals which can function independently appears to be a common feature of bHLH proteins. Nuclear import of murine MyoD is mediated by two short sequences present in the basic helix 1 region (amino acids 100–112 and 131–135 [2009]). These sequences are conserved in all four myogenic bHLH proteins from different species. Similarly, a Tal1 protein lacking a basic domain (which includes a nuclear localization signal) is still localized to the nucleus, and this may be due to a second domain in the N-terminal region [1389] or to dimerization with a bHLH partner containing an intact nuclear localization signal [1554].

Transactivation domains of HLH proteins

Activation domains of transcription factors are presumed to engage the basal transcriptional machinery in some way. Although several generic classes of transactivation domain have been identified (e.g. stretches of acidic amino acids or glutamine-rich or serine/threonine-rich regions), many are novel or unique and uncovered only by the questionable experimental artifice of fusing them to a modular DNA-binding domain within an artificial test system. By this criterion, transactivation domains of the bHLH and bHLHZ proteins have been experimentally identified in several bHLH and bHLHZ transcription factors (Table 4). Two transactivation domains have been mapped to a conserved region in E12/E47, HEB and Daughterless bHLH proteins which have the potential to form helical structures [826, 1345, 1761]. Amino acid substitutions in conserved hydrophobic residues within these motifs abolish transactivation activity [826, 1759]. There is also evidence that one of these domains (AD2) shows cell type preference *in vivo* when microinjected as a fusion protein with a heterologous DNA-binding domain [1343]. The N-terminal transactivation domain of TFE3 is also predicted to form a negatively charged amphipathic helix [134], suggesting that it might be related to the transactivation domains of E12/E47. In this regard, it is of interest that a similar motif present in ALF1A protein (= murine HEB protein) is extended by an insertion of 24 amino acids in ALF1B [1193] yet no difference has been observed between ALF1A and ALF1B in their transactivation activity from a heterologous promoter. However, as indicated above, such artificial assays may not reflect accurately the activity of these proteins on bona fide promoters *in vivo*. Moreover, the loop–helix structure is not the only determinant of transcriptional activity in ALF1 proteins and it may act to mediate interactions with other transcriptional regulatory proteins [826, 1193].

The N-terminal third of c-Myc, when fused to the DNA-binding domain of Gal4, can activate transcription from a reporter gene containing Gal4-binding

Table 4 Activation and repression domains

Protein	Effect	Region	Reference
c-Myc	Activation	*N* terminus	551
c-Myc	Repression	122–140	646
N-Myc	Activation	13–84	278
v-Myc	Activation	*N* terminus	364
USF	Activation	15–59 and 93–159	572
TFE3	Activation	1–126, *C* terminus	134, 1348
E12, E47	Activation	1–426 loop–helix (259–366), helix (1–99)	471, 826, 1761
ITF2	Activation	1-451 loop–helix (292–362)	472, 826
HEB	Activation	loop–helix (352–421)	826
Da	Activation	loop–helix (295–387)	826
MyoD	Activation	*N*-terminal 53 residues	1073
Tal1	Activation	117–175	895
AhR, Arnt	Activation	Glutamine-rich *C* terminus of AhR (580-797) and Arnt (714-789)	1540, 1641, 1677, 1719, 1740, 1952, 2045, 2155
Hes5	Repression	Proline-rich region	70

This table lists HLH proteins whose activation/repression domains have been identified. Amino acid numbering is the same as shown in the protein sequence alignment (see the Appendix).

sites [551]. By this assay, the transactivation domain of human c-Myc appears subdivisible into independent regions [551]. The first region, amino acids 1–41, includes a section with high glutamine content and a short acidic section. The second region, amino acids 42–103, includes a highly conserved 21 amino acid section (43–63) previously identified as Myc homology box 1 [60] that is rich in proline residues. Conserved within this homology box are two critical residues (threonine at position 58 and serine at position 62) that may modulate the transactivation activity of c-Myc in response to phosphorylation [1267, 1284, 1288]. Interestingly, mutations in this second transactivation region of c-Myc occur in many cell lines derived from Burkitt's lymphomas and may contribute to carcinogenic progression [1258]. The third region, amino acids 104–143, also contains a stretch of amino acids (128–141) strikingly conserved in all Myc proteins and has been termed 'Myc homology box 2' [60]. However, box 2 bears no resemblance to any other characterized transactivation domains [551]. Mutagenesis studies demonstrate that the tripartite *N*-terminal 'transactivation' region of c-Myc is required for all observed Myc biological functions including cotransformation [974], autoregulation [794], inhibition of differentiation [385], and the induction of cell cycle progression and of apoptosis

[356]. The *N*-terminal region of the Myc protein also interacts with components of the basal transcriptional machinery such as TBP [1232, 1239] and TFII-I [879]. Competition assays with v-Myc indicate that the transactivation domain of MyoD may interact with the same or similar components [709] and, interestingly, overexpression of Myc inhibits skeletal muscle differentiation [1485] and antagonizes MyoD function in NIH3T3 cells [713], although this may depend on the host cell type [1467]. In addition, interactions between the Myc *N* terminus and the products of the *rb* gene and p107 genes have been observed, although the physiological significance of these interactions is unclear [138, 1230, 1247, 1248].

The transactivation domain of USF resembles that of c-Myc. Analysis of the transactivation activity of USF–Gal4 fusion proteins containing various portions of USF[43] on Gal4-responsive reporter genes indicates a bipartite structure [572] in the *N*-terminal half of human USF, one located between residues 15 and 59 and another between residues 93 and 156. Both regions are required for full transactivation. As with Myc, these regions are rich in serine and threonine residues, raising the potential for modulation of the transactivation activity by phosphorylation. Similar clusters of serine and threonine residues are also present in other bHLH proteins, for example

ITF1 and ITF2 [927], and most probably also reside within transactivation domains.

Although a number of HLH proteins [1214] (Table 4) can *repress* the transcriptional activity of reporter constructs, regions of the protein responsible for this trans-repression activity have not been mapped.

Post-translational modifications of HLH proteins

Many, if not all, HLH proteins are targets for phosphorylation and, in many cases, phosphorylated forms have been detected *in vivo*. Significantly, phosphorylation sites are often conserved between homologues from different species and are located in regions of the protein shown to be essential for functional activity as a transcription factor (Table 5). Some well-studied examples are described below.

Myc proteins are phosphorylated *in vivo* on serine and threonine but not tyrosine [1267, 1269, 1277, 1278, 1279, 1284, 1288, 1289] and this phosphorylation may account for some of the observed size

heterogeneity of Myc proteins on denaturing polyacrylamide gel electrophoresis [24]. Myc proteins can serve as substrates *in vitro* for phosphorylation by casein kinase II [1269, 1278] and phosphopeptide mapping indicates that casein kinase II phosphorylates c-Myc *in vivo* [1278, 1284]. Hyperphosphorylation of c-Myc occurs during mitosis [1277], and the reduced ability of hyperphosphorylated c-Myc to bind nonspecifically to double-stranded DNA has led to the suggestion that hyperphosphorylation during the M phase may serve to release c-Myc from chromatin during chromosome condensation [1277]. Significantly, the phosphorylation state of critical residues in the *N*-terminal portion of c-Myc can modulate its transactivation potential (see below). In addition, c-Myc and Max can be phosphorylated *in vitro* by Mxi2, a mitogen-activated protein kinase related to the p38 member of the ERK family [2179].

In yeast the transcription of Pho5, which encodes a secreted acid phosphatase, is regulated by the bHLH protein Pho4. Pho5 is repressed when yeast are grown in phosphate-rich medium, probably as a result of negative regulation of Pho4 by phosphorylation [2174].

Table 5 Phosphorylation sites in HLH proteins

Protein	Kinase	Site(s)	Effect(s)	References
c-Myc (human)	p34^{cdc2}, MAP-K, CKII, GSK-3α, ERK2	T58, S62	Individual and combined effects on transactivation and transformation	1259, 1267, 1270, 1271, 1277, 1278, 1279, 1284, 1288, 1290, 2161, 2167
N-Myc	CKII	Acidic central, S367	Unknown	1268, 1269
L-Myc	GSK-3	Unknown	Unknown	1266, 1286, 1287
Max (human)	CKII	S11	↓ DNA binding of homodimer	1260, 1262, 1274, 2161
E12, E47, HEB	PKA PKC	Unknown	↓ Myogenic activity of heterodimers	1275, 1276, 2173
E47	CKII	S449 and/or S464	↓ DNA binding of homodimer	2169
MyoD	Unknown	Serine(s)	↓ DNA binding of homodimer	1275, 1276, 1282
	PKA	Unknown	↓ Transactivation	1292
Tal1	ERK1	Serine(s), S122	Unknown	1265, 2162
Tal2	ERK1	Serine(s), S100	Unknown	1293
Hen1	Unknown	Serine(s)	Unknown	1165
AhR	PKC	368-605 and 636-759	↓ DNA binding activity	1388
Arnt	PKC	unknown	↓ Association with AhR	1388, 2170
Pho4	Pho80/Pho85 cyclin–cdk	S100, S114, S128, S152, S223	↓ Transactivation	2174

HLH proteins with known phosphorylation sites are listed, together with the kinase responsible and any observed effect (↓, decreased activity). Amino acid numbers refer to the sequences shown in the protein sequence alignment in the Appendix.

Sequence-specific DNA binding by HLH proteins

Virtually all bHLH and bHLHZ proteins bind specifically to a consensus hexameric DNA sequence (CANNTG) known as the E box. E box sequences are often palindromic and contain identical half-sites, each of which may be bound by one component of the dimer. Although the central dinucleotides of the E box are usually GC or CG, exceptions have been noted. The preferred E box sequences bound by known HLH proteins are summarized in Table 3. It is of note that several independent HLH factors within one species often bind the same sequence, implying the existence of mechanisms for regulating precisely which HLH protein is bound to the E box in the control region of a given gene at any one time. Sometimes, this involves differential expression of iso-specific factors within specific cell lineages. Often, however, several bHLH/bHLHZ factors coexist within a cell. One possible mechanism dictating specificity of binding may reside in additional sequence specificities flanking the consensus E box element. Such a possibility was investigated for c-Myc, Max and USF, and revealed that, although the USF and Max homodimers and the Myc/Max heterodimer all bind oligonucleotides containing the core hexamer CACGTG in vitro, the c-Myc/Max heterodimer is specifically unable to bind the core when it is flanked by a 5′ T or a 3′ A (TCACGTGA; see Table 3), and this precludes transactivation by c-Myc from such sites in vivo [1160, 1203]. Thus, USF and Max homodimers bind more promiscuously than c-Myc/Max heterodimers to sequences containing CACGTG, and this raises the possibility that USF and Max homodimers may influence the activity of additional genes that are not c-Myc/Max targets. A further possibility is that specific cellular factors may regulate the DNA-binding properties of bHLH proteins. For example, an unidentified cellular factor is required for efficient DNA binding by the MyoD/E47 heterodimer but not by either homodimer [1206].

Dimerization partners

Dimerization is a prerequisite for sequence–specific DNA binding by several classes of transcription factors. Examples of both homo- and heterodimerization occur – with precise dimerization specificity dependent upon the protein in question. Whereas some bHLH and bHLHZ proteins can form both homodimers and heterodimers (e.g. MyoD and Max), others appear exclusively as homodimers (e.g. USF) or heterodimers (e.g. Myc and Mad). The dimerization specificities of various bHLH and bHLHZ proteins are summarized in Table 6, and some are discussed in detail below.

bHLH proteins belonging to the MyoD family activate muscle-specific genes through interaction with E boxes in their control regions. Originally, MyoD was thought to exist either as homo-oligomers or as MyoD/Id hetero-oligomers in proliferating, undifferentiated myoblasts [1226]. However, it now seems most probable that the DNA-binding activity of the myogenic HLH proteins is dependent upon heterodimerization with ubiquitously expressed bHLH proteins such as E12, E47 and HEB [1222]. Consistent with this, antisense inhibition of E12 expression blocks muscle-specific gene expression [1236], arguing for a requirement for E12 in myogenic determination. Detailed analysis of the interaction between various mutants of MyoD in which single residues in the HLH region were substituted identifies at least seven key pairs of residues that stabilize the MyoD/E12 heterodimer [1249]. Id is thought to block MyoD function by sequestering E12/E47 proteins into inactive heterodimers, although Id will also interact with MyoD family members [1226]. For Id proteins to function effectively they must efficiently compete with the binding of tissue-specific bHLH proteins (such as MyoD and Tal1) to the ubiquitously expressed E proteins. Consistent with this, Id proteins exhibit greater affinity for E proteins than Tal1 or MyoD when expressed in a yeast two-hybrid protein interaction assay [1555, 2128]. Mutants of Tal1 with

increased affinity for the E2-2 protein have been selected from a library of randomly mutated bHLH sequences [2128]. Not surprisingly these mutants have amino acid changes in helix 1 and helix 2. In helix 1, glycine at position 205 is changed to glutamic acid (G205E), the position of which is common to many other bHLH proteins (including MyoD, MRF4, myogenin, E12, E47, HEB, Daughterless and Twist), and which may form an intermolecular electrostatic bond with a basic residue in helix 2 [1249]. In helix 2, M233I increases the hydrophobicity at the dimerization interface. The Tal1 mutant with the highest affinity for E2-2, N204D/K225E, represents non-conservative changes in the most highly conserved residues in the HLH family. However, the N204D/K225E mutant binds E2-2 with high affinity, and it is suggested that loss of an intramolecular hydrogen bond (between helix 1 and helix 2) is compensated for by gain of an additional intermolecular ionic bond [2128].

The situation with MyoD and E12/E47 has parallels in *Drosophila* neurogenesis and sex determination. Members of the Achaete–Scute protein complex probably function as obligate heterodimers with Daughterless in the regulation of *Drosophila* neural-specific and sex-determining genes. Moreover, activity of *Drosophila* neurogenic and sex-determination factors, like mammalian myogenic determination factors, is inhibited through sequestration of Daughterless into inactive complexes by the Extra-macrochaetae HLH protein, which lacks a basic (DNA-binding) domain. This mode of regulation is discussed in more detail in the next section.

By analogy to the tissue-specific gene regulation of myogenesis and neurogenesis by heterodimerization between ubiquitously expressed (class A) and cell-type-restricted (class B) bHLH proteins, a similar mechanism might be envisaged for the B cell-specific transcription of immunoglobulin genes. However,

Table 6 Heterodimeric partners

Protein	Heterodimer partner	References
Max	c-Myc	168, 169, 1186, 1217, 1244
	N-Myc	1256
	L-Myc	168
	Mad1, 3, 4	1214, 1624
	Mxi1	1257
TFE3	TFEB	377
	TFEC	1123
E12/E47	MyoD family	1219, 1222, 1223, 1236, 1237, 1238, 1242, 1249, 1251
	Mash1, Mash2	1182
	Tal1	1180
	Hen1	1165
	Id2	1251
	Thing1	1470, 1468, 1608
	Thing2	1470, 1468, 1608
	bHLH-EC2	1395
	Scleraxis	1469
	MATH1	1324
	MATH2	1933
Daughterless	Achaete–Scute family	1221
	Emc	32
	Atonal	1645
Arnt	Ah receptor	692, 1603
	HIF-1α	1603, 2024
	Sim	1603, 1953
Hes5	Mash1	79
Emc	Achaete–Scute proteins	32, 344, 391
Id1	MyoD	1226, 243

The known dimeric combinations of HLH proteins *in vitro* are shown.

there is at present no evidence for expression of any cell-type-restricted bHLH proteins in B cells. Rather, it seems that transcription of immunoglobulin μ and κ chains is dependent upon homo- and hetero-dimerization entirely of class A proteins encoded by the *E2A* and *E2-2* genes. However, it is clear that the observed B-cell-specific activity of E boxes in the μE5 and κE2 enhancers is also modulated by other, identified, factors. It remains to be determined why class A dimers operate in B cells but not in other cell types.

In those HLH proteins that also possess a leucine zipper (bHLHZ) the leucine zipper is required for efficient dimerization [90, 874, 974, 1234]. A major insight into the relative contributions of the HLH and leucine zipper towards dimerization has come from mutagenesis studies of the Myc bHLHZ protein. All the known biological functions of c-Myc require an intact basic HLHZ region, indicating that both sequence–specific DNA-binding and dimerization are prerequisites for c-Myc function. Moreover, inter-action between c-Myc and Max is absolutely dependent upon the integrity of both HLH and zipper domains in each protein. Substitution of c-Myc helix 1 or helix 2 with analogous sequences derived from E12 (E12 does not associate with Max) significantly impairs or abolishes dimerization with Max. In contrast, substitu-tions within the loop between the two helices have no deleterious effect on dimerization [291]. Thus, both helices are required for efficient dimerization whereas the loop is not. None the less, in studies in which the entire c-Myc HLH was replaced by the analogous HLH region from TFEB, interaction with Max was compromised yet still occurred through the c-Myc zipper [291]. Similar results have been obtained for TFE3, USF and AP4 [874, 1215, 1234]. These studies all suggest that the zipper acts as a dominant interface of dimerization specificity, a notion supported by the fact that deletion of the c-Myc zipper, or its replace-ment with a heterologous zipper, totally abolishes dimerization with Max [291]. Yet other data indicate that c-Myc helix 2 and the zipper actually comprise a single extended helix [846]. As with the leucine zipper, one side of this extended helix 2 zipper is a hydrophobic face by virtue of the critical 4,3 spacing of hydrophobic residues along it, and this hydrophobic surface provides the dimerization interface. Not surprisingly, therefore, disruption of the 4,3 register by a three amino acid insertion between the HLH and the zipper abolishes dimerization with wild-type Max. However, if both proteins have such insertions they once again interact efficiently [291]. These data are all consistent with mutational analyses of Max, which suggest that helix 1 and helix 2 are both required for DNA binding by the homodimer and that hetero-dimerization with Myc is dependent on a functional zipper domain [846]. Although leucine zipper dimerization is mediated by the interaction of two hydrophobic surfaces, the crystal structure of the GCN4 leucine zipper suggests that dimerization specificity between zippers is, in part, specified by the nature of residues lying at the **e** and **g** positions of the helix [1147, 1150, 1151]. Residues at position **e** on one zipper are usually of opposite charge to residues at position **g** on the other, so facilitating the interaction. Consistent with this notion, complementary Myc and Max mutants with reciprocally exchanged charged amino acids at the **e** and **g** positions in their leucine zippers are unable to associate with their wild-type counterparts yet form stable DNA-binding heterodimers *in vitro* and *in vivo* [90] (see Fig. 4).

Why should there exist two classes of bHLH protein, one with an additional leucine zipper and one without? One possible reason may be that the leucine zipper in bHLHZ proteins may act to suppress promiscuous interactions with bHLH proteins. Deletion of the AP4 leucine zipper generates a truncated molecule that can now interact with E12 *in vitro* [1234]. Although any *in vivo* significance of this observation is doubtful, it injects a note of caution that studies using deletion mutants of bHLHZ proteins may reveal unpredictable and unphysiological interactions. TFE3, TFEB, USF and FIP (Fos-interacting protein, see below) all possess an insertion of three amino acids between the HLH and zipper which adjusts the register of hydrophobic residues by one turn of the helix and may further restrict dimerization, in this case with other bHLHZ proteins. Another possible reason for the additional zipper domain in bHLHZ proteins may be that the isolated helix–loop–helix domains of bHLHZ proteins (unlike those of bHLH proteins) appear generally to be unable to form stable DNA-binding dimers in solution. Indeed, analysis of the HLH sequences of bHLHZ proteins indicates that only a few potentially attractive pairs of residues exist between the monomers [1249]. The additional leucine zipper in bHLHZ proteins may therefore be required for their efficient dimerization and function.

In general, bHLH and bHLHZ proteins interact with members of their own class. However, some exceptions to this are known (Table 7). The bHLHZ protein FIP [1218] (identical to USF2 [950, 1202])

was isolated from a HeLa cDNA expression library through its interaction with a fragment of the c-Fos protein (a member of the bZIP family of transcription factors which interacts with other bZIP proteins, see review [30]) comprising the basic domain and leucine zipper [1218]. The USF2 zipper mediates interaction with the c-Fos protein leucine zipper, and stimulation of an AP-1 reporter is observed upon cotransfection of c-*fos* and *USF2* into F9 embryonal carcinoma cells. In response to antigen stimulation of mast cells, complexes containing Fos and USF2 bind to both a TPA-response element (an AP1 site also bound by Fos/Jun dimers [30]) and a FIP-binding site (FBS, which contains the E box consensus CACGTG [1716, 1717]). Binding of these complexes in response to antigen stimulation appears to be regulated by the effects of PKC-β on the synthesis and DNA-binding activity of USF2. The physiological significance of the complexity generated by different protein–protein and protein–DNA interactions has still to be elucidated. Another example of interaction between a bHLH and a bZIP protein is the observed physical interaction between the HLH domain of MyoD and the leucine zipper of c-Jun *in vitro* [1216]. However, this interaction is observed even when the MyoD loop region is deleted and may be due to nonspecific association of amphipathic helices promoted, or stabilized, by the cross-linking reagents used in these experiments. Moreover, no interaction between c-Jun and MyoD has been detected using a two-hybrid system, suggesting that such interactions either involve only a small proportion of the available proteins or are extremely unstable *in vivo* [1223, 1227]. Although such experiments argue against direct interaction between MyoD proteins and c-Jun *in vivo*, c-Jun does inhibit MyoD and myogenin-induced transcription of muscle-specific genes. However, this inhibition may not operate through direct interaction between c-Jun and MyoD proteins but may involve competition between the transactivation domains of c-Jun and MyoD for essential auxiliary factors [647]. In addition to c-Jun, inhibition of MyoD action by the c-Fos and JunB bZip proteins and by the bHLHZ protein c-Myc has also been noted [1695]. Adenovirus *E1A* gene products (E1A$_{12S}$ and E1A$_{13S}$) also inhibit differentiation of skeletal myocytes, suggesting that E1A,

Table 7 Other potential interacting proteins

HLH protein	Interacting protein	Interaction domains	Effect	Reference
c-Myc	Rb	Myc *N* terminus, 13–178		278, 1232, 1247, 1248, 1322
	p107	41–178 of Myc, 'pocket' region of p107	Transactivation	138, 1230
	TBP	Myc *N* terminus		1232, 1239
	TFII-I			879
	YY1	250–439 of Myc, 201–343 of YY1	Modulation of YY1 transcriptional activity	1250
	Nmi	bHLHZ of Myc, putative coiled coil of Nmi	Unknown	2120a
	α-Tubulin	48–134 of c-Myc	Regulation of Myc subcellular location?	2120
	Mxi2	*C* terminus of Myc	Phosphorylation of Myc	2179
	ERK2	1–100 of Myc	Phosphorylation of Myc S62	2167
	AP2	bHLHZ of Myc, 203–437 of AP2	↓ Myc transactivation	1547
N–Myc	Nmi	bHLHZ of Myc, putative coiled coil of Nmi	Unknown	2120a
Max	Mxi2		Phosphorylation of Max	2179
Mad1, Mad2, Mad4, Mxi1	mSin3A, mSin3B	Mad and Mxi1 *N*-terminal domains, paired amphipathic helices of mSin3	Co-repressor of transactivation	1361, 1624, 2146
USF2 (FIP)	c-Fos	Zipper of USF2, bZIP of Fos		1218
Mi	Rb	Not known	↓ Mi function	2157
E12	Ca^{2+}-loaded calmodulin	HLH of E12	↓ DNA binding	1224
	E1A$_{12S}$	bHLH of E12, *N* terminus of E1A	Repression of target genes	1253
Myogenin	E1A$_{12S}$	bHLH of myogenin, *N* terminus of E1A	Repression of target genes	1253
MyoD	c-Jun	HLH of MyoD, leucine zipper of Jun	↓ MyoD function	1216, 1227
	Rb	bHLH of MyoD, 'pocket' region of Rb	↑ MyoD function	432
	MEF2A	A114, T115 and K124 of MyoD, MADS domain of MEF2A	Cooperative DNA binding and activation	1663, 1786
Tal1, Tal2	RBTN1, RBTN2	bHLH of Tal1 and 2, LIM domain of RBTN1 and 2		2151
Lyl1	RBTN1, RBTN2	bHLH of Lyl1, LIM domain of RBTN1 and -2		2151
Mash1	MEF2A	bHLH of Mash1, MADS domain of MEF2A	Cooperative transactivation	2138
AhR	hsp90	230–421 of AhR	Inactive cytoplasmic AhR	1465

Table 7 Continued

HLH protein	Interacting protein	Interaction domains	Effect	Reference
AhR/Arnt	Sp1	HLH-PAS of AhR/Arnt, Zn finger of SP1	Cooperative activation of target genes	1678
Maize B	Maize C1	1–244 of B	↑ Activation of reporter gene	409
Hairy, E(spl), Deadpan	Groucho	WRPW of bHLH protein, 251–414 of Groucho	Repression of HLH target genes	1838
Id2	Rb, p107, p130	HLH of Id2	Inhibition of Rb growth suppressive activity	504, 1699

HLH proteins which interact with other proteins are listed. Where known, the interacting domains and any observed effects are indicated (↑, increased activity; ↓ decreased activity). Amino acid numbering is the same as shown in the protein sequence alignment (Appendix).

too, modulates the activity of the myogenic bHLH proteins. *N*-terminal sequences of E1A bind to myogenin *in vitro* [1253], but this interaction has not been duplicated *in vivo*. The mammalian Notch protein represses activation of MyoD/E12 target genes by interacting with a co-activator which itself can interact with the MyoD bHLH region [583]. The recent discovery that MyoD and myogenin interact directly with Rb [432] and that cyclin D1 inhibits transactivation by MyoD suggests mechanisms whereby the control of myogenesis and cell cycle progression can be coupled [842]. Thus, in all cases in which heterotypic factors modulate action of the bHLH myogenic proteins, the mechanism by which this inhibition occurs is obscure. None the less, the abilities of the c-Fos, c-Jun, JunB, Myc, E1A and Rb proteins to modulate the activities of myogenic HLH proteins *in vivo* [647] exemplifies the multiple layers of complexity involved in regulating gene transcription.

In summary, although dimerization between bHLH or bHLHZ proteins is specific, it can occur with one of several different partners, thereby giving rise to a potentially large number of dimer combinations. However, these dimerization interactions are not promiscuous and not all bHLH proteins can interact with each other. The specificity of interaction resides within the sequence (and consequently the three-dimensional structure) of the α-helical regions. None the less, the potentially large combinatorial range of dimers provides a mechanism for generating sufficient diversity to regulate many different transcriptional programmes.

Regulation of target genes by HLH proteins

The activities of bHLH and bHLHZ proteins are modulated by a variety of mechanisms. First, as outlined above, many HLH proteins can dimerize with more than one partner (including themselves), and both the DNA-binding specificity and activity of a particular HLH protein can be influenced by the identity of its dimeric partner. Second, phosphorylation modulates the affinity of DNA binding and the activity of the activation/repression domain(s) of some dimers. Third, there is evidence that the activity of some HLH proteins depends on their ability to recruit accessory factors. These issues are discussed in detail below.

Dynamic networks of HLH proteins

Whilst some bHLH and bHLHZ proteins are unable to homodimerize (e.g. Myc [90, 1186, 1225]), others are functionally active as homodimers but this activity can be modulated through hetero-dimerization with other partners. Clearly, the availability of differing monomeric subunits within a cell is a major factor in dictating which particular types of heterodimer, each with its own particular complement of activities and specificities, will form. Consistent with this idea, strict spatial and temporal expression of many HLH proteins is observed during myogenesis, neurogenesis and haematopoiesis. For example, expression of the myogenic HLH proteins such as MyoD, myogenin, MRF4 and Myf5 is restricted to muscle cell lineages. None the less, as already discussed, these tissue-specific (class B) HLH proteins are active as heterodimers with members of the ubiquitously expressed (class A) HLH proteins.

In the case of the myogenic determination factors, dimerization occurs with members of the ubiquitously expressed E12/E47 family of bHLH proteins. Significantly, the preferred DNA-binding site of the MyoD/E47 heterodimer differs from that preferred by the E47 homodimer [1164]. In *Drosophila*, members of the Achaete–Scute family of bHLH proteins are

expressed in a temporally and spatially regulated fashion during neural development and form hetero-dimers with a ubiquitously expressed bHLH protein, Daughterless. Related class B HLH proteins involved in vertebrate neurogenesis exhibit similarly restricted patterns of expression. Expression of several mammalian bHLH proteins is restricted to haematopoietic lineages where they are presumably involved in the determination and/or maintenance of differentiated haematopoietic cell types. Thus, patterns of expression of bHLH proteins are critical in the determination and maintenance of cell lineages.

The Myc proteins and their obligatory interaction with Max provides an example of an analogous network involving bHLHZ proteins (Fig. 6). N-Myc and L-Myc exhibit limited tissue-specific expression whilst the c-Myc protein is expressed in mature cells that retain a proliferative capacity (e.g. mesenchyme, epithelial and lymphoid cells, hepatocytes). Expression of c-Myc correlates with the proliferative state of the cell (reviewed in [25]) and, at least in fibroblasts, is absolutely dependent upon the presence of mitogenic growth factors [299, 1065]. Withdrawal of growth factors triggers rapid and synchronous down-regulation of c-*myc* expression in cells irrespective of their position in the cell cycle. The rapid disappearance of the c-Myc protein is a consequence of the extremely short half-life of both c-*myc* mRNA and protein [299, 1065]. It has been suggested that down-regulation of the c-Myc protein is a critical signal that triggers a cell to withdraw from the cycle and undergo growth arrest [25]. Recent data suggest that the contribution of c-Myc to cell cycle regulation involves modulation of cyclin expression [452, 525, 805, 1371, 1473, 1955, 1960]. Deregulated expression of c-Myc blocks growth arrest in response to mitogen deprivation or the antiproliferative effects of cytokines such as interferon or TGF-β. Intriguingly, in addition to promoting cell cycle progression, expression of c-Myc also triggers apoptosis (programmed cell

Expression

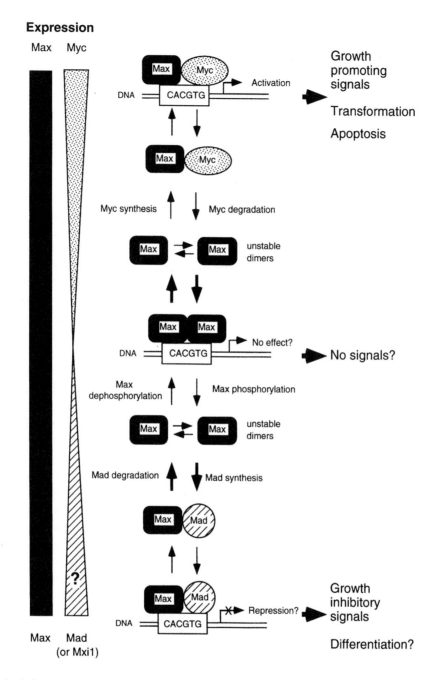

Figure 6

The Myc network. A diagram representing the biochemical equilibria between different CACGTG-binding complexes formed by c-Myc, Max, Mad and Mxi1 and their proposed biological effects is given. The different Max variants are not distinguished since no major functional differences between them have been unequivocally established (see text for details). Since the steady-state level of Max appears to be constant, the intracellular concentration of c-Myc is proposed to be the principal regulator of c-Myc/Max activity. Mad/Max and Mxi1/Max are proposed to have an opposite effect to c-Myc/Max and the levels of Mad and Mxi1 may be regulated in an inverse fashion to c-Myc. The overall biological effect of these complexes may be regulated by their differing affinities for each other and by post-translational regulation of their respective DNA-binding activities. For simplicity only Mad is shown, but this should not be taken to indicate that other members of the Mad family, including Mxi1, necessarily behave in the same way.

death) in cells deprived of specific survival factors [356, 363]. Perhaps paradoxically, both induction of cell cycle progression *and* of apoptosis are the result of the action of Myc as a transcription factor in modulating target genes. However, because few bona fide Myc target genes have been identified to date, it remains unclear precisely how Myc exerts its biological effects. Myc proteins do not form homodimers but, instead, hetero-dimerize with the bHLHZ protein Max. Whereas c-*myc* mRNA and protein are short lived, *max* RNA [154, 846] and protein [1217] are extremely stable. Moreover, levels of Max protein are invariant throughout the cell cycle [1217] and are not regulated by serum mitogens [154, 1049, 1217]. DNA binding and transcriptional activation by c-Myc are both absolutely dependent upon association with Max [1161, 1213]. Furthermore, the role of c-Myc in cell cycle progression, differentiation and apoptosis all require dimerization with Max [90, 91] (reviewed in [3]). The ratio of Myc/Max versus Max/Max complexes is thus likely to be a crucial determinant of Myc activity within cells. In summary, therefore, Max appears to fulfil a role somewhat analogous to that provided for class B bHLH proteins by the ubiquitously expressed (class A) bHLH proteins described above. However, the situation *in vivo* is likely to be yet more complex. For example, c-Myc interacts with a zinc finger-containing transcription factor, Yin-Yang-1 (YY1), *in vitro* and *in vivo* when coexpressed in yeast [1250], and in cotransfection studies, c-Myc interferes with both the transcriptional repressor and activator functions of YY1. These results indicate that Myc modulates the activity of YY1 [1250] and perhaps vice versa. Max interferes with the Myc–YY1 interaction *in vitro*, suggesting that any interaction between Myc and YY1 *in vivo* is also regulated by the relative concentrations of Myc and Max.

Max homodimers bind to the same DNA sequence as Myc/Max heterodimers but do not transactivate *in vitro* [431, 591, 592, 1213]. Consistent with this, Max appears to have no transactivation domain [552] and overexpression of Max represses the Myc-dependent transcription of a reporter gene [591, 1213]. As Max repression of c-Myc function is relieved by overexpression of Myc, it probably operates through competition with c-Myc/Max heterodimers for access to DNA-binding sites.

In addition to Myc proteins, four related bHLHZ proteins, Mad1 [1214], Mad3 [1624], Mad4 [1624] and Mxi1 [1257], also dimerize with Max, and these heterodimers bind the same core sequence (CACGTG) as Myc/Max heterodimers. Mad and Mxi1 may therefore interfere with Myc function either by sequestering Max or by direct competition for DNA target sites. Unlike Myc/Max dimers, which activate transcription, or Max/Max homodimers which are transcriptionally silent, Mad/Max heterodimers actively repress the transcriptional activity of reporter constructs [1214, 2061]. In addition, both Mad and Mxi1 are able to suppress cotransformation of rat embryo cells by c-*myc* and activated *ras* alleles [610, 1624, 1681, 2146]. Mutant Mad and Mxi1 proteins with deletions in the basic domain exhibit only mild suppressive effects in *myc/ras* co-transformation suggesting that occupation of common DNA binding sites plays a more significant role in suppression of Myc transforming activity than titration of the partner Max. During differentiation of certain myeloid cell lines *in vitro* [3, 116, 618, 620, 791, 1483, 1623, 1624], and in certain tissues *in vivo* [315, 732, 1054, 1448, 1623, 1624, 2010], expression of *mad* and *mxi1* is elevated, c-*myc* declines and *max* remains relatively constant. This suggests that activity of a set of genes responsive to these transcription factors can be rapidly modulated simply by relative changes in the intracellular concentration of Myc and Mad (or Mxi1). Such a putative Myc/Max/Mad/Mxi1 network is illustrated in Fig. 6. It is further possible that different Max-containing dimers exhibit differing preferences for nucleotides flanking the core CACGTG. For example, the Myc/Max heterodimer exhibits a more restricted selection of binding sites than Max homodimers *in vitro* [1203], although the significance of this awaits the characterization of bona fide gene targets.

Regulation of HLH activity by dimerization with inhibitory HLH proteins

A distinct class of HLH proteins has been described whose members act as negative regulators of other

HLH proteins. These inhibitory proteins have one important feature in common: all lack a functional DNA-binding domain. For example, the HLH protein Id1 lacks any basic region adjacent to the HLH. However, Id1 dimerizes with a number of bHLH proteins, including MyoD and E12/E47, and attenuates their function via sequestration into dimers that cannot bind DNA. For example, the presence of Id proteins can alter the transcriptional potential of Tal1 heterodimers [492]. In the absence of Id, E47/E47 homodimers may form and, since the Tal1/E47 heterodimer has a weaker transactivation activity than E47/E47, Tal1 can repress transcription by recruiting E47. On the other hand, Tal1 can activate transcription because Tal1/E47 heterodimers are more resistant to negative regulation by Id proteins. Id1 is expressed at varying levels in many cell lines and tissues, including cell lines from a number of lineages that can be induced to undergo terminal differentiation *in vitro*. During terminal differentiation, Id1 levels decrease giving rise to the notion that Id1 can act as an *i*nhibitor of *d*ifferentiation (hence 'Id' [142, 143, 529, 590, 745, 944, 1487, 1701]). For example, Id1 inhibits muscle differentiation by associating with members of the E12 family and preventing them from forming the active myogenic MyoD/E12 heterodimers [529, 1243]. As a consequence, overexpression of Id1 will suppress transactivation of the muscle creatine kinase enhancer by MyoD [143], and can prevent the high rate of neonatal mortality observed in transgenic mice that overexpress myogenin in differentiated postmitotic muscle fibres [1570]. In addition, constitutive expression of Id1 in the lymphoid cells of transgenic mice results in a severe defect in B cell development [1968], implying that down-regulation of Id1 transcription is essential for B cell development. The fact that the Id1 transgenic animals have a very similar phenotype to E2A-deficient mice [1366, 2080] suggests that the primary targets of Id1 protein at early stages in B cell development are likely to be the products of the E2A gene.

Thus far, three further Id-related HLH proteins have been described: all lack a basic DNA-binding domain. They are Id2 [1204], Id3 (also known as mouse HLH462 [241] and human HLHIR21 [302] or Heir-1 [345]) and Id4 [866]. Like Id1 (formerly known as plain 'Id'), expression of Id2 is inversely correlated with cell differentiation, and it is probable that all of the Id proteins can serve as inhibitors of cellular differentiation. In nearly all eukaryotic tissues cell differentiation is associated with decreased proliferation [43, 85]. Consistent with this, Id1, Id2 and Id3 are rapidly induced by serum stimulation of quiescent human [454, 1692] and murine [127] fibroblasts and entry into S-phase is delayed or inhibited by antisense oligonucleotides or antibodies specific for *Id* [127, 1854]. This suggests a model whereby Id proteins sequester growth-suppressing HLH proteins into inactive, non-DNA binding complexes [1854]. Other data suggest that Id proteins may directly inhibit the activity of the Rb protein and/or the related proteins p107 and p130 [504, 1699]. Whereas depletion of a single Id protein by antisense oligonucleotides partially inhibits DNA synthesis, depletion of additional Id proteins with a combination of antisense oligonucleotides results in almost complete inhibition of DNA synthesis suggesting a degree of functional redundancy amongst Id family proteins. There, are, however, differences in patterns of expression of the various Id proteins. For example, whereas Id1 and Id3 are both widely expressed [1510, 1884], Id2 expression is highest during neural development [162] and Id4 expression is up-regulated during murine embryogenesis and is highest in the brain, testis and kidney of adult mice [866, 1832, 1884]. Id3 is expressed throughout the pre-B and B cell stages of B lymphoid development but is down-regulated in plasma cells, which correlates with the temporal activation of the IgH 3′ enhancer by E12/E47 during later stages [1774]. Recent evidence suggests that Id2 expression is regulated by bHLH proteins through E box clusters in the 5′ regulatory region [1810].

In *Drosophila*, expression of the *extramacrochaetae* gene (*emc*) is required to establish the normal spatial pattern of sensory organs. Its product, Emc, is also an HLH protein with no DNA-binding domain [344, 391]. Emc acts to suppress sensory organ development in specific regions of the body surface by antagonizing the function of the neurogenic bHLH proteins, Achaete and Scute. Emc and Hairy act together negatively to regulate morphogenetic furrow progression and neuronal differentiation in the *Drosophila* eye, which is partly dependent on the proneural HLH protein, Atonal [1415, 1645, 1646]. By analogy to the Id proteins, the Emc protein is thought to sequester Daughterless (and possibly Achaete and Scute themselves) into non-functional dimers, preventing the formation of the active Daughterless/Achaete and Daughterless/Scute dimers.

There is also evidence that Ca^{2+}-loaded calmodulin can inhibit the DNA-binding activity of some bHLH proteins by direct interaction with their HLH domains [1224]. However, the interaction has only been demonstrated *in vitro*, and a direct link between free intracellular Ca^{2+} levels and transcriptional regulation by bHLH proteins *in vivo* has not been shown.

The inhibitory HLH proteins discussed above clearly lack anything homologous to a basic DNA-binding domain. However, several other inhibitory HLH proteins have been identified in which a basic region is present but altered. For example, the *Drosophila* Hairy and Enhancer of split proteins, and members of the rat Hes protein family possess basic regions which are disrupted by a proline residue (see Fig. 2). Proteins of this group do not bind an E box efficiently but bind the so-called N box (CACNAG). Hairy also binds the non-canonical site, CACGCC, which is present in the *achaete* gene [1821]. Mutation of this site blocks Hairy-mediated repression of *achaete* transcription in cultured *Drosophila* cells and the transfection of an *achaete* gene carrying the same mutation creates ectopic sensory hair organs in flies similar to those seen in mutants of Hairy [1821]. Like Emc, Hairy antagonizes the function of Achaete and Scute, resulting in the readily observable phenotypic patterns of sensory bristles which originally gave these genes their names.

Post-translational regulation of HLH proteins

Phosphorylation appears to regulate activity of some HLH proteins at three levels (Table 5). First, phosphorylation can determine the subcellular location. The transcription of Pho5 is under the control of the bHLH protein Pho4. It is tightly repressed when *S. cerevisiae* is grown in phosphate-rich medium, and it is induced more than 100-fold when yeast is starved of phosphate. The transcriptional activity of Pho4 correlates with its phosphorylation state. In a phosphate-rich medium the Pho80–Pho85 cyclin/CDK complex phosphorylates Pho4 which remains in the cytoplasm, and Pho5 transcription is repressed [2174]. When starved of phosphate the Pho80–Pho85 complex is down-regulated by the cdk inhibitor Pho81 [1604, 1916], Pho4 is hypophosphorylated and localized to the nucleus, and Pho5 is induced [2174]. Thus, the phosphorylation state governs the activity of Pho4 by altering its subcellular location. In addition, nuclear import of MyoD requires cAMP-dependent protein kinase although this does not appear to involve the direct phosphorylation of MyoD [1291]. Second, phosphorylation can influence the DNA-binding affinity of an HLH dimer. For example, Max proteins are phosphorylated at a consensus casein kinase II site (serine at amino acid 11), and this inhibits DNA binding by the Max/Max homodimer but not the Myc/Max or Mad/Max heterodimers [1214, 1260, 1274, 2161]. Consistent with this, N-terminal phosphorylation of Max compromises its ability to interfere negatively with Myc-induced transcription and transformation [1274]. Similarly, phosphorylation of MyoD or E47 inhibits the DNA-binding activity of the homodimers but not the MyoD/E47 heterodimers [41, 1282, 2169]. Third, phosphorylation can modulate activity of the transactivation domain. Dimerization with E12 potentiates phosphorylation of myogenin at sites within its transactivation domain. Mutations at these sites result in enhanced transcriptional activity of myogenin, suggesting that E12 diminishes the transcriptional activity of the heterodimer without affecting DNA binding [1294]. Phosphorylation of two residues in the transactivation domain of c-Myc (T58 and S62) may regulate c-Myc transformation and/or transactivation activity [178, 1267, 1279, 1284, 1288], possibly in a cell cycle regulated manner [1289]. Myc proteins carrying mutations adjacent to one of these sites (T58) have altered functional (but not physical) interactions with p107 protein complexes, fail to be phosphorylated at T58 and transactivate weakly [1605]. These data, however, have not been confirmed by others [1951]. Mutation of T58 in retroviral v-Myc proteins [1837] and in human Burkitt's [830, 1106, 1258, 1359, 1391] and AIDS-related [1390, 1452] lymphomas appears to be associated with enhanced transforming activity and tumourigenicity. There is also evidence that T58 may also be modified by O-linked N-acetylglucosamine [1449, 2163]. It is, however, unclear what the biological significance of reciprocal glycosylation and phosphorylation of T58 is for Myc functions.

HLH proteins also interact with accessory factors that are required for, or modify, their activity. For example, expression of immunoglobulin genes is repressed in non-lymphoid cells by a repressor that binds the μE5 sequence in the IgH enhancer [395, 2118]. Over-expression of ITF1 in non-lymphoid cells relieves this repression by two mechanisms. First, binding of ITF1 to the μE5 leads to transcriptional activation. Second, the binding of ITF1 physically displaces a repressor that normally blocks the stimulatory activity of TFE3 and which binds the adjacent μE3 site [395, 883]. Since TFE3 and MyoD can only stimulate enhancer activity in the presence of E12 or ITF1 (or, experimentally, in the absence of a μE5 site) this exemplifies a mechanism in which gene expression is regulated by the availability of neighbouring, or overlapping, E boxes, each specific for different HLH protein dimers. MyoD and E12 bind similar E box elements in the MCK and IgH enhancers. However, MyoD fails to activate the IgH enhancer as a result of specific inhibition of MyoD activity via cis-acting inhibitory sequences present in the enhancer [2118]. Surprisingly, inhibition of MyoD is mediated by only 4 bp flanking the μE5 E box. Repression of MyoD appears to be directed to the bHLH region since deletion of other regions has little effect on repression at the μE5 enhancer. Furthermore, repression can be overcome by replacing the MyoD bH1 with that from E12, suggesting that E12 can inactivate the μE5 repressor. Intriguingly, three conserved amino acids in the bH1 region of the myogenic proteins (A114, T115 and K124 of human MyoD) which can confer myogenic activity to E12 [1170] are required for the interaction with the MADS domain of MEF2 proteins [1663]. MEF2 proteins cooperate with myogenic bHLH proteins to activate muscle-specific genes, possibly by stabilizing the DNA binding of each other at colinear binding sites, and it is tempting to speculate that MEF2 proteins are involved in displacing or inactivating the μE5 repressor.

There is also circumstantial evidence that the transactivation activity of c-Myc may require interaction with at least one further protein [709, 856]. The B-Myc protein shares homology with the transactivation domain of c-Myc yet lacks a DNA-binding domain. B-Myc inhibits transformation and transcriptional activation by c-Myc, suggesting that B-Myc may regulate c-Myc activity by interacting with a common adapter protein(s) required by c-Myc to contact the basal transcriptional machinery [856]. The c-Myc protein has been shown to interact with both the TATA-binding protein [1232, 1239] and with a factor involved in transcription from initiator elements [879]. The region of the c-Myc protein required for this interaction (amino acids 122–140) is conserved amongst Myc family members but is not required for transactivation [646]. Rather, this region is required for repression of basal promoters containing initiator elements [646]. Interestingly, this region of c-Myc, which also interacts with TBP, overlaps with a region that mediates interaction with both the Rb protein (in vitro) [1232, 1247, 1248] and with p107 [138, 1230]. Rb and p107 inhibit c-Myc transactivation suggesting that they modulate c-Myc transcriptional activity by interacting with the transactivation domain [138, 1322]. However, the relevance of interactions between p105^{Rb} and p107 and c-Myc in vivo is unclear.

There is also evidence that Myc interacts with a further nuclear factor(s) that is required for transformation by Myc [1414]. Deletion or point mutation (at position W136) of an evolutionarily conserved region (amino acids 129–145 of human c-Myc) inactivates the transformation activity of Myc while retaining the ability to transactivate reporters. Whereas expression of the wild-type c-Myc N terminus (amino acids 1–262) inhibits cell transformation by both Myc and adenovirus E1A genes, deletion of amino acids 129–145 eliminates this activity, suggesting that this region mediates interaction with a specific nuclear factor(s) which is required for transformation [1414].

In addition, the transcriptional activity of c-Myc is negatively regulated by the transcription factor AP-2 via two distinct mechanisms [1547]. First, high-affinity AP-2 binding sites overlap E box sequences in two transcriptional targets of Myc, ornithine decarboxylase and prothymosin-α. *In vitro*, AP-2 competes with, and can displace, Max homodimers and Myc/Max heterodimers from the Myc-responsive E box. Conversely, Myc/Max is unable to displace AP-2. Second, AP-2 can impair DNA binding by Myc/Max and inhibit transactivation by Myc even in the absence of an overlapping AP-2 site. This effect appears to be mediated by a direct interaction between the bHLHZ of Myc (but not Max or Mad) and the *C*-terminal region of AP-2 (amino acids 203–437), which includes the potential DNA binding and dimerization domains of AP-2. This interaction does not preclude association with Max. It is possible that the interaction of Myc with AP-2 may provide further combinatorial potential for the integration of signals from different pathways that converge on individual genes.

In maize, the anthocyanin pathway involves cooperation between two classes of proteins, the bHLH R/B proteins and the C1/Pl proteins [409], and this interaction is not dependent on the HLH domain. It seems likely that the B proteins (which possesses no innate transactivation activity) bind DNA and then bind the C1 protein and recruit its transactivation domain. HLH proteins also recruit co-repressors. For example, members of the Mad family of bHLHZ proteins recruit the co-repressor mSin3 and repress transcription from specific binding sites which are activated by Myc/Max heterodimers [1361, 1624, 1870, 2146].

Acknowledgement

We would like to thank Alex Whittaker and Mike Mitchell for help in compiling the sequence alignment shown in the Appendix, and Helen Urry for secretarial assistance.

Bibliography

References up to and including second edition†

Reviews

1. **Alitalo, K., P. Koskinen, T. P. Makela, K. Saksela, L. Sistonen, and R. Winqvist.** 1987. myc oncogenes: activation and amplification. *Biochim. Biophys. Acta* **907**: 1–32.

2. **Alt, F. W., R. DePinho, K. Zimmerman, E. Legouy, K. Hatton, P. Ferrier, A. Tesfaye, G. Yancopoulos, and P. Nisen.** 1986. The human myc gene family. *Cold Spring Harb. Symp. Quant. Biol.* **51 Pt 2**: 931–941.

3*. **Amati, B. and H. Land.** 1994. Myc–Max–Mad: a transcription factor network controlling cell cycle progression, differentiation and death. *Curr. Opin. Cell Biol.* **4**: 102–108.

4. **Barinaga, M.** 1991. Dimers direct development. *Science* **251**: 1176–1177.

5*. **Baxevanis, A. D. and C. R. Vinson.** 1993. Interactions of coiled coils in transcription factors: where is the specificity? *Curr. Opin. Genet. Dev.* **3**: 278–285.

6. **Bishop, J. M., M. Eilers, A. L. Katzen, T. Kornberg, G. Ramsay, and S. Schirm.** 1991. MYB and MYC in the cell cycle. *Cold Spring Harb. Symp. Quant. Biol.* **56**: 99–107.

7. **Buckingham, M.** 1992. Making muscle in mammals. *Trends Genet.* **8**: 144–148.

8*. **Buckingham, M.** 1994. Molecular biology of muscle development. *Cell* **78**: 15–21.

9*. **Campuzano, S. and J. Modolell.** 1992. Patterning of the *Drosophila* nervous system: the achaete–scute gene complex. *Trends Genet.* **8**: 202–208.

10. **Cline, T. W.** 1989. The affairs of daughterless and the promiscuity of developmental regulators. *Cell* **59**: 231–234.

11. **Cole, M. D.** 1986. The myc oncogene: its role in transformation and differentiation. *Annu. Rev. Genet.* **20**: 361–384.

12. **Cole, M. D.** 1990. The myb and myc nuclear oncogenes as transcriptional activators. *Curr. Opin. Cell Biol.* **2**: 502–508.

13. **Cole, M. D.** 1991. Myc meets its Max. *Cell* **65**: 715–716.

14. **Collum, R. G. and F. W. Alt.** 1990. Are myc proteins transcription factors? *Cancer Cells* **2**: 69–75.

15. **Cory, S., S. Gerondakis, L. M. Corcoran, O. Bernard, E. Webb, and J. M. Adams.** 1984. Activation of the c-myc oncogene in B and T lymphoid tumors. *Curr. Top. Microbiol. Immunol.* **113**: 161–165.

16. **da Silva, A. C. and F. C. Reinach.** 1991. Calcium binding induces conformational changes in muscle regulatory proteins. *Trends Biochem. Sci.* **16**: 53–57.

17. **Dang, C. V.** 1991. c-myc oncoprotein function. *Biochim. Biophys. Acta* **1072**: 103–113.

18. **Davis, A. and A. Bradley.** 1993. Mutation of N-myc in mice: what does the phenotype tell us? *Bioessays* **15**: 273–275.

19. **DePinho, R. A., N. Schreiber Agus, and F. W. Alt.** 1991. myc family oncogenes in the development of normal and neoplastic cells. *Adv. Cancer Res.* **57**: 1–46.

20. **Eisenman, R. N. and S. R. Hann.** 1984. myc-Encoded proteins of chickens and men. *Curr. Top. Microbiol. Immunol.* **113**: 192–197.

21. **Emerson, C. P.** 1990. Myogenesis and developmental control genes. *Curr. Opin. Cell Biol.* **2**: 1065–1075.

22*. **Emerson, C. P. J.** 1993. Skeletal myogenesis: genetics and embryology to the fore. *Curr. Opin. Genet. Dev.* **3**: 265–274.

23. **Emerson, C. P. J.** 1993. Embryonic signals for skeletal myogenesis: arriving at the beginning. *Curr. Opin. Cell Biol.* **5**: 1057–1064.

24. **Evan, G. I., D. C. Hancock, T. D. Littlewood, and N. S. Gee.** 1986. Characterisation of human myc proteins. *Curr. Top. Microbiol. Immunol.* **132**: 362–374.

25. **Evan, G. I. and T. D. Littlewood.** 1993. The role of c-myc in cell growth. *Curr. Opin. Genet. Dev.* **3**: 44–49.

26. **Garrell, J. and S. Campuzano.** 1991. The helix–loop–helix domain: a common motif for bristles, muscles and sex. *Bioessays* **13**: 493–498.

27. **Garte, S. J.** 1993. The c-myc oncogene in tumor progression. *Crit. Rev. Oncog.* **4**: 435–449.

28. **Green, A. R. and C. G. Begley.** 1992. SCL and related hemopoietic helix–loop–helix transcription factors. *Int. J. Cell Cloning* **10**: 269–276.

29. **Harrington, E. A., A. Fanidi, and G. I. Evan.** 1994. Oncogenes and cell death. *Curr. Opin. Cell Biol.* **4**: 120–129.

30. **Hurst, H. C.** 1994. Transcription Factors 1:bZIP Proteins. *Protein Profile* **1**: 123–168.

31. **Ingvarsson, S.** 1990. The myc gene family proteins and their role in transformation and differentiation. *Semin. Cancer Biol.* **1**: 359–369.

32*. **Jan, Y. N. and L. Y. Jan.** 1993. HLH proteins, fly neurogenesis, and vertebrate myogenesis. *Cell* **75**: 827–830.

* Key references.
† See p. 100 for new references for this edition.

33. **Johnson, E. F.** 1991. A partnership between the dioxin receptor and a basic helix–loop–helix protein. *Science* **252**: 924–925.

34. **Kadesch, T.** 1992. Helix-loop-helix proteins in the regulation of immunoglobulin gene transcription. *Immunol. Today* **13**: 31–36.

35*. **Kadesch, T.** 1993. Consequences of heteromeric interactions among helix–loop– helix proteins. *Cell Growth Differ.* **4**: 49–55.

36. **Kato, G. J. and C. V. Dang.** 1992. Function of the c-Myc oncoprotein. *FASEB. J.* **6**: 3065–3072.

37. **Kelly, K. and U. Siebenlist.** 1986. The regulation and expression of c-myc in normal and malignant cells. *Annu. Rev. Immunol.* **4**: 317–338.

38. **Kingston, R. E.** 1989. Transcription control and differentiation: the HLH family, c-myc and C/EBP. *Curr. Opin. Cell Biol.* **1**: 1081–1087.

39. **Koskinen, P. J. and K. Alitalo.** 1993. Role of myc amplification and overexpression in cell growth, differentiation and death. *Semin. Cancer Biol.* **4**: 3–12.

40. **Laird Offringa, I. A.** 1992. What determines the instability of c-myc proto-oncogene mRNA? *Bioessays* **14**: 119–124.

41. **Lassar, A. and A. Munsterberg.** 1994. Wiring diagrams: regulatory circuits and the control of skeletal myogenesis. *Curr. Opin. Cell Biol.* **6**: 432–442.

42. **Lee, W. M.** 1989. The myc family of nuclear proto-oncogenes. *Cancer Treat. Res.* **47**: 37–71.

43. **Li, L. and E. N. Olson.** 1992. Regulation of muscle cell growth and differentiation by the MyoD family of helix–loop–helix proteins. *Adv. Cancer Res.* **58**: 95–119.

44. **Littlewood, T. D. and G. I. Evan.** 1990. The role of myc oncogenes in cell growth and differentiation. *Adv. Dent. Res.* **4**: 69–79.

45. **Luscher, B. and R. N. Eisenman.** 1990. New light on Myc and Myb. Part II. Myb. *Genes Dev.* **4**: 2235–2241.

46. **Luscher, B. and R. N. Eisenman.** 1990. New light on Myc and Myb. Part I. Myc. *Genes Dev.* **4**: 2025–2035.

47. **Marcu, K. B., S. A. Bossone, and A. J. Patel.** 1992. myc function and regulation. *Annu. Rev. Biochem.* **61**: 809–860.

48. **Marsden, B. J., G. S. Shaw, and B. D. Sykes.** 1990. Calcium binding proteins. Elucidating the contributions to calcium affinity from an analysis of species variants and peptide fragments. *Biochem. Cell Biol.* **68**: 587–601.

49. **Meichle, A., A. Philipp, and M. Eilers.** 1992. The functions of Myc proteins. *Biochim. Biophys. Acta* **1114**: 129–146.

50. **Olson, E. N.** 1990. MyoD family: a paradigm for development? *Genes Dev.* **4**: 1454–1461.

51. **Olson, E. N.** 1993. Regulation of muscle transcription by the MyoD family. The heart of the matter. *Circ. Res.* **72**: 1–6.

52*. **Olson, E. N. and W. H. Klein.** 1994. bHLH factors in muscle development: dead lines and commitments, what to leave in and what to leave out. *Genes Dev.* **8**: 1–8.

53. **Parkhurst, S. M. and P. M. Meneely.** 1994. Sex determination and dosage compensation: lessons from flies and worms. *Science* **264**: 924–932.

54. **Penn, L. J., E. M. Laufer, and H. Land.** 1990. C-MYC: evidence for multiple regulatory functions. *Semin. Cancer Biol.* **1**: 69–80.

55. **Peterson, C. A.** 1991. MyoD and more. Gene Expression in Neuromuscular Development: a Keystone Symposium, Keystone, CO, USA, January 24–30, 1991. *New Biol.* **3**: 442–445.

56. **Prendergast, G. C. and E. B. Ziff.** 1992. A new bind for Myc. *Trends Genet.* **8**: 91–96.

57. **Rabbitts, T. H., R. Baer, M. Davis, A. Forster, P. H. Hamlyn, and S. Malcolm.** 1984. The c-myc gene paradox in Burkitt's lymphoma chromosomal translocation. *Curr. Top. Microbiol. Immunol.* **113**: 166–171.

58. **Robertson, M.** 1990. Gene regulation. More to muscle than MyoD. *Nature* **344**: 378–379.

59. **Saksela, K.** 1990. myc genes and their deregula-tion in lung cancer. *J. Cell Biochem.* **42**: 153–180.

60. **Schwab, M.** 1988. The *myc*-box oncogenes. In *The Oncogene Handbook.* E.P. Reddy, A.M. Skalka, and T. Curran, editors. Elsevier Science, Germany. 381–391.

61. **Spencer, C. A. and M. Groudine.** 1991. Control of c-myc regulation in normal and neoplastic cells. *Adv. Cancer Res.* **56**: 1–48.

62. **Tapscott, S. J., R. L. Davis, A. B. Lassar, and H. Weintraub.** 1990. MyoD: a regulatory gene of skeletal myogenesis. *Adv. Exp. Med. Biol.* **280**: 3–5.

63. **Tapscott, S. J. and H. Weintraub.** 1991. MyoD and the regulation of myogenesis by helix–loop– helix proteins. *J. Clin. Invest.* **87**: 1133–1138.

64. **Torres, R., N. Schreiber Agus, S. D. Morgenbesser, and R. A. DePinho.** 1992. Myc and Max: a putative transcriptional complex in search of a cellular target. *Curr. Opin. Cell Biol.* **4**: 468–474.

65. **Vaessin, H., M. Caudy, E. Bier, L. Y. Jan, and Y. N. Jan.** 1990. Role of helix–loop–helix proteins in *Drosophila* neurogenesis. *Cold Spring Harb. Symp. Quant. Biol.* **55**: 239–245.

66. **Visvader, J. and C. G. Begley.** 1991. Helix-loop-helix genes translocated in lymphoid leukemia. *Trends Biochem. Sci.* **16**: 330–333.

67*. **Weintraub, H.** 1993. The MyoD family and myogenesis: redundancy, networks, and thresholds. *Cell* **75**: 1241–1244.

68. **Weintraub, H., R. Davis, S. Tapscott, M. Thayer, M. Krause, R. Benezra, T. K. Blackwell, D. Turner, R. Rupp, S. Hollenberg** *et al.* 1991. The myoD gene family: nodal point during specification of the muscle cell lineage. *Science* **251**: 761−766.

69. **Wright, W. E.** 1992. Muscle basic helix−loop−helix proteins and the regulation of myogenesis. *Curr. Opin. Genet. Dev.* **2**: 243−248.

70. **Yang, J. Q., J. F. Mushinski, L. W. Stanton, P. D. Fahrlander, P. C. Tesser, and K. B. Marcu.** 1984. Modes of c-myc oncogene activation in murine plasmacytomas. *Curr. Top. Microbiol. Immunol.* **113**: 146−153.

71. **Zimmerman, K. and F. W. Alt.** 1990. Expression and function of myc family genes. *Crit. Rev. Oncog.* **2**: 75−95.

Sequences, expression and functions of HLH proteins

72. **Adami, G. and L. E. Babiss.** 1992. Evidence that USF can interact with only a single general transcription complex at one time. *Mol. Cell Biol.* **12**: 1630−1638.

73. **Adams, J. M., S. Gerondakis, E. Webb, L. M. Corcoran, and S. Cory.** 1983. Cellular myc oncogene is altered by chromosome translocation to an immunoglobulin locus in murine plasmacytomas and is rearranged similarly in human Burkitt lymphomas. *Proc. Natl Acad. Sci. USA* **80**: 1982−1986.

74. **Adams, J. M., A. W. Harris, C. A. Pinkert, L. M. Corcoran, W. S. Alexander, S. Cory, R. D. Palmiter, and R. L. Brinster.** 1985. The c-myc oncogene driven by immunoglobulin enhancers induces lymphoid malignancy in transgenic mice. *Nature* **318**: 533−538.

75. **Adams, J. M., H. Houston, J. Allen, T. Lints, and R. Harvey.** 1992. The hematopoietically expressed vav proto-oncogene shares homology with the dbl GDP-GTP exchange factor, the bcr gene and a yeast gene (CDC24) involved in cytoskeletal organization. *Oncogene* **7**: 611−618.

76. **Afar, D. E., A. Goga, J. McLaughlin, O. N. Witte, and C. L. Sawyers.** 1994. Differential complementation of Bcr-Abl point mutants with c-Myc. *Science* **264**: 424−426.

77. **Aghib, D. F. and J. M. Bishop.** 1991. A $3'$ truncation of myc caused by chromosomal translocation in a human T-cell leukemia is tumorigenic when tested in established rat fibroblasts. *Oncogene* **6**: 2371−2375.

78. **Aghib, D. F., J. M. Bishop, S. Ottolenghi, A. Guerrasio, A. Serra, and G. Saglio.** 1990. A $3'$ truncation of MYC caused by chromosomal translocation in a human T-ccll leukemia increases mRNA stability. *Oncogene* **5**: 707−711.

79. **Akazawa, C., Y. Sasai, S. Nakanishi, and R. Kageyama.** 1992. Molecular characterization of a rat negative regulator with a basic helix−loop−helix structure predominantly expressed in the developing nervous system. *J. Biol. Chem.* **267**: 21879−21885.

80. **Akeson, R. and R. Bernards.** 1990. N-myc down regulates neural cell adhesion molecule expression in rat neuroblastoma. *Mol. Cell Biol.* **10**: 2012−2016.

81. **Akiyama, K., N. Kanda, M. Yamada, K. Tadokoro, T. Matsunaga, and Y. Nishi.** 1994. Megabase-scale analysis of the origin of N-myc amplicons in human neuroblastomas. *Nucleic Acids Res.* **22**: 187−193.

82. **Akiyama, K. and Y. Nishi.** 1991. Cloning and physical mapping of DNA sequences encompassing a region in N-myc amplicons of a human neuroblastoma cell line. *Nucleic Acids Res.* **19**: 6887−6894.

83. **al Moustafa, A. E., B. Quatannens, F. Dieterlen Lievre, and S. Saule.** 1992. Tumorigenic effects mediated in the avian embryo by one or more oncogenes associated with v-myc. *Oncogene* **7**: 1667−1670.

84. **Alberta, J. A., K. Rundell, and C. D. Stiles.** 1994. Identification of an activity that interacts with the $3'$-untranslated region of c-myc mRNA and the role of its target sequence in mediating rapid mRNA degradation. *J. Biol. Chem.* **269**: 4532−4538.

85. **Alema, S. and F. Tato.** 1987. Interaction of retroviral oncogenes with the differentiation program of myogenic cells. *Adv. Cancer Res.* **49**: 1−28.

86. **Algarra, I., S. Silva, and H. G. Ljunggren.** 1993. MHC class I expression on prelymphomatous and lymphomatous B-cells is not inhibited by an E mu-myc transgene. *Eur. J. Cancer* **29A**: 238−241.

87. **Alitalo, K., J. M. Bishop, D. H. Smith, E. Y. Chen, W. W. Colby, and A. D. Levinson.** 1983. Nucleotide sequence to the v-myc oncogene of avian retrovirus MC29. *Proc. Natl Acad. Sci. USA* **80**: 100−104.

88. **Alitalo, K., G. Ramsay, J. M. Bishop, S. O. Pfeifer, W. W. Colby, and A. D. Levinson.** 1983. Identification of nuclear proteins encoded by viral and cellular myc oncogenes. *Nature* **306**: 274−277.

89*. **Alonso, M. C. and C. V. Cabrera.** 1988. The achaete-scute gene complex of *Drosophila melanogaster* comprises four homologous genes. *EMBO J.* **7**: 2585−2591.

90*. **Amati, B., M. W. Brooks, N. Levy, T. D. Littlewood, G. I. Evan, and H. Land.** 1993. Oncogenic activity of the c-Myc protein requires dimerization with Max. *Cell* **72**: 233−245.

91. **Amati, B., T. D. Littlewood, G. I. Evan, and H. Land.** 1993. The c-Myc protein induces cell cycle progression and apoptosis through dimerization with Max. *EMBO J.* **12**: 5083−5087.

92. **Amin, C., A. J. Wagner, and N. Hay.** 1993. Sequence-specific transcriptional activation by Myc and repression by Max. *Mol. Cell Biol.* **13**: 383−390.

93. **Anand, G., D. N. Shapiro, P. S. Dickman, and E. V. Prochownik.** 1994. Rhabdomyosarcomas do not contain mutations in the DNA binding domains of myogenic transcription factors. *J. Clin. Invest.* **93**: 5—9.

94. **Andersson, K. B., A. Deggerdal, C. Skjonsberg, E. B. Smeland, and H. K. Blomhoff.** 1993. Constitutive expression of c-myc does not relieve cAMP-mediated growth arrest in human lymphoid Reh cells. *J. Cell Physiol.* **157**: 61—69.

95. **Apel, T. W., J. Mautner, A. Polack, G. W. Bornkamm, and D. Eick.** 1992. Two antisense promoters in the immunoglobulin mu-switch region drive expression of c-myc in the Burkitt's lymphoma cell line BL67. *Oncogene* **7**: 1267—1271.

96. **Aplan, P. D., C. G. Begley, V. Bertness, M. Nussmeier, A. Ezquerra, J. Coligan, and I. R. Kirsch.** 1990. The SCL gene is formed from a transcriptionally complex locus. *Mol. Cell Biol.* **10**: 6426—6435.

97. **Aplan, P. D., D. P. Lombardi, G. H. Reaman, H. N. Sather, G. D. Hammond, and I. R. Kirsch.** 1992. Involvement of the putative hematopoietic transcription factor SCL in T-cell acute lymphoblastic leukemia. *Blood* **79**: 1327—1333.

98. **Aplan, P. D., K. Nakahara, S. H. Orkin, and I. R. Kirsch.** 1992. The SCL gene product: a positive regulator of erythroid differentiation. *EMBO J.* **11**: 4073—4081.

99. **ar Rushdi, A., K. Nishikura, J. Erikson, R. Watt, G. Rovera, and C. M. Croce.** 1983. Differential expression of the translocated and the untranslocated c-myc oncogene in Burkitt lymphoma. *Science* **222**: 390—393.

100. **Arends, M. J., A. H. McGregor, N. J. Toft, E. J. Brown, and A. H. Wyllie.** 1993. Susceptibility to apoptosis is differentially regulated by c-myc and mutated Ha-ras oncogenes and is associated with endonuclease availability. *Br. J. Cancer* **68**: 1127—1133.

101. **Argaut, C., M. Rigolet, M. E. Eladari, and F. Galibert.** 1991. Cloning and nucleotide sequence of the chimpanzee c-myc gene. *Gene* **97**: 231—237.

102. **Armand, P., A. C. Knapp, A. J. Hirsch, E. F. Wieschaus, and M. D. Cole.** 1994. A novel basic helix—loop—helix protein is expressed in muscle attachment sites of the *Drosophila* epidermis. *Mol. Cell Biol.* **14**: 4145—4154.

103. **Armelin, H. A., M. C. Armelin, K. Kelly, T. Stewart, P. Leder, B. H. Cochran, and C. D. Stiles.** 1984. Functional role for c-myc in mitogenic response to platelet-derived growth factor. *Nature* **310**: 655—660.

104. **Armstrong, B. C. and G. W. Krystal.** 1992. Isolation and characterization of complementary DNA for N-cym, a gene encoded by the DNA strand opposite to N-myc. *Cell Growth Differ.* **3**: 385—390.

105. **Arnold, H. H. and T. Braun.** 1993. The role of Myf-5 in somatogenesis and the development of skeletal muscles in vertebrates. *J. Cell Sci.* **104**: 957—960.

106. **Arnold, H. H., T. Braun, E. Bober, A. Buchberger, B. Winter, and A. Salminen.** 1992. Regulation of myogenin expression in normal and transformed myogenic cell lines. *Symp. Soc. Exp. Biol.* **46**: 37—51.

107. **Aronheim, A., H. Ohlsson, C. W. Park, T. Edlund, and M. D. Walker.** 1991. Distribution and characterization of helix—loop—helix enhancer-binding proteins from pancreatic beta cells and lymphocytes. *Nucleic Acids Res.* **19**: 3893—3899.

108. **Aronheim, A., R. Shiran, A. Rosen, and M. D. Walker.** 1993. Cell-specific expression of helix—loop—helix transcription factors encoded by the E2A gene. *Nucleic Acids Res.* **21**: 1601—1606.

109. **Asai, A., Y. Miyagi, A. Sugiyama, Y. Nagashima, H. Kanemitsu, M. Obinata, K. Mishima, and Y. Kuchino.** 1994. The s-Myc protein having the ability to induce apoptosis is selectively expressed in rat embryo chondrocytes. *Oncogene* **9**: 2345—2352.

110. **Asakura, A., A. Fujisawa Sehara, T. Komiya, and Y. Nabeshima.** 1993. MyoD and myogenin act on the chicken myosin light-chain 1 gene as distinct transcriptional factors. *Mol. Cell Biol.* **13**: 7153—7162.

111. **Asker, C., M. Steinitz, K. Andersson, J. Sumegi, G. Klein, and S. Ingvarsson.** 1989. Nucleotide sequence of the rat Bmyc gene. *Oncogene* **4**: 1523—1527.

112. **Askew, D. S., J. N. Ihle, and J. L. Cleveland.** 1993. Activation of apoptosis associated with enforced myc expression in myeloid progenitor cells is dominant to the suppression of apoptosis by interleukin-3 or erythropoietin. *Blood* **82**: 2079—2087.

113. **Asselin, C., A. Nepveu, and K. B. Marcu.** 1989. Molecular requirements for transcriptional initiation of the murine c-myc gene. *Oncogene* **4**: 549—558.

114. **Auvinen, M., A. Paasinen, L. C. Andersson, and E. Holtta.** 1992. Ornithine decarboxylase activity is critical for cell transformation. *Nature* **360**: 355—358.

115. **Axelson, H., C. K. Panda, and G. Klein.** 1994. Three exceptional IgH/myc-translocation-carrying rat immunocytomas have breakpoints 50 to 80 kb 5′ of c-myc. *Int. J. Cancer* **56**: 418—421.

116*. **Ayer, D. E. and R. N. Eisenman.** 1993. A switch from Myc:Max to Mad:Max heterocomplexes accompanies monocyte/macrophage differentiation. *Genes Dev.* **7**: 2110—2119.

117. **Babiss, L. E. and J. M. Friedman.** 1990. Regulation of N-myc gene expression: use of an adenovirus vector to demonstrate posttranscriptional control. *Mol. Cell Biol.* **10**: 6700—6708.

118. **Bading, H. and K. Moelling.** 1990. Transcriptional down-regulation of c-myc expression by protein synthesis-dependent and -independent pathways in a human T lymphoblastic tumor cell line. *Cell Growth Differ.* **1**: 113−117.

119. **Baer, M. R., P. Augustinos, and A. J. Kinniburgh.** 1992. Defective c-myc and c-myb RNA turnover in acute myeloid leukemia cells. *Blood* **79**: 1319−1326.

120. **Baer, R.** 1993. TAL1, TAL2 and LYL1:a family of basic helix−loop−helix proteins implicated in T cell acute leukaemia. *Semin. Cancer Biol.* **4**: 341−347.

121. **Baker, R. E. and D. C. Masison.** 1990. Isolation of the gene encoding the *Saccharomyces cerevisiae* centromere-binding protein CP1. *Mol. Cell Biol.* **10**: 2458−2467.

122. **Ball, D. W., C. G. Azzoli, S. B. Baylin, D. Chi, S. Dou, H. Donis Keller, A. Cumaraswamy, M. Borges, and B. D. Nelkin.** 1993. Identification of a human achaete−scute homolog highly expressed in neuroendocrine tumors. *Proc. Natl Acad. Sci. USA* **90**: 5648−5652.

123. **Ball, D. W., D. Compton, B. D. Nelkin, S. B. Baylin, and A. de Bustros.** 1992. Human calcitonin gene regulation by helix−loop−helix recognition sequences. *Nucleic Acids Res.* **20**: 117−123.

124. **Bar Ner, M., L. T. Messing, C. M. Cultraro, M. J. Birrer, and S. Segal.** 1992. Regions within the c-Myc protein that are necessary for transformation are also required for inhibition of differentiation of murine erythroleukemia cells. *Cell Growth Differ.* **3**: 183−190.

125. **Bar Ner, M., L. T. Messing, and S. Segal.** 1992. Inhibition of murine erythroleukemia cell differentiation by normal and partially deleted c-myc genes. *Immunobiology* **185**: 150−158.

126. **Barker, K. A. and P. E. Newburger.** 1990. Relationships between the cell cycle and the expression of c-myc and transferrin receptor genes during induced myeloid differentiation. *Exp. Cell Res.* **186**: 1−5.

127. **Barone, M. V., R. Pepperkok, F. A. Peverali, and L. Philipson.** 1994. Id proteins control growth induction in mammalian cells. *Proc. Natl Acad. Sci. USA* **91**: 4985−4988.

128. **Barrett, J., M. J. Birrer, G. J. Kato, H. Dosaka Akita, and C. V. Dang.** 1992. Activation domains of L-Myc and c-Myc determine their transforming potencies in rat embryo cells. *Mol. Cell Biol.* **12**: 3130−3137.

129. **Barth, J. L., R. A. Worrell, J. M. Crawford, J. Morris, and R. Ivarie.** 1993. Isolation, sequence, and characterization of the bovine myogenic factor-encoding gene myf-5. *Gene* **127**: 185−191.

130. **Bartlett, P. F., H. H. Reid, K. A. Bailey, and O. Bernard.** 1988. Immortalization of mouse neural precursor cells by the c-myc oncogene. *Proc. Natl Acad. Sci. USA* **85**: 3255−3259.

131. **Batsche, E., M. Lipp, and C. Cremisi.** 1994. Transcriptional repression and activation in the same cell type of the human c-MYC promoter by the retinoblastoma gene protein: antagonisation of both effects by SV40 T antigen. *Oncogene* **9**: 2235−2243.

132. **Battey, J., C. Moulding, R. Taub, W. Murphy, T. Stewart, H. Potter, G. Lenoir, and P. Leder.** 1983. The human c-myc oncogene: structural consequences of translocation into the IgH locus in Burkitt lymphoma. *Cell* **34**: 779−787.

133. **Bauknecht, T., P. Angel, M. Kohler, F. Kommoss, G. Birmelin, A. Pfleiderer, and E. Wagner.** 1993. Gene structure and expression analysis of the epidermal growth factor receptor, transforming growth factor-alpha, myc, jun, and metallothionein in human ovarian carcinomas. Classification of malignant phenotypes. *Cancer* **71**: 419−429.

134. **Beckmann, H., L. K. Su, and T. Kadesch.** 1990. TFE3:a helix−loop−helix protein that activates transcription through the immunoglobulin enhancer muE3 motif. *Genes Dev.* **4**: 167−179.

135. **Begley, C. G., P. D. Aplan, S. M. Denning, B. F. Haynes, T. A. Waldmann, and I. R. Kirsch.** 1989. The gene SCL is expressed during early hematopoiesis and encodes a differentiation-related DNA-binding motif. *Proc. Natl Acad. Sci. USA* **86**: 10128−10132.

136. **Begley, C. G., S. Lipkowitz, V. Gobel, K. A. Mahon, V. Bertness, A. R. Green, N. M. Gough, and I. R. Kirsch.** 1992. Molecular characterization of NSCL, a gene encoding a helix−loop−helix protein expressed in the developing nervous system. *Proc. Natl Acad. Sci. USA* **89**: 38−42.

137. **Begley, C. G., J. Visvader, A. R. Green, P. D. Aplan, D. Metcalf, I. R. Kirsch, and N. M. Gough.** 1991. Molecular cloning and chromosomal localization of the murine homolog of the human helix−loop−helix gene SCL. *Proc. Natl Acad. Sci. USA* **88**: 869−873.

138*. **Beijersbergen, R. L., E. M. Hijmans, L. Zhu, and R. Bernards.** 1994. Interaction of c-Myc with the pRb-related protein p107 results in inhibition of c-Myc-mediated transactivation. *EMBO J.* **13**: 4080−4086.

139. **Beimling, P., T. Benter, T. Sander, and K. Moelling.** 1985. Isolation and characterization of the human cellular myc gene product. *Biochemistry* **24**: 6349−6355.

140. **Bello Fernandez, C. and J. L. Cleveland.** 1992. c-myc transactivates the ornithine decarboxylase gene. *Curr. Top. Microbiol. Immunol.* **182**: 445−452.

141. **Bello Fernandez, C., G. Packham, and J. L. Cleveland.** 1993. The ornithine decarboxylase gene is a transcriptional target of c-Myc. *Proc. Natl Acad. Sci. USA* **90**: 7804−7808.

142. **Benezra, R., R. L. Davis, A. Lassar, S. Tapscott, M. Thayer, D. Lockshon, and H. Weintraub.** 1990. Id: a negative regulator of helix−loop−helix DNA binding proteins. Control of terminal myogenic differentiation. *Ann. N. Y. Acad. Sci.* **599**: 1−11.

143*. **Benezra, R., R. L. Davis, D. Lockshon, D. L. Turner, and H. Weintraub.** 1990. The protein Id: a negative regulator of helix−loop−helix DNA binding proteins. *Cell* **61**: 49−59.

144. **Bengal, E., O. Flores, P. N. Rangarajan, A. Chen, H. Weintraub, and I. M. Verma.** 1994. Positive control mutations in the MyoD basic region fail to show cooperative DNA binding and transcriptional activation *in vitro*. *Proc. Natl Acad. Sci. USA* **91**: 6221−6225.

145. **Bennett, M. R., S. Anglin, J. R. McEwan, R. Jagoe, A. C. Newby, and G. I. Evan.** 1994. Inhibition of vascular smooth muscle cell proliferation *in vitro* and *in vivo* by c-myc antisense oligodeoxynucleotides. *J. Clin. Invest.* **93**: 820−828.

146. **Bennett, M. R., G. I. Evan, and A. C. Newby.** 1994. Deregulated expression of the c-myc oncogene abolishes inhibition of proliferation of rat vascular smooth muscle cells by serum reduction, interferon-gamma, heparin, and cyclic nucleotide analogues and induces apoptosis. *Circ. Res.* **74**: 525−536.

147. **Bentley, D. L., W. L. Brown, and M. Groudine.** 1989. Accurate, TATA box-dependent polymerase III transcription from promoters of the c-myc gene in injected *Xenopus* oocytes. *Genes Dev.* **3**: 1179−1189.

148. **Bentley, D. L. and M. Groudine.** 1986. Novel promoter upstream of the human c-myc gene and regulation of c-myc expression in B-cell lymphomas. *Mol. Cell Biol.* **6**: 3481−3489.

149. **Bentley, D. L. and M. Groudine.** 1986. A block to elongation is largely responsible for decreased transcription of c-myc in differentiated HL60 cells. *Nature* **321**: 702−706.

150. **Bentley, D. L. and M. Groudine.** 1988. Sequence requirements for premature termination of transcription in the human c-myc gene. *Cell* **53**: 245−256.

151. **Benton, B. K., M. S. Reid, and H. Okayama.** 1993. A *Schizosaccharomyces pombe* gene that promotes sexual differentiation encodes a helix−loop−helix protein with homology to MyoD. *EMBO J.* **12**: 135−143.

152. **Benvenisty, N., A. Leder, A. Kuo, and P. Leder.** 1992. An embryonically expressed gene is a target for c-Myc regulation via the c-Myc-binding sequence. *Genes Dev.* **6**: 2513−2523.

153. **Berben, G., M. Legrain, V. Gilliquet, and F. Hilger.** 1990. The yeast regulatory gene PHO4 encodes a helix−loop helix motif. *Yeast* **6**: 451−454.

154. **Berberich, S., N. Hyde DeRuyscher, P. Espenshade, and M. Cole.** 1992. max encodes a sequence-specific DNA-binding protein and is not regulated by serum growth factors. *Oncogene* **7**: 775−779.

155. **Bernard, O., O. Azogui, N. Lecointe, F. Mugneret, R. Berger, C. J. Larsen, and D. Mathieu Mahul.** 1992. A third tal-1 promoter is specifically used in human T cell leukemias. *J. Exp. Med.* **176**: 919−925.

156. **Bernard, O., S. Cory, S. Gerondakis, E. Webb, and J. M. Adams.** 1983. Sequence of the murine and human cellular myc oncogenes and two modes of myc transcription resulting from chromosome translocation in B lymphoid tumours. *EMBO J.* **2**: 2375−2383.

157. **Bernard, O., N. Lecointe, P. Jonveaux, M. Souyri, M. Mauchauffe, R. Berger, C. J. Larsen, and D. Mathieu Mahul.** 1991. Two site-specific deletions and t(1;14) translocation restricted to human T-cell acute leukemias disrupt the 5′ part of the tal-1 gene. *Oncogene* **6**: 1477−1488.

158. **Bernards, R.** 1991. N-myc disrupts protein kinase C-mediated signal transduction in neuroblastoma. *EMBO J.* **10**: 1119−1125.

159. **Bernards, R., S. K. Dessain, and R. A. Weinberg.** 1986. N-myc amplification causes down-modulation of MHC class I antigen expression in neuroblastoma. *Cell* **47**: 667−674.

160. **Bernstein, P. L., D. J. Herrick, R. D. Prokipcak, and J. Ross.** 1992. Control of c-myc mRNA half-life *in vitro* by a protein capable of binding to a coding region stability determinant. *Genes Dev.* **6**: 642−654.

161. **Bier, E., H. Vaessin, S. Younger Shepherd, L. Y. Jan, and Y. N. Jan.** 1992. deadpan, an essential pan-neural gene in *Drosophila*, encodes a helix−loop−helix protein similar to the hairy gene product. *Genes Dev.* **6**: 2137−2151.

162. **Biggs, J., E. V. Murphy, and M. A. Israel.** 1992. A human Id-like helix−loop−helix protein expressed during early development. *Proc. Natl Acad. Sci. USA* **89**: 1512−1516.

163. **Biro, S., Y. M. Fu, Z. X. Yu, and S. E. Epstein.** 1993. Inhibitory effects of antisense oligodeoxynucleotides targeting c-myc mRNA on smooth muscle cell proliferation and migration. *Proc. Natl Acad. Sci. USA* **90**: 654−658.

164. **Birrer, M. J., L. Raveh, H. Dosaka, and S. Segal.** 1989. A transfected L-myc gene can substitute for c-myc in blocking murine erythroleukemia differentiation. *Mol. Cell Biol.* **9**: 2734−2737.

165. **Birrer, M. J., S. Segal, J. S. DeGreve, F. Kaye, E. A. Sausville, and J. D. Minna.** 1988. L-myc cooperates with ras to transform primary rat embryo fibroblasts. *Mol. Cell Biol.* **8**: 2668−2673.

166. **Bissonnette, R. P., F. Echeverri, A. Mahboubi, and D. R. Green.** 1992. Apoptotic cell death induced by c-myc is inhibited by bcl-2. *Nature* **359**: 552−554.

167. **Bister, K., C. Trachmann, H. W. Jansen, B. Schroeer, and T. Patschinsky.** 1987. Structure of mutant and wild-type MC29 v-myc alleles and biochemical properties of their protein products. *Oncogene* **1**: 97–109.

168. **Blackwood, E. M. and R. N. Eisenman.** 1991. Max: a helix–loop–helix zipper protein that forms a sequence-specific DNA-binding complex with Myc. *Science* **251**: 1211–1217.

169. **Blackwood, E. M., L. Kretzner, and R. N. Eisenman.** 1992. Myc and Max function as a nucleoprotein complex. *Curr. Opin. Genet. Dev.* **2**: 227–235.

170. **Blanchard, J. M., M. Piechaczyk, C. Dani, J. C. Chambard, A. Franchi, J. Pouyssegur, and P. Jeanteur.** 1985. c-myc gene is transcribed at high rate in G0-arrested fibroblasts and is post-transcriptionally regulated in response to growth factors. *Nature* **317**: 443–445.

171. **Block, N. E. and J. B. Miller.** 1992. Expression of MRF4, a myogenic helix–loop–helix protein, produces multiple changes in the myogenic program of BC3H-1 cells. *Mol. Cell Biol.* **12**: 2484–2492.

172. **Blondel, B., N. Talbot, G. R. Merlo, C. Wychowski, H. Yokozaki, E. M. Valverius, D. S. Salomon, and R. H. Bassin.** 1990. Efficient induction of focus formation in a subclone of NIH3T3 cells by c-myc and its inhibition by serum and by growth factors. *Oncogene* **5**: 857–865.

173. **Bober, E., G. E. Lyons, T. Braun, G. Cossu, M. Buckingham, and H. H. Arnold.** 1991. The muscle regulatory gene, Myf-6, has a biphasic pattern of expression during early mouse development. *J. Cell Biol.* **113**: 1255–1265.

174. **Bonham, L., K. MacKenzie, S. Wood, P. B. Rowe, and G. Symonds.** 1992. Both myeloproliferative disease and leukemia are induced by transplantation of bone marrow cells expressing v-myc. *Oncogene* **7**: 2219–2229.

175. **Bonnieu, A., P. Roux, L. Marty, P. Jeanteur, and M. Piechaczyk.** 1990. AUUUA motifs are dispensable for rapid degradation of the mouse c-myc RNA. *Oncogene* **5**: 1585–1588.

176. **Borkhardt, A., R. Repp, J. Harbott, C. Keller, F. Berner, J. Ritterbach, and F. Lampert.** 1992. Frequency and DNA sequence of tal-1 rearrangement in children with T-cell acute lymphoblastic leukemia. *Ann. Hematol.* **64**: 305–308.

177. **Borkhardt, A., R. Repp, J. Harbott, J. Kreuder, and F. Lampert.** 1993. Quantification of leukaemic cells based on heteroduplex formation of tal-1 gene sequences after PCR coamplification. *Br. J. Haematol.* **83**: 39–44.

178. **Born, T. L., J. A. Frost, A. Schonthal, G. C. Prendergast, and J. R. Feramisco.** 1994. c-Myc cooperates with activated ras to induce the cdc2 promoter. *Mol. Cell Biol.* **14**: 5710–5718.

179. **Bossone, S. A., C. Asselin, A. J. Patel, and K. B. Marcu.** 1992. MAZ, a zinc finger protein, binds to c-MYC and C2 gene sequences regulating transcriptional initiation and termination. *Proc. Natl Acad. Sci. USA* **89**: 7452–7456.

180. **Bossone, S. A., A. J. Patel, C. Asselin, and K. B. Marcu.** 1992. Cloning and characterization of DNA binding factors which bind sequences required for proper c-myc initiation. *Curr. Top. Microbiol. Immunol.* **182**: 425–433.

181. **Bradley, J. F., P. G. Rothberg, M. Ladanyi, and R. S. Chaganti.** 1993. Hypermutation of the MYC gene in diffuse large cell lymphomas with translocations involving band 8q24. *Genes Chromosom. Cancer* **7**: 128–130.

182. **Braun, M. J., P. L. Deininger, and J. W. Casey.** 1985. Nucleotide sequence of a transduced myc gene from a defective feline leukemia provirus. *J. Virol.* **55**: 177–183.

183. **Braun, T., E. Bober, and H. H. Arnold.** 1992. Inhibition of muscle differentiation by the adenovirus E1a protein: repression of the transcriptional activating function of the HLH protein Myf-5. *Genes Dev.* **6**: 888–902.

184. **Braun, T., E. Bober, G. Buschhausen Denker, S. Kohtz, K. H. Grzeschik, H. H. Arnold, and S. K. Kotz.** 1989. Differential expression of myogenic determination genes in muscle cells: possible autoactivation by the *Myf* gene products. *EMBO J.* **8**: 3617–3625.

185. **Braun, T., E. Bober, G. Buschhausen-Denker, S. Kohtz, K. -H. Grzeschik, and H. Henning Arnold.** 1990. Differential expression of myogenic determination genes in muscle cells: possible autoactivation by the *Myf* gene products (corrigendum). *EMBO J.* **9**: 592.

186. **Braun, T., E. Bober, B. Winter, N. Rosenthal, and H. H. Arnold.** 1990. Myf-6, a new member of the human gene family of myogenic determination factors: evidence for a gene cluster on chromosome 12. *EMBO J.* **9**: 821–831.

187. **Braun, T., G. Buschhausen Denker, E. Bober, E. Tannich, and H. H. Arnold.** 1989. A novel human muscle factor related to but distinct from MyoD1 induces myogenic conversion in 10T1/2 fibroblasts. *EMBO J.* **8**: 701–709.

188. **Braun, T., M. A. Rudnicki, H. H. Arnold, and R. Jaenisch.** 1992. Targeted inactivation of the muscle regulatory gene Myf-5 results in abnormal rib development and perinatal death. *Cell* **71**: 369–382.

189. **Breit, T. M., A. Beishuizen, W. D. Ludwig, E. J. Mol, H. J. Adriaansen, E. R. van Wering, and J. J. van Dongen.** 1993. tal-1 deletions in T-cell acute lymphoblastic leukemia as PCR target for detection of minimal residual disease. *Leukemia* **7**: 2004–2011.

190. **Breit, T. M., E. J. Mol, I. L. Wolvers Tettero, W. D. Ludwig, E. R. van Wering, and J. J. van Dongen.** 1993. Site-specific deletions involving the tal-1 and sil genes are restricted to cells of the T cell receptor alpha/beta lineage: T cell receptor delta gene deletion mechanism affects multiple genes. *J. Exp. Med.* **177**: 965–977.

191. **Breit, T. M., I. L. M. Wolvers-Tettero, and J. J. M. van Dongen.** 1994. Lineage specific demethylation of *tal*-1 gene breakpoint region determines the frequency of *tal*-1 deletions in ab lineage T-cells. *Oncogene* **9**: 1847–1853.

192. **Bresnick, E. H. and G. Felsenfeld.** 1993. Evidence that the transcription factor USF is a component of the human beta-globin locus control region heteromeric protein complex. *J. Biol. Chem.* **268**: 18824–18834.

193. **Brewer, G. and J. Ross.** 1988. Poly(A) shortening and degradation of the $3'$ A + U-rich sequences of human c-myc mRNA in a cell-free system. *Mol. Cell Biol.* **8**: 1697–1708.

194. **Brewer, G. and J. Ross.** 1989. Regulation of c-myc mRNA stability *in vitro* by a labile destabilizer with an essential nucleic acid component. *Mol. Cell Biol.* **9**: 1996–2006.

195. **Broad, T. E., D. J. Burkin, C. Jones, P. E. Lewis, H. A. Ansari, and P. D. Pearce.** 1993. Mapping of MYF5, C1R, MYHL, TPI1, IAPP, A2MR and RNR onto sheep chromosome 3q. *Anim. Genet.* **24**: 415–419.

196. **Brodeur, G. M., R. C. Seeger, M. Schwab, H. E. Varmus, and J. M. Bishop.** 1984. Amplification of N-myc in untreated human neuroblastomas correlates with advanced disease stage. *Science* **224**: 1121–1124.

197. **Brondyk, W. H., F. A. Boeckman, and W. E. Fahl.** 1991. N-myc oncogene enhances mitogenic responsiveness of diploid human fibroblasts to growth factors but fails to immortalize. *Oncogene* **6**: 1269–1276.

198. **Brown, L., J. T. Cheng, Q. Chen, M. J. Siciliano, W. Crist, G. Buchanan, and R. Baer.** 1990. Site-specific recombination of the tal-1 gene is a common occurrence in human T cell leukemia. *EMBO J.* **9**: 3343–3351.

199. **Brown, L., R. Espinosa, M. M. Le Beau, M. J. Siciliano, and R. Baer.** 1992. HEN1 and HEN2:a subgroup of basic helix–loop–helix genes that are coexpressed in a human neuroblastoma. *Proc. Natl Acad. Sci. USA* **89**: 8492–8496.

200. **Buchberger, A., K. Ragge, and H-H. Arnold.** 1994. The myogenin gene is activated during myocyte differentiation by pre-existing, not newly synthesized transcription factor MEF-2. *J. Biol. Chem.* **269**: 17289–17296.

201. **Buckingham, M., D. Houzelstein, G. Lyons, M. Ontell, M. O. Ott, and D. Sassoon.** 1992. Expression of muscle genes in the mouse embryo. *Symp. Soc. Exp. Biol.* **46**: 203–217.

202. **Buckler, A. J., T. L. Rothstein, and G. E. Sonenshein.** 1990. Transcriptional control of c-myc gene expression during stimulation of murine B lymphocytes. *J. Immunol.* **145**: 732–736.

203. **Bunch, R. T., L. F. Povirk, M. S. Orr, J. K. Randolph, F. A. Fornari, and D. A. Gewirtz.** 1994. Influence of amsacrine (m-AMSA) on bulk and gene-specific DNA damage and c-myc expression in MCF-7 breast tumor cells. *Biochem. Pharmacol.* **47**: 317–329.

204. **Bunte, T., P. Donner, E. Pfaff, B. Reis, I. Greiser Wilke, H. Schaller, and K. Moelling.** 1984. Inhibition of DNA binding of purified p55v-myc *in vitro* by antibodies against bacterially expressed myc protein and a synthetic peptide. *EMBO J.* **3**: 1919–1924.

205. **Buonanno, A., L. Apone, M. I. Morasso, R. Beers, H. R. Brenner, and R. Eftimie.** 1992. The MyoD family of myogenic factors is regulated by electrical activity: isolation and characterization of a mouse Myf-5 cDNA. *Nucleic Acids Res.* **20**: 539–544.

206. **Burbach, K. M., A. Poland, and C. A. Bradfield.** 1992. Cloning of the Ah-receptor cDNA reveals a distinctive ligand-activated transcription factor. *Proc. Natl Acad. Sci. USA* **89**: 8185–8189.

207. **Bustelo, X. R., K-L. Suen, K. Leftheris, C. A. Meyers, and M. Barbacid.** 1994. Vav cooperates with Ras to transform rodent fibroblasts but is not a Ras GDP/GTP exchange factor. *Oncogene* **9**: 2405–2413.

208*. **Cabrera, C. V., A. Martinez Arias, and M. Bate.** 1987. The expression of three members of the achaete–scute gene complex correlates with neuroblast segregation in *Drosophila*. *Cell* **50**: 425–433.

209. **Cai, M. and R. W. Davis.** 1990. Yeast centromere binding protein CBF1, of the helix–loop–helix protein family, is required for chromosome stability and methionine prototrophy. *Cell* **61**: 437–446.

210. **Campbell, V. W., D. Davin, S. Thomas, D. Jones, J. Roesel, R. Tran Patterson, C. A. Mayfield, B. Rodu, D. M. Miller, and R. A. Hiramoto.** 1994. The G–C specific DNA binding drug, mithramycin, selectively inhibits transcription of the C-MYC and C-HA-RAS genes in regenerating liver. *Am. J. Med. Sci.* **307**: 167–172.

211. **Campisi, J., H. E. Gray, A. B. Pardee, M. Dean, and G. E. Sonenshein.** 1984. Cell-cycle control of c-myc but not c-ras expression is lost following chemical transformation. *Cell* **36**: 241–247.

212. **Campuzano, S., L. Carramolino, C. V. Cabrera, M. Ruiz Gomez, R. Villares, A. Boronat, and J. Modolell.** 1985. Molecular genetics of the achaete–scute gene complex of *D. melanogaster*. *Cell* **40**: 327–338.

213. **Care, A., L. Cianetti, A. Giampaolo, N. M. Sposi, V. Zappavigna, F. Mavilio, G. Alimena, S. Amadori, F. Mandelli, and C. Peschle.** 1986. Translocation of c-myc into the immunoglobulin heavy-chain locus in human acute B-cell leukemia. A molecular analysis. *EMBO J.* **5**: 905–911.

214. **Carr, C. S. and P. A. Sharp.** 1990. A helix–loop–helix protein related to the immunoglobulin E box-binding proteins. *Mol. Cell Biol.* **10**: 4384–4388.

215. **Carthew, R. W., L. A. Chodosh, and P. A. Sharp.** 1985. An RNA polymerase II transcription factor binds to an upstream element in the adenovirus major late promoter. *Cell* **43**: 439–448.

216. **Carthew, R. W., L. A. Chodosh, and P. A. Sharp.** 1987. The major late transcription factor binds to and activates the mouse metallothionein I promoter. *Genes Dev.* **1**: 973–980.

217. **Caruso, M., F. Martelli, A. Giordano, and A. Felsani.** 1993. Regulation of MyoD gene transcription and protein function by the transforming domains of the adenovirus E1A oncoprotein. *Oncogene* **8**: 267–278.

218. **Carver, L. A., J. B. Hogenesch, and C. A. Bradfield.** 1994. Tissue specific expression of the rat Ah-receptor and ARNT mRNAs. *Nucleic Acids Res.* **22**: 3038–3044.

219. **Caterina, J. J., D. J. Ciavatta, D. Donze, R. R. Behringer, and T. M. Townes.** 1994. Multiple elements in human beta-globin locus control region 5′ HS 2 are involved in enhancer activity and position-independent, transgene expression. *Nucleic Acids Res.* **22**: 1006–1011.

220. **Caudy, M., E. H. Grell, C. Dambly Chaudiere, A. Ghysen, L. Y. Jan, and Y. N. Jan.** 1988. The maternal sex determination gene daughterless has zygotic activity necessary for the formation of peripheral neurons in *Drosophila*. *Genes Dev.* **2**: 843–852.

221*. **Caudy, M., H. Vassin, M. Brand, R. Tuma, L. Y. Jan, and Y. N. Jan.** 1988. daughterless, a *Drosophila* gene essential for both neurogenesis and sex determination, has sequence similarities to myc and the achaete–scute complex. *Cell* **55**: 1061–1067.

222. **Cavalieri, F. and M. Goldfarb.** 1988. N-myc proto-oncogene expression can induce DNA replication in Balb/c 3T3 fibroblasts. *Oncogene* **2**: 289–291.

223. **Celano, P., C. M. Berchtold, D. L. Kizer, A. Weeraratna, B. D. Nelkin, S. B. Baylin, and R. A. J. Casero.** 1992. Characterization of an endogenous RNA transcript with homology to the antisense strand of the human c-myc gene. *J. Biol. Chem.* **267**: 15092–15096.

224. **Cerni, C., E. Mougneau, M. Zerlin, M. Julius, K. B. Marcu, and F. Cuzin.** 1986. c-myc and functionally related oncogenes induce both high rates of sister chromatid exchange and abnormal karyotypes in rat fibroblasts. *Curr. Top. Microbiol. Immunol.* **132**: 193–201.

225. **Chaganti, S. R., J. Mitra, and J. LoBue.** 1992. Detection of canine homologs of human MYC, BCL2, IGH, and TCRB genes by Southern blot analysis. *Cancer Genet. Cytogenet.* **62**: 9–14.

226. **Chakraborty, T., T. Brennan, and E. Olson.** 1991. Differential trans-activation of a muscle-specific enhancer by myogenic helix–loop–helix proteins is separable from DNA binding. *J. Biol. Chem.* **266**: 2878–2882.

227. **Champeme, M. H., I. Bieche, A. Latil, K. Hacene, and R. Lidereau.** 1992. Association between restriction fragment length polymorphism of the L-myc gene and lung metastasis in human breast cancer. *Int. J. Cancer* **50**: 6–9.

228. **Chang, L. A., T. Smith, P. Pognonec, R. G. Roeder, and H. Murialdo.** 1992. Identification of USF as the ubiquitous murine factor that binds to and stimulates transcription from the immunoglobulin lambda 2-chain promoter. *Nucleic Acids Res.* **20**: 287–293.

229. **Charron, J., B. A. Malynn, P. Fisher, V. Stewart, L. Jeannotte, S. P. Goff, E. J. Robertson, and F. W. Alt.** 1992. Embryonic lethality in mice homozygous for a targeted disruption of the N-myc gene. *Genes Dev.* **6**: 2248–2257.

230. **Chen, L., M. Krause, B. Draper, H. Weintraub, and A. Fire.** 1992. Body-wall muscle formation in *Caenorhabditis elegans* embryos that lack the MyoD homolog hlh-1. *Science* **256**: 240–243.

231. **Chen, Q., J. T. Cheng, L. H. Tasi, N. Schneider, G. Buchanan, A. Carroll, W. Crist, B. Ozanne, M. J. Siciliano, and R. Baer.** 1990. The tal gene undergoes chromosome translocation in T cell leukemia and potentially encodes a helix–loop–helix protein. *EMBO J.* **9**: 415–424.

232. **Chen, Q., C. Y. Yang, J. T. Tsan, Y. Xia, A. H. Ragab, S. C. Peiper, A. Carroll, and R. Baer.** 1990. Coding sequences of the tal-1 gene are disrupted by chromosome translocation in human T cell leukemia. *J. Exp. Med.* **172**: 1403–1408.

233. **Chen, T. M. and V. Defendi.** 1992. Functional interaction of p53 with HPV18 E6, c-myc and H-ras in 3T3 cells. *Oncogene* **7**: 1541–1547.

234. **Cheng, G. H. and A. I. Skoultchi.** 1989. Rapid induction of polyadenylated H1 histone mRNAs in mouse erythroleukemia cells is regulated by c-myc. *Mol. Cell Biol.* **9**: 2332–2340.

235. **Chernavsky, A. C., A. V. Valerani, and J. A. Burdman.** 1993. Haloperidol and oestrogens induce c-myc and c-fos expression in the anterior pituitary gland of the rat. *Neurol. Res.* **15**: 339–343.

236. **Chisholm, O., P. Stapleton, and G. Symonds.** 1992. Constitutive expression of exogenous myc in myelomonocytic cells: acquisition of a more transformed phenotype and inhibition of differentiation induction. *Oncogene* **7**: 1827–1836.

237. **Chisholm, O. and G. Symonds.** 1992. An *in vitro* fibroblast model system to study myc-driven tumour progression. *Int. J. Cancer* **51**: 149–158.

238. **Chodosh, L. A., R. W. Carthew, J. G. Morgan, G. R. Crabtree, and P. A. Sharp.** 1987. The adenovirus major late transcription factor activates the rat gamma-fibrinogen promoter. *Science* **238**: 684–688.

239. **Choi, J., M. L. Costa, C. S. Mermelstein, C. Chagas, S. Holtzer, and H. Holtzer.** 1990. MyoD converts primary dermal fibroblasts, chondroblasts, smooth muscle, and retinal pigmented epithelial cells into striated mononucleated myoblasts and multinucleated myotubes. *Proc. Natl Acad. Sci. USA* **87**: 7988–7992.

240. **Christensen, T. H., H. Prentice, R. Gahlmann, and L. Kedes.** 1993. Regulation of the human cardiac/slow-twitch troponin C gene by multiple, cooperative, cell-type-specific, and MyoD-responsive elements. *Mol. Cell Biol.* **13**: 6752–6765.

241. **Christy, B. A., L. K. Sanders, L. F. Lau, N. G. Copeland, N. A. Jenkins, and D. Nathans.** 1991. An Id-related helix–loop–helix protein encoded by a growth factor-inducible gene. *Proc. Natl Acad. Sci. USA* **88**: 1815–1819.

242. **Clark, J., P. J. Rocques, T. Braun, E. Bober, H. H. Arnold, C. Fisher, C. Fletcher, K. Brown, B. A. Gusterson, R. L. Carter** *et al.* 1991. Expression of members of the myf gene family in human rhabdomyosarcomas. *Br. J. Cancer* **64**: 1039–1042.

243. **Clark, T. G., J. Morris, M. Akamatsu, R. McGraw, and R. Ivarie.** 1990. A bovine homolog to the human myogenic determination factor myf-**5**:sequence conservation and 3′ processing of transcripts. *Nucleic Acids Res.* **18**: 3147–3153.

244. **Classon, M., M. Henriksson, G. Klein, and J. Sumegi.** 1990. The effect of myc proteins on SV40 replication in human lymphoid cells. *Oncogene* **5**: 1371–1376.

245. **Classon, M., M. Henriksson, J. Sumegi, G. Klein, and M. L. Hammaskjold.** 1987. Elevated c-myc expression facilitates the replication of SV40 DNA in human lymphoma cells. *Nature* **330**: 272–274.

246. **Classon, M., A. Wennborg, M. Henriksson, and G. Klein.** 1993. Analysis of c-Myc domains involved in stimulating SV40 replication. *Gene* **133**: 153–161.

247. **Cleveland, J. L., M. Dean, J. Y. Wang, A. M. Hedge, J. N. Ihle, and U. R. Rapp.** 1988. Abrogation of IL-3 dependence of myeloid FDC-P1 cells by tyrosine kinase oncogenes is associated with induction of c-myc. *Curr. Top. Microbiol. Immunol.* **141**: 300–309.

248. **Cleveland, J. L., M. Huleihel, P. Bressler, U. Siebenlist, L. Akiyama, R. N. Eisenman, and U. R. Rapp** 1988. Negative regulation of c-myc transcription involves myc family proteins. *Oncogene Res.* **3**: 357–375.

249. **Cline, T. W.** 1983. The interaction between daughterless and sex-lethal in triploids: a lethal sex-transforming maternal effect linking sex determination and dosage compensation in *Drosophila melanogaster*. *Dev. Biol.* **95**: 260–274.

250. **Cogswell, J. P., P. C. Cogswell, W. M. Kuehl, A. M. Cuddihy, T. M. Bender, U. Engelke, K. B. Marcu, and J. P. Ting.** 1993. Mechanism of c-myc regulation by c-Myb in different cell lineages. *Mol. Cell Biol.* **13**: 2858–2869.

251. **Cohn, S. L., H. Salwen, M. W. Quasney, N. Ikegaki, J. M. Cowan, C. V. Herst, R. H. Kennett, S. T. Rosen, J. A. DiGiuseppe, and G. M. Brodeur.** 1990. Prolonged N-myc protein half-life in a neuroblastoma cell line lacking N-myc amplification. *Oncogene* **5**: 1821–1827.

252. **Colby, W. W., E. Y. Chen, D. H. Smith, and A. D. Levinson.** 1983. Identification and nucleotide sequence of a human locus homologous to the v-myc oncogene of avian myelocytomatosis virus MC29. *Nature* **301**: 722–725.

253. **Collins, J. F., P. Herman, C. Schuch, and G. C. J. Bagby.** 1992. c-myc antisense oligonucleotides inhibit the colony-forming capacity of Colo 320 colonic carcinoma cells. *J. Clin. Invest.* **89**: 1523–1527.

254. **Collins, S. and M. Groudine.** 1982. Amplification of endogenous myc-related DNA sequences in a human myeloid leukaemia cell line. *Nature* **298**: 679–681.

255. **Collum, R. G., D. F. Clayton, and F. W. Alt.** 1991. Structure and expression of canary myc family genes. *Mol. Cell Biol.* **11**: 1770–1776.

256. **Colmenares, C., J. K. Teumer, and E. Stavnezer.** 1991. Transformation-defective v-ski induces MyoD and myogenin expression but not myotube formation. *Mol. Cell Biol.* **11**: 1167–1170.

257. **Compere, S. J., P. Baldacci, A. H. Sharpe, T. Thompson, H. Land, and R. Jaenisch.** 1989. The ras and myc oncogenes cooperate in tumor induction in many tissues when introduced into midgestation mouse embryos by retroviral vectors. *Proc. Natl Acad. Sci. USA* **86**: 2224–2228.

258. **Coppola, J. A. and M. D. Cole.** 1986. Constitutive c-myc oncogene expression blocks mouse erythroleukaemia cell differentiation but not commitment. *Nature* **320**: 760–763.

259. **Coppola, J. A., J. M. Parker, G. D. Schuler, and M. D. Cole.** 1989. Continued withdrawal from the cell cycle and regulation of cellular genes in mouse erythroleukemia cells blocked in differentiation by the c-myc oncogene. *Mol. Cell Biol.* **9**: 1714–1720.

260. **Corcoran, L. M., J. M. Adams, A. R. Dunn, and S. Cory.** 1984. Murine T lymphomas in which the cellular myc oncogene has been activated by retroviral insertion. *Cell* **37**: 113–122.

261. **Cordle, S. R., E. Henderson, H. Masuoka, P. A. Weil, and R. Stein.** 1991. Pancreatic beta-cell-type-specific transcription of the insulin gene is mediated by basic helix−loop−helix DNA-binding proteins. *Mol. Cell Biol.* **11**: 1734−1738.

262. **Corneliussen, B., A. Thornell, B. Hallberg, and T. Grundstrom.** 1991. Helix-loop-helix transcriptional activators bind to a sequence in glucocorticoid response elements of retrovirus enhancers. *J. Virol.* **65**: 6084−6093.

263. **Craig, R. W., H. L. Buchan, C. I. Civin, and M. B. Kastan.** 1993. Altered cytoplasmic/nuclear distribution of the c-myc protein in differentiating ML-1 human myeloid leukemia cells. *Cell Growth Differ.* **4**: 349−357.

264. **Crescenzi, M., T. P. Fleming, A. B. Lassar, H. Weintraub, and S. A. Aaronson.** 1990. MyoD induces growth arrest independent of differentiation in normal and transformed cells. *Proc. Natl Acad. Sci. USA* **87**: 8442−8446.

265. **Crews, S. T., J. B. Thomas, and C. S. Goodman.** 1988. The *Drosophila* single-minded gene encodes a nuclear protein with sequence similarity to the per gene product. *Cell* **52**: 143−151.

266. **Cronmiller, C. and T. W. Cline.** 1986. The relationship of relative gene dose to the complex phenotype of the daughterless locus in *Drosophila*. *Dev. Genet.* **7**: 205−221.

267. **Cronmiller, C. and T. W. Cline.** 1987. The *Drosophila* sex determination gene daughterless has different functions in the germ line versus the soma. *Cell* **48**: 479−487.

268. **Cronmiller, C. and C. A. Cummings.** 1993. The daughterless gene product in *Drosophila* is a nuclear protein that is broadly expressed throughout the organism during development. *Mech. Dev.* **42**: 159−169.

269. **Cronmiller, C., P. Schedl, and T. W. Cline.** 1988. Molecular characterization of daughterless, a *Drosophila* sex determination gene with multiple roles in development. *Genes Dev.* **2**: 1666−1676.

270. **Crook, T., I. Greenfield, J. Howard, and M. Stanley.** 1990. Alterations in growth properties of human papilloma virus type 16 immortalised human cervical keratinocyte cell line correlate with amplification and overexpression of c-myc oncogene. *Oncogene* **5**: 619−622.

271. **Crossen, P. E., M. J. Morrison, and B. M. Colls.** 1994. Increased frequency of the S allele of the L-myc oncogene in non-Hodgkin's lymphoma. *Br. J. Cancer* **69**: 759−761.

272. **Crouch, D. H., F. Fisher, W. Clark, P. S. Jayaraman, C. R. Goding, and D. A. Gillespie.** 1993. Gene-regulatory properties of Myc helix−loop−helix/leucine zipper mutants: Max-dependent DNA binding and transcriptional activation in yeast correlates with transforming capacity. *Oncogene* **8**: 1849−1855.

273. **Cserjesi, P. and E. N. Olson.** 1991. Myogenin induces the myocyte-specific enhancer binding factor MEF-2 independently of other muscle-specific gene products. *Mol. Cell Biol.* **11**: 4854−4862.

274. **Cubas, P., J. F. de Celis, S. Campuzano, and J. Modolell.** 1991. Proneural clusters of achaete−scute expression and the generation of sensory organs in the *Drosophila* imaginal wing disc. *Genes Dev.* **5**: 996−1008.

275*. **Cubas, P., J. Modolell, and M. Ruiz-Gomez.** 1994. The helix−loop−helix extramacrochaetae protein is required for proper specification of many cell types in the *Drosophila* embryo. *Development* **120**: 2555−2565.

276. **Cummings, C. A. and C. Cronmiller.** 1994. The daughterless gene functions together with Notch and Delta in the control of ovarian follicle development in *Drosophila*. *Development* **120**: 381−394.

277. **Cusella De Angelis, M. G., G. Lyons, C. Sonnino, L. De Angelis, E. Vivarelli, K. Farmer, W. E. Wright, M. Molinaro, M. Bouche, M. Buckingham** *et al.* 1992. MyoD, myogenin independent differentiation of primordial myoblasts in mouse somites. *J. Cell Biol.* **116**: 1243−1255.

278. **Cziepluch, C., A. Wenzel, J. Schurmann, and M. Schwab.** 1993. Activation of gene transcription by the amino terminus of the N-Myc protein does not require association with the protein encoded by the retinoblastoma suppressor gene RB1. *Oncogene* **8**: 2833−2838.

279. **Dahllof, B.** 1990. Down-regulation of MHC class I antigens is not a general mechanism for the increased tumorigenicity caused by c-myc amplification. *Oncogene* **5**: 433−435.

280. **Dalla Favera, R., E. P. Gelmann, S. Martinotti, G. Franchini, T. S. Papas, R. C. Gallo, and F. Wong Staal.** 1982. Cloning and characterization of different human sequences related to the onc gene (v-myc) of avian myelocytomatosis virus (MC29). *Proc. Natl Acad. Sci. USA* **79**: 6497−6501.

281. **Dang, C. V., C. Dolde, M. L. Gillison, and G. J. Kato.** 1992. Discrimination between related DNA sites by a single amino acid residue of Myc-related basic-helix−loop−helix proteins. *Proc. Natl Acad. Sci. USA* **89**: 599−602.

282. **Dang, C. V. and W. M. Lee.** 1988. Identification of the human c-myc protein nuclear translocation signal. *Mol. Cell Biol.* **8**: 4048−4054.

283. **Dang, C. V. and W. M. Lee.** 1989. Nuclear and nucleolar targeting sequences of c-erb-Λ, c-myb, N-myc, p53, HSP70, and HIV tat proteins. *J. Biol. Chem.* **264**: 18019−18023.

284. **Dang, C. V., M. McGuire, M. Buckmire, and W. M. Lee.** 1989. Involvement of the 'leucine zipper' region in the oligomerization and transforming activity of human c-myc protein. *Nature* **337**: 664−666.

285. **Dani, C., J. M. Blanchard, M. Piechaczyk, S. El Sabouty, L. Marty, and P. Jeanteur.** 1984. Extreme instability of myc mRNA in normal and transformed human cells. *Proc. Natl Acad. Sci. USA* **81**: 7046–7050.

286. **Darling, D., M. Tavassoli, M. H. Linskens, and F. Farzaneh.** 1989. DMSO induced modulation of c-myc steady-state RNA levels in a variety of different cell lines. *Oncogene* **4**: 175–179.

287. **Darnbrough, C. and C. MacDonald.** 1991. Enhanced growth characteristics of hybridoma cells infected with myc- and ras-containing retroviruses. *Exp. Cell Res.* **195**: 263–268.

288. **Davenport, E. A. and E. J. Taparowsky.** 1992. Basal levels of max are sufficient for the cotransformation of C3H10T1/2 cells by ras and myc. *Exp. Cell Res.* **202**: 532–540.

289. **Davidoff, A. N. and B. V. Mendelow.** 1993. Puromycin-elicited c-myc mRNA superinduction precedes apoptosis in HL-60 leukaemic cells. *Anticancer Res.* **13**: 2257–2260.

290. **Davis, A. C., M. Wims, G. D. Spotts, S. R. Hann, and A. Bradley.** 1993. A null c-myc mutation causes lethality before 10.5 days of gestation in homozygotes and reduced fertility in heterozygous female mice. *Genes Dev.* **7**: 671–682.

291*. **Davis, L. J. and T. D. Halazonetis.** 1993. Both the helix–loop–helix and the leucine zipper motifs of c-Myc contribute to its dimerization specificity with Max. *Oncogene* **8**: 125–132.

292. **Davis, M., S. Malcolm, and T. H. Rabbitts.** 1984. Chromosome translocation can occur on either side of the c-myc oncogene in Burkitt lymphoma cells. *Nature* **308**: 286–288.

293*. **Davis, R. L., H. Weintraub, and A. B. Lassar.** 1987. Expression of a single transfected cDNA converts fibroblasts to myoblasts. *Cell* **51**: 987–1000.

294. **Davis, T. L., A. B. Firulli, and A. J. Kinniburgh.** 1989. Ribonucleoprotein and protein factors bind to an H-DNA-forming c-myc DNA element: possible regulators of the c-myc gene. *Proc. Natl Acad. Sci. USA* **86**: 9682–9686.

295. **De Greve, J., J. Battey, J. Fedorko, M. Birrer, G. Evan, F. Kaye, E. Sausville, and J. Minna.** 1988. The human L-myc gene encodes multiple nuclear phosphoproteins from alternatively processed mRNAs. *Mol. Cell Biol.* **8**: 4381–4388.

296. **Dean, M., J. Cleveland, H. Y. Kim, J. Campisi, R. A. Levine, J. N. Ihle, and U. Rapp.** 1988. Deregulation of the c-myc and N-myc genes in transformed cells. *Curr. Top. Microbiol. Immunol.* **141**: 216–222.

297. **Dean, M., J. L. Cleveland, U. R. Rapp, and J. N. Ihle.** 1987. Role of myc in the abrogation of IL3 dependence of myeloid FDC-P1 cells. *Oncogene Res.* **1**: 279–296.

298. **Dean, M., R. A. Levine, and J. Campisi.** 1986. c-myc regulation during retinoic acid-induced differentiation of F9 cells is posttranscriptional and associated with growth arrest. *Mol. Cell Biol.* **6**: 518–524.

299. **Dean, M., R. A. Levine, W. Ran, M. S. Kindy, G. E. Sonenshein, and J. Campisi.** 1986. Regulation of c-myc transcription and mRNA abundance by serum growth factors and cell contact. *J. Biol. Chem.* **261**: 9161–9166.

300. **Dean, R., S. S. Kim, and D. Delgado.** 1986. Expression of c-myc oncogene in human fibroblasts during *in vitro* senescence. *Biochem. Biophys. Res. Commun.* **135**: 105–109.

301. **Dechesne, C. A., Q. Wei, J. Eldridge, L. Gannoun-Zaki, P. Millasseau, L. Bougueleret, D. Caterina, and B. M. Paterson.** 1994. E-box- and MEF-2-independent muscle-specific expression, positive autoregulation, and cross-activation of the chicken *MyoD* (*CMD1*) promoter reveal an indirect regulatory pathway. *Mol. Cell Biol.* **14**: 5474–5486.

302. **Deed, R. W., S. M. Bianchi, G. T. Atherton, D. Johnston, M. Santibanez Koref, J. J. Murphy, and J. D. Norton.** 1993. An immediate early human gene encodes an Id-like helix–loop–helix protein and is regulated by protein kinase C activation in diverse cell types. *Oncogene* **8**: 599–607.

303. **Degols, G., J. P. Leonetti, N. Mechti, and B. Lebleu.** 1991. Antiproliferative effects of antisense oligonucleotides directed to the RNA of c-myc oncogene. *Nucleic Acids Res.* **19**: 945–948.

304. **Delidakis, C. and S. Artavanis Tsakonas.** 1992. The Enhancer of split E(spl) locus of *Drosophila* encodes seven independent helix–loop–helix proteins. *Proc. Natl Acad. Sci. USA* **89**: 8731–8735.

305. **DePinho, R., L. Mitsock, K. Hatton, P. Ferrier, K. Zimmerman, E. Legouy, A. Tesfaye, R. Collum, G. Yancopoulos, P. Nisen et al.** 1987. Myc family of cellular oncogenes. *J. Cell Biochem.* **33**: 257–266.

306. **DePinho, R. A., K. S. Hatton, A. Tesfaye, G. D. Yancopoulos, and F. W. Alt.** 1987. The human myc gene family: structure and activity of L-myc and an L-myc pseudogene. *Genes Dev.* **1**: 1311–1326.

307. **DePinho, R. A., E. Legouy, L. B. Feldman, N. E. Kohl, G. D. Yancopoulos, and F. W. Alt.** 1986. Structure and expression of the murine N-myc gene. *Proc. Natl Acad. Sci. USA* **83**: 1827–1831.

308. **DesJardins, E. and N. Hay.** 1993. Repeated CT elements bound by zinc finger proteins control the absolute and relative activities of the two principal human c-myc promoters. *Mol. Cell Biol.* **13**: 5710–5724.

309. **Dildrop, R., A. Ma, K. Zimmerman, E. Hsu, A. Tesfaye, R. DePinho, and F. W. Alt.** 1989. IgH enhancer-mediated deregulation of N-myc gene expression in transgenic mice: generation of lymphoid neoplasias that lack c-myc expression. *EMBO J.* **8**: 1121–1128.

310. **Dildrop, R., K. Zimmerman, R. A. DePinho, G. D. Yancopoulos, A. Tesfaye, and F. W. Alt.** 1988. Differential expression of myc-family genes during development: normal and deregulated N-myc expression in transgenic mice. *Curr. Top. Microbiol. Immunol.* **141**: 100−109.

311. **Dmitrovsky, E., W. M. Kuehl, G. F. Hollis, I. R. Kirsch, T. P. Bender, and S. Segal.** 1986. Expression of a transfected human c-myc oncogene inhibits differentiation of a mouse erythroleukaemia cell line. *Nature* **322**: 748−750.

312. **Dominguez, M. and S. Campuzano.** 1993. asense, a member of the *Drosophila* achaete−scute complex, is a proneural and neural differentiation gene. *EMBO J.* **12**: 2049−2060.

313. **Dony, C., M. Kessel, and P. Gruss.** 1985. Post-transcriptional control of myc and p53 expression during differentiation of the embryonal carcinoma cell line F9. *Nature* **317**: 636−639.

314. **Dotto, G. P., M. Z. Gilman, M. Maruyama, and R. A. Weinberg.** 1986. c-myc and c-fos expression in differentiating mouse primary keratinocytes. *EMBO J.* **5**: 2853−2857.

315. **Downs, K. M., G. R. Martin, and J. M. Bishop.** 1989. Contrasting patterns of myc and N-myc expression during gastrulation of the mouse embryo. *Genes Dev.* **3**: 860−869.

316. **Doyle, K., Y. Zhang, R. Baer, and M. Bina.** 1994. Distinguishable patterns of protein−DNA interactions involving complexes of basic helix−loop−helix proteins. *J. Biol. Chem.* **269**: 12099−12105.

317. **Dufort, D., M. Drolet, and A. Nepveu.** 1993. A protein binding site from the murine c-myc promoter contributes to transcriptional block. *Oncogene* **8**: 165−171.

318. **Duncan, M., E. M. DiCicco Bloom, X. Xiang, R. Benezra, and K. Chada.** 1992. The gene for the helix−loop−helix protein, Id, is specifically expressed in neural precursors. *Dev. Biol.* **154**: 1−10.

319. **Duncan, R., L. Bazar, G. Michelotti, T. Tomonaga, H. Krutzsch, M. Avigan, and D. Levens.** 1994. A sequence-specific, single-strand binding protein activates the far upstream element of c-myc and defines a new DNA-binding motif. *Genes Dev.* **8**: 465−480.

320. **Dunn, B. K., T. Cogliati, C. M. Cultraro, M. Bar-Ner, and S. Segal.** 1994. Regulation of murine Max (Myn) parallels the regulation of c-Myc in differentiating murine erythroleukemia cells. *Cell Growth Differ.* **5**: 847−854.

321. **Dunnick, W., J. Baumgartner, L. Fradkin, and C. Schultz.** 1984. DNA sequences involved in the rearrangement and expression of the murine c-myc gene. *Curr. Top. Microbiol. Immunol.* **113**: 154−160.

322. **During, F., H. Gerhold, and K. H. Seifart.** 1990. Transcription factor USF from duck erythrocytes transactivates expression of the histone H5 gene *in vitro* by interacting with an intragenic sequence. *Nucleic Acids Res.* **18**: 1225−1231.

323. **Dutta, S. K. and M. Verma.** 1993. C-myc, c-fos, and c-ras coding sequences are conserved from yeast to mammals. *Cancer Biochem. Biophys.* **13**: 181−185.

324. **Dutton, E. K., A. M. Simon, and S. J. Burden.** 1993. Electrical activity-dependent regulation of the acetylcholine receptor delta-subunit gene, MyoD, and myogenin in primary myotubes. *Proc. Natl Acad. Sci. USA* **90**: 2040−2044.

325. **Duyao, M. P., D. J. Kessler, D. B. Spicer, and G. E. Sonenshein.** 1990. Binding of NF-KB-like factors to regulatory sequences of the c-myc gene. *Curr. Top. Microbiol. Immunol.* **166**: 211−220.

326. **Duyao, M. P., D. J. Kessler, D. B. Spicer, and G. E. Sonenshein.** 1992. Transactivation of the c-myc gene by HTLV-1 tax is mediated by NFkB. *Curr. Top. Microbiol. Immunol.* **182**: 421−424.

327. **Dyson, P. J., T. D. Littlewood, A. Forster, and T. H. Rabbitts.** 1985. Chromatin structure of transcriptionally active and inactive human c-myc alleles. *EMBO J.* **4**: 2885−2891.

328. **Dyson, P. J. and T. H. Rabbitts.** 1985. Chromatin structure around the c-myc gene in Burkitt lymphomas with upstream and downstream translocation points. *Proc. Natl Acad. Sci. USA* **82**: 1984−1988.

329. **Edelhoff, S., D. E. Ayer, A. S. Zervos, E. Steingrimsson, N. A. Jenkins, N. G. Copeland, R. N. Eisenman, R. Brent, and C. M. Disteche.** 1994. Mapping of two genes encoding members of a distinct subfamily of MAX interacting proteins: MAD to human chromosome 2 and mouse chromosome 6, and MXI1 to human chromosome 10 and mouse chromosome 19. *Oncogene* **9**: 665−668.

330. **Edmondson, D. G. and E. N. Olson.** 1989. A gene with homology to the myc similarity region of MyoD1 is expressed during myogenesis and is sufficient to activate the muscle differentiation program. [published erratum appears in *Genes Dev.* 1990 Aug; 4(8): 1450] *Genes Dev.* **3**: 628−640.

331. **Edmondson, D. G. and E. N. Olson.** 1990. A gene with homology to the myc similarity region of MyoD1 is expressed during myogenesis and is sufficient to activate the muscle differentiation program. *Genes Dev.* **4**: 1450.

332. **Edmondson, D. G. and E. N. Olson.** 1993. Helix−loop−helix proteins as regulators of muscle-specific transcription. *J. Biol. Chem.* **268**: 755−758.

333. **Eftimie, R., H. R. Brenner, and A. Buonanno.** 1991. Myogenin and MyoD join a family of skeletal muscle genes regulated by electrical activity. *Proc. Natl Acad. Sci. USA* **88**: 1349−1353.

334. **Egorov, E. E., N. F. Sullivan, C. Cremisi, and L. Lyne.** 1994. Activity of c-myc protein is necessary in the first 6 hours of the prereplicative period for 3T3 Swiss cells. *Mol. Biol. Mosk.* **28**: 127−136.

335. **Eick, D.** 1990. Elongation and maturation of c-myc RNA is inhibited by differentiation inducing agents in HL60 cells. *Nucleic Acids Res.* **18**: 1199−1205.

336. **Eick, D. and G. W. Bornkamm.** 1989. Expression of normal and translocated c-myc alleles in Burkitt's lymphoma cells: evidence for different regulation. *EMBO J.* **8**: 1965−1972.

337. **Eick, D., M. Piechaczyk, B. Henglein, J. M. Blanchard, B. Traub, E. Kofler, S. Wiest, G. M. Lenoir, and G. W. Bornkamm.** 1985. Aberrant c-myc RNAs of Burkitt's lymphoma cells have longer half-lives. *EMBO J.* **4**: 3717−3725.

338. **Eilers, M., D. Picard, K. R. Yamamoto, and J. M. Bishop.** 1989. Chimaeras of myc oncoprotein and steroid receptors cause hormone-dependent transformation of cells. *Nature* **340**: 66−68.

339. **Eilers, M., S. Schirm, and J. M. Bishop.** 1991. The MYC protein activates transcription of the alpha-prothymosin gene. *EMBO J.* **10**: 133−141.

340. **Einat, M. and A. Kimchi.** 1988. Transfection of fibroblasts with activated c-myc confers resistance to antigrowth effects of interferon. *Oncogene* **2**: 485−491.

341. **Einat, M., D. Resnitzky, and A. Kimchi.** 1985. Close link between reduction of c-myc expression by interferon and, G0/G1 arrest. *Nature* **313**: 597−600.

342. **Eisenman, R. N., C. Y. Tachibana, H. D. Abrams, and S. R. Hann.** 1985. V-myc- and c-myc-encoded proteins are associated with the nuclear matrix. *Mol. Cell Biol.* **5**: 114−126.

343. **Eladari, M. E., K. Mohammad Ali, C. Argaut, and F. Galibert.** 1992. Gibbon and marmoset c-myc nucleotide sequences. *Gene* **116**: 231−243.

344*. **Ellis, H. M., D. R. Spann, and J. W. Posakony.** 1990. extramacrochaetae, a negative regulator of sensory organ development in *Drosophila*, defines a new class of helix−loop−helix proteins. *Cell* **61**: 27−38.

345. **Ellmeier, W., A. Aguzzi, E. Kleiner, R. Kurzbauer, and A. Weith.** 1992. Mutually exclusive expression of a helix−loop−helix gene and N-myc in human neuroblastomas and in normal development. *EMBO J.* **11**: 2563−2571.

346. **Ema, M., K. Sogawa, N. Watanabe, Y. Chujoh, N. Matsushita, O. Gotoh, Y. Funae, and Y. Fujii Kuriyama.** 1992. cDNA cloning and structure of mouse putative Ah receptor. *Biochem. Biophys. Res. Commun.* **184**: 246−253.

347. **Endo, T. and B. Nadal Ginard.** 1986. Transcriptional and posttranscriptional control of c-myc during myogenesis: its mRNA remains inducible in differentiated cells and does not suppress the differentiated phenotype. *Mol. Cell Biol.* **6**: 1412−1421.

348. **Enrietto, P. J.** 1986. Molecular analysis of myc gene mutants. *Curr. Top. Microbiol. Immunol.* **132**: 231−236.

349. **Erickson, J. W. and T. W. Cline.** 1991. Molecular nature of the *Drosophila* sex determination signal and its link to neurogenesis. *Science* **251**: 1071−1074.

350. **Erickson, J. W. and T. W. Cline.** 1993. A bZIP protein, Sisterless-a, collaborates with bHLH transcription factors early in *Drosophila* development to determine sex. *Genes Dev.* **7**: 1688−1702.

351. **Erikson, J., A. ar Rushdi, H. L. Drwinga, P. C. Nowell, and C. M. Croce.** 1983. Transcriptional activation of the translocated c-myc oncogene in burkitt lymphoma. *Proc. Natl Acad. Sci. USA* **80**: 820−824.

352. **Erikson, J., K. Nishikura, A. ar Rushdi, J. Finan, B. Emanuel, G. Lenoir, P. C. Nowell, and C. M. Croce.** 1983. Translocation of an immunoglobulin kappa locus to a region 3′ of an unrearranged c-myc oncogene enhances c-myc transcription. *Proc. Natl Acad. Sci. USA* **80**: 7581−7585.

353. **Etiemble, J., C. Degott, C. A. Renard, G. Fourel, B. Shamoon, L. Vitvitski Trepo, T. Y. Hsu, P. Tiollais, C. Babinet, and M. A. Buendia.** 1994. Liver-specific expression and high oncogenic efficiency of a c-myc transgene activated by woodchuck hepatitis virus insertion. *Oncogene* **9**: 727−737.

354. **Evan, G. I. and D. C. Hancock.** 1985. Studies on the interaction of the human c-myc protein with cell nuclei: p62c-myc as a member of a discrete subset of nuclear proteins. *Cell* **43**: 253−261.

355. **Evan, G. I., J. P. Moore, J. M. Ibson, C. M. Waters, D. C. Hancock, and T. D. Littlewood.** 1988. Immunological probes in the analysis of myc protein expression. *Curr. Top. Microbiol. Immunol.* **141**: 189−201.

356. **Evan, G. I., A. H. Wyllie, C. S. Gilbert, T. D. Littlewood, H. Land, M. Brooks, C. M. Waters, L. Z. Penn, and D. C. Hancock.** 1992. Induction of apoptosis in fibroblasts by c-myc protein. *Cell* **69**: 119−128.

357. **Evans, J. L., T. L. Moore, W. M. Kuehl, T. Bender, and J. P. Ting.** 1990. Functional analysis of c-Myb protein in T-lymphocytic cell lines shows that it trans-activates the c-myc promoter. *Mol. Cell Biol.* **10**: 5747−5752.

358. **Evans, S. M. and T. X. O'Brien.** 1993. Expression of the helix−loop−helix factor Id during mouse embryonic development. *Dev. Biol.* **159**: 485−499.

359. **Evans, S. M., B. A. Walsh, C. B. Newton, J. S. Thorburn, P. D. Gardner, and M. van Bilsen.** 1993. Potential role of helix loop−helix proteins in cardiac gene expression. *Circ. Res.* **73**: 569−578.

360. **Facchini, L. M., S. Chen, and L. J. Z. Penn.** 1994. Dysfunction of the Myc-induced apoptosis mechanism accompanies c-*myc* activation in the tumorigenic L929 cell line. *Cell Growth Differ.* **5**: 637–646.

361. **Fahrlander, P. D., M. Piechaczyk, and K. B. Marcu.** 1985. Chromatin structure of the murine c-myc locus: implications for the regulation of normal and chromosomally translocated genes. *EMBO J.* **4**: 3195–3202.

362. **Fahrlander, P. D., J. Sumegi, J. Q. Yang, F. Wiener, K. B. Marcu, and G. Klein.** 1985. Activation of the c-myc oncogene by the immunoglobulin heavy-chain gene enhancer after multiple switch region-mediated chromosome rearrangements in a murine plasmacytoma. *Proc. Natl Acad. Sci. USA* **82**: 3746–3750.

363. **Fanidi, A., E. A. Harrington, and G. I. Evan.** 1992. Cooperative interaction between c-myc and bcl-2 proto-oncogenes. *Nature* **359**: 554–556.

364. **Farina, S. F., J. L. Huff, and J. T. Parsons.** 1992. Mutations within the 5' half of the avian retrovirus MC29 v-myc gene alter or abolish transformation of chicken embryo fibroblasts and macrophages. *J. Virol.* **66**: 2698–2708.

365. **Farquharson, C., J. E. Hesketh, and N. Loveridge.** 1992. The proto-oncogene c-myc is involved in cell differentiation as well as cell proliferation: studies on growth plate chondrocytes in situ. *J. Cell Physiol.* **152**: 135–144.

366. **Feder, J. N., L. Y. Jan, and Y. N. Jan.** 1993. A rat gene with sequence homology to the *Drosophila* gene hairy is rapidly induced by growth factors known to influence neuronal differentiation. *Mol. Cell Biol.* **13**: 105–113.

367. **Feo, S., A. ar Rushdi, K. Huebner, J. Finan, P. C. Nowell, B. Clarkson, and C. M. Croce.** 1985. Suppression of the normal mouse c-myc oncogene in human lymphoma cells. *Nature* **313**: 493–495.

368. **Feo, S., C. Di Liegro, T. Jones, M. Read, and M. Fried.** 1994. The DNA region around the c-myc gene and its amplification in human tumour cell lines. *Oncogene* **9**: 955–961.

369. **Ferrari, S., B. Calabretta, R. Battini, S. C. Cosenza, T. A. Owen, K. J. Soprano, and R. Baserga.** 1988. Expression of c-myc and induction of DNA synthesis by platelet-poor plasma in human diploid fibroblasts. *Exp. Cell Res.* **174**: 25–33.

370. **Ferreiro, B., P. Skoglund, A. Bailey, R. Dorsky, and W. A. Harris.** 1993. XASH1, a *Xenopus* homolog of achaete–scute: a proneural gene in anterior regions of the vertebrate CNS. *Mech. Dev.* **40**: 25–36.

371. **Figge, J., T. Webster, T. F. Smith, and E. Paucha.** 1988. Prediction of similar transforming regions in simian virus 40 large T, adenovirus E1A, and myc oncoproteins. *J. Virol.* **62**: 1814–1818.

372. **Filmus, J. and R. N. Buick.** 1985. Relationship of c-myc expression to differentiation and proliferation of HL-60 cells. *Cancer Res.* **45**: 822–825.

373. **Finger, L. R., J. Kagan, G. Christopher, J. Kurtzberg, M. S. Hershfield, P. C. Nowell, and C. M. Croce.** 1989. Involvement of the TCL5 gene on human chromosome 1 in T-cell leukemia and melanoma. *Proc. Natl Acad. Sci. USA* **86**: 5039–5043.

374. **Finver, S. N., K. Nishikura, L. R. Finger, F. G. Haluska, J. Finan, P. C. Nowell, and C. M. Croce.** 1988. Sequence analysis of the MYC oncogene involved in the t(8;14)(q24;q11) chromosome translocation in a human leukemia T-cell line indicates that putative regulatory regions are not altered. *Proc. Natl Acad. Sci. USA* **85**: 3052–3056.

375. **Firulli, A. B., D. C. Maibenco, and A. J. Kinniburgh.** 1994. Triplex forming ability of a c-myc promoter element predicts promoter strength. *Arch. Biochem. Biophys.* **310**: 236–242.

376. **Fischer, G., S. C. Kent, L. Joseph, D. R. Green, and D. W. Scott.** 1994. Lymphoma models for B cell activation and tolerance. X. Anti-mu-mediated growth arrest and apoptosis of murine B cell lymphomas is prevented by the stabilization of myc. *J. Exp. Med.* **179**: 221–228.

377. **Fisher, D. E., C. S. Carr, L. A. Parent, and P. A. Sharp.** 1991. TFEB has DNA-binding and oligomerization properties of a unique helix–loop–helix/leucine-zipper family. *Genes Dev.* **5**: 2342–2352.

378. **Fitzgerald, T. J., G. A. Neale, S. C. Raimondi, and R. M. Goorha.** 1991. c-tal, a helix–loop–helix protein, is juxtaposed to the T-cell receptor-beta chain gene by a reciprocal chromosomal translocation: t(1;7)(p32;q35). *Blood* **78**: 2686–2695.

379. **Fougerousse, F., R. Meloni, C. Roudaut, and J. S. Beckmann.** 1992. Tetranucleotide repeat polymorphism at the human N-MYC gene (MYCN). *Nucleic Acids Res.* **20**: 1165.

380. **Fourel, G., P. Tiollais, and M. A. Buendia.** 1990. Nucleotide sequence of the woodchuck N-myc gene (WN-myc1). *Nucleic Acids Res.* **18**: 4918.

381. **Fourel, G., C. Transy, B. C. Tennant, and M. A. Buendia.** 1992. Expression of the woodchuck N-myc2 retroposon in brain and in liver tumors is driven by a cryptic N-myc promoter. *Mol. Cell Biol.* **12**: 5336–5344.

382. **Fourel, G., C. Trepo, L. Bougueleret, B. Henglein, A. Ponzetto, P. Tiollais, and M. A. Buendia.** 1990. Frequent activation of N-myc genes by hepadnavirus insertion in woodchuck liver tumours. *Nature* **347**: 294–298.

383. **Franco del Amo, F., M. Gendron Maguire, P. J. Swiatek, and T. Gridley.** 1993. Cloning, sequencing and expression of the mouse mammalian achaete–scute homolog 1 (MASH1). *Biochim. Biophys. Acta* **1171**: 323–327.

384. **Freytag, S. O.** 1988. Enforced expression of the c-myc oncogene inhibits cell differentiation by precluding entry into a distinct predifferentiation state in G0/G1. *Mol. Cell Biol.* **8**: 1614–1624.

385. **Freytag, S. O., C. V. Dang, and W. M. Lee.** 1990. Definition of the activities and properties of c-myc required to inhibit cell differentiation. *Cell Growth Differ.* **1**: 339–343.

386. **Freytag, S. O. and T. J. Geddes.** 1992. Reciprocal regulation of adipogenesis by Myc and C/EBP alpha. *Science* **256**: 379–382.

387. **Frykberg, L., T. Graf, and B. Vennstrom.** 1987. The transforming activity of the chicken c-myc gene can be potentiated by mutations. *Oncogene* **1**: 415–422.

388. **Fujisawa Sehara, A., Y. Nabeshima, T. Komiya, T. Uetsuki, and A. Asakura.** 1992. Differential transactivation of muscle-specific regulatory elements including the myosin light chain box by chicken MyoD, myogenin, and MRF4. *J. Biol. Chem.* **267**: 10031–10038.

389. **Fundele, R., E. Bober, H. H. Arnold, M. Grim, R. Bender, J. Wilting, and B. Christ.** 1994. Early skeletal muscle development proceeds normally in parthenogenetic mouse embryos. *Dev. Biol.* **161**: 30–36.

390. **Galibert, M. D., Y. Miyagoe, and T. Meo.** 1993. E-box activator of the C4 promoter is related to but distinct from the transcription factor upstream stimulating factor. *J. Immunol.* **151**: 6099–6109.

391*. **Garrell, J. and J. Modolell.** 1990. The *Drosophila* extramacrochaetae locus, an antagonist of proneural genes that, like these genes, encodes a helix–loop–helix protein. *Cell* **61**: 39–48.

392. **Gaubatz, S., A. Meichle, and M. Eilers.** 1994. An E-box element localized in the first intron mediates regulation of the prothymosin gene by c-*myc*. *Mol. Cell Biol.* **14**: 3853–3862.

393. **Gazin, C., S. Dupont de Dinechin, A. Hampe, J. M. Masson, P. Martin, D. Stehelin, and F. Galibert.** 1984. Nucleotide sequence of the human c-myc locus: provocative open reading frame within the first exon. *EMBO J.* **3**: 383–387.

394. **Gazitt, Y., G. W. Erdos, and R. J. Cohen.** 1993. Ultrastructural localization and fluctuation in the level of the proliferating cell nuclear antigen and myc oncoproteins in synchronized neuroblastoma cells. *Cancer Res.* **53**: 1899–1905.

395. **Genetta, T., D. Ruczinsky, and T. Kadesch.** 1994. Displacement of an E-box-binding repressor by basic helix–loop–helix proteins: implications for B-cell specificity of the immunoglobulin heavy-chain enhancer. *Mol. Cell Biol.* **14**: 6153–6163.

396. **Geraudie, J., M. J. Monnot, J. P. Muller, and J. Hourdry.** 1993. Effects of denervation on the expression of c-myc proto-oncogene during forelimb regeneration of *Xenopus laevis* froglets. *Prog. Clin. Biol. Res.* 383B: 683–693.

397. **German, M. S., M. A. Blanar, C. Nelson, L. G. Moss, and W. J. Rutter.** 1991. Two related helix–loop–helix proteins participate in separate cell-specific complexes that bind the insulin enhancer. *Mol. Endocrinol.* **5**: 292–299.

398. **German, M. S., J. Wang, R. B. Chadwick, and W. J. Rutter.** 1992. Synergistic activation of the insulin gene by a LIM-homeo domain protein and a basic helix–loop–helix protein: building a functional insulin minienhancer complex. *Genes Dev.* **6**: 2165–2176.

399. **Ghrist, B. F. and R. P. Ricciardi.** 1986. How reliable is amino acid sequence homology in predicting similarity of structure and function of c-myc and Ad12 E1A oncogenic proteins? *J. Mol. Evol.* **23**: 177–181.

400. **Ghysen, A. and C. Dambly Chaudiere.** 1988. From DNA to form: the achaete–scute complex. *Genes Dev.* **2**: 495–501.

401. **Giacca, M., M. I. Gutierrez, S. Menzo, F. D. Di Fagagna, and A. Falaschi.** 1992. A human binding site for transcription factor USF/MLTF mimics the negative regulatory element of human immunodeficiency virus type 1. *Virology* **186**: 133–147.

402. **Giallongo, A., E. Appella, R. Ricciardi, G. Rovera, and C. M. Croce.** 1983. Identification of the c-myc oncogene product in normal and malignant B cells. *Science* **222**: 430–432.

403. **Gibson, A. W., R. Ye, R. N. Johnston, and L. W. Browder.** 1992. A possible role for c-Myc oncoproteins in post-transcriptional regulation of ribosomal RNA. *Oncogene* **7**: 2363–2367.

404. **Gibson, T. J., P. R. Sibbald, and P. Rice.** 1991. Rop/helix–loop–helix similarity letter. *DNA Seq.* **1**: 213–215.

405. **Girdlestone, J.** 1993. An HLA-B regulatory element binds a factor immunologically related to the upstream stimulation factor. *Immunogenetics* **38**: 430–436.

406. **Glackin, C. A., E. J. Murray, and S. S. Murray.** 1992. Doxorubicin inhibits differentiation and enhances expression of the helix–loop–helix genes Id and mTwi in mouse osteoblastic cells. *Biochem. Int.* **28**: 67–75.

407. **Gobel, V., S. Lipkowitz, C. A. Kozak, and I. R. Kirsch.** 1992. NSCL-2: a basic domain helix–loop–helix gene expressed in early neurogenesis. *Cell Growth Differ.* **3**: 143–148.

408. **Godeau, F., H. Persson, H. E. Gray, and A. B. Pardee.** 1986. C-myc expression is dissociated from DNA synthesis and cell division in *Xenopus* oocyte and early embryonic development. *EMBO J.* **5**: 3571–3577.

409. **Goff, S. A., K. C. Cone, and V. L. Chandler.** 1992. Functional analysis of the transcriptional activator encoded by the maize B gene: evidence for a direct functional interaction between two classes of regulatory proteins. *Genes Dev.* **6**: 864–875.

410. **Goff, S. A., T. M. Klein, B. A. Roth, M. E. Fromm, K. C. Cone, J. P. Radicella, and V. L. Chandler.** 1990. Transactivation of anthocyanin biosynthetic genes following transfer of B regulatory genes into maize tissues. *EMBO J.* **9**: 2517–2522.

411. **Golay, J., G. Cusmano, and M. Introna.** 1992. Independent regulation of c-myc, B-myb, and c-myb gene expression by inducers and inhibitors of proliferation in human B lymphocytes. *J. Immunol.* **149**: 300–308.

412. **Goldfarb, A. N., S. Goueli, D. Mickelson, and J. M. Greenberg.** 1992. T-cell acute lymphoblastic leukemia—the associated gene SCL/tal codes for a 42-Kd nuclear phosphoprotein. *Blood* **80**: 2858–2866.

413. **Goldfarb, A. N., M. L. Wolf, and J. M. Greenberg.** 1992. Expression of a chimeric helix–loop–helix gene, Id-SCL, in K562 human leukemic cells is associated with nuclear segmentation. *Am. J. Pathol.* **141**: 1125–1137.

414. **Goldhamer, D. J., A. Faerman, M. Shani, and C. P. J. Emerson.** 1992. Regulatory elements that control the lineage-specific expression of myoD. *Science* **256**: 538–542.

415. **Gomez Casares, M. T., M. D. Delgado, A. Lerga, P. Crespo, A. F. Quincoces, C. Richard, and J. Leon.** 1993. Down-regulation of c-myc gene is not obligatory for growth inhibition and differentiation of human myeloid leukemia cells. *Leukemia* **7**: 1824–1833.

416. **Gonda, T. J. and D. Metcalf.** 1984. Expression of myb, myc and fos proto-oncogenes during the differentiation of a murine myeloid leukaemia. *Nature* **310**: 249–251.

417. **Gonzalez Crespo, S. and M. Levine.** 1993. Interactions between dorsal and helix–loop–helix proteins initiate the differentiation of the embryonic mesoderm and neuroectoderm in *Drosophila. Genes Dev.* **7**: 1703–1713.

418. **Gonzalez, F., S. Romani, P. Cubas, J. Modolell, and S. Campuzano.** 1989. Molecular analysis of the asense gene, a member of the achaete–scute complex of *Drosophila melanogaster*, and its novel role in optic lobe development. *EMBO J.* **8**: 3553–3562.

419. **Goodrich, D. W. and W. H. Lee.** 1992. Abrogation by c-myc of G1 phase arrest induced by RB protein but not by p53. *Nature* **360**: 177–179.

420. **Goodrich, J., R. Carpenter, and E. S. Coen.** 1992. A common gene regulates pigmentation pattern in diverse plant species. *Cell* **68**: 955–964.

421. **Goruppi, S., S. Gustincich, C. Brancolini, W. M. F. Lee, and C. Schneider.** 1994. Dissection of c-*myc* domains involved in S phase induction of NIH3T3 fibroblasts. *Oncogene* **9**: 1537–1544.

422. **Goswami, S. K., Y. Y. Zhao, M. A. Siddiqui, and A. Kumar.** 1993. MyoD transactivates angiotensinogen promoter in fibroblast C3H10T1/2 cells. *Cell Mol. Biol. Res.* **39**: 125–130.

423. **Grand, R. J., P. S. Lecane, S. Roberts, M. L. Grant, D. P. Lane, L. S. Young, C. W. Dawson, and P. H. Gallimore.** 1993. Overexpression of wild-type p53 and c-Myc in human fetal cells transformed with adenovirus early region 1. *Virology* **193**: 579–591.

424. **Green, A. R., E. Salvaris, and C. G. Begley.** 1991. Erythroid expression of the 'helix–loop–helix' gene, SCL. *Oncogene* **6**: 475–479.

425. **Greenberg, M. E., A. L. Hermanowski, and E. B. Ziff.** 1986. Effect of protein synthesis inhibitors on growth factor activation of c-fos, c-myc, and actin gene transcription. *Mol. Cell Biol.* **6**: 1050–1057.

426. **Gregor, P. D., M. Sawadogo, and R. G. Roeder.** 1990. The adenovirus major late transcription factor USF is a member of the helix–loop–helix group of regulatory proteins and binds to DNA as a dimer. *Genes Dev.* **4**: 1730–1740.

427. **Greil, R., P. Loidl, B. Fasching, and H. Huber.** 1992. Differential expression of c-myc-mRNA and c-MYC-protein during terminal neoplastic B-cell differentiation. *Curr. Top. Microbiol. Immunol.* **182**: 215–221.

428. **Griep, A. E. and H. F. DeLuca.** 1986. Decreased c-myc expression is an early event in retinoic acid-induced differentiation of F9 teratocarcinoma cells. *Proc. Natl Acad. Sci. USA* **83**: 5539–5543.

429. **Griep, A. E. and H. Westphal.** 1988. Antisense Myc sequences induce differentiation of F9 cells. *Proc. Natl Acad. Sci. USA* **85**: 6806–6810.

430. **Grignani, F., L. Lombardi, G. Inghirami, L. Sternas, K. Cechova, and R. Dalla Favera.** 1990. Negative autoregulation of c-myc gene expression is inactivated in transformed cells. *EMBO J.* **9**: 3913–3922.

431*. **Gu, W., K. Cechova, V. Tassi, and R. Dalla Favera.** 1993. Opposite regulation of gene transcription and cell proliferation by c-Myc and Max. *Proc. Natl Acad. Sci. USA* **90**: 2935–2939.

432*. **Gu, W., J. W. Schneider, G. Condorelli, S. Kaushal, V. Mahdavi, and B. Nadal Ginard.** 1993. Interaction of myogenic factors and the retinoblastoma protein mediates muscle cell commitment and differentiation. *Cell* **72**: 309–324.

433. **Guilhot, S., B. Petridou, S. Syed Hussain, and F. Galibert.** 1988. Nucleotide sequence $3'$ to the human c-myc oncogene; presence of a long inverted repeat. *Gene* **72**: 105–108.

434. **Guillemot, F. and A. L. Joyner.** 1993. Dynamic expression of the murine Achaete–Scute homologue Mash-1 in the developing nervous system. *Mech. Dev.* **42**: 171–185.

435. **Guillemot, F., L. C. Lo, J. E. Johnson, A. Auerbach, D. J. Anderson, and A. L. Joyner.** 1993. Mammalian achaete–scute homolog 1 is required for the early development of olfactory and autonomic neurons. *Cell* **75**: 463–476.

436. **Gulbins, E., K. M. Coggeshall, G. Baier, S. Katzav, P. Burn, and A. Altman.** 1993. Tyrosine kinase-stimulated guanine nucleotide exchange activity of Vav in T cell activation. *Science* **260**: 822–825.

437. **Gulbins, E., K. M. Coggeshall, G. Baier, D. Telford, C. Langlet, G. Baier-Bitterlich, N. Bonnefoy-Berard, P. Burn, A. Wittinghofer, and A. Altman.** 1994. Direct stimulation of Vav guanine nucleotide exchange activity for Ras by phorbol esters and diglycerides. *Mol. Cell Biol.* **14**: 4749–4758.

438. **Gulbins, E., K. M. Coggeshall, C. Langlet, G. Baier, N. Bonnefoy Berard, P. Burn, A. Wittinghofer, S. Katzav, and A. Altman.** 1994. Activation of Ras *in vitro* and in intact fibroblasts by the Vav guanine nucleotide exchange protein. *Mol. Cell Biol.* **14**: 906–913.

439. **Gulbins, E., C. Langlet, G. Baier, N. Bonnefoy Berard, E. Herbert, A. Altman, and K. M. Coggeshall.** 1994. Tyrosine phosphorylation and activation of Vav GTP/GDP exchange activity in antigen receptor-triggered B cells. *J. Immunol.* **152**: 2123–2129.

440. **Gusse, M., J. Ghysdael, G. Evan, T. Soussi, and M. Mechali.** 1989. Translocation of a store of maternal cytoplasmic c-myc protein into nuclei during early development. *Mol. Cell Biol.* **9**: 5395–5403.

441. **Gutierrez, C., Z. S. Guo, W. Burhans, M. L. DePamphilis, J. Farrell Towt, and G. Ju.** 1988. Is c-myc protein directly involved in DNA replication? *Science* **240**: 1202–1203.

442. **Gutierrez, C., Z. S. Guo, J. Farrell Towt, G. Ju, and M. L. DePamphilis.** 1987. c-myc protein and DNA replication: separation of c-myc antibodies from an inhibitor of DNA synthesis. *Mol. Cell Biol.* **7**: 4594–4598.

443. **Haider, S. R., W. Wang, and S. J. Kaufman.** 1994. SV40 T antigen inhibits expression of MyoD and myogenin, up-regulates Myf-5, but does not affect early expression of desmin or alpha 7 integrin during muscle development. *Exp. Cell Res.* **210**: 278–286.

444. **Hall, D. J.** 1990. Regulation of c-myc transcription *in vitro*:dependence on the guanine-rich promoter element ME1a1. *Oncogene* **5**: 47–54.

445. **Hann, S. R., H. D. Abrams, L. R. Rohrschneider, and R. N. Eisenman.** 1983. Proteins encoded by v-myc and c-myc oncogenes: identification and localization in acute leukemia virus transformants and bursal lymphoma cell lines. *Cell* **34**: 789–798.

446. **Hann, S. R. and R. N. Eisenman.** 1984. Proteins encoded by the human c-myc oncogene: differential expression in neoplastic cells. *Mol. Cell Biol.* **4**: 2486–2497.

447. **Hann, S. R., M. W. King, D. L. Bentley, C. W. Anderson, and R. N. Eisenman.** 1988. A non-AUG translational initiation in c-myc exon 1 generates an N-terminally distinct protein whose synthesis is disrupted in Burkitt's lymphomas. *Cell* **52**: 185–195.

448. **Hann, S. R., K. Sloan Brown, and G. D. Spotts.** 1992. Translational activation of the non-AUG-initiated c-myc 1 protein at high cell densities due to methionine deprivation. *Genes Dev.* **6**: 1229–1240.

449. **Hann, S. R., C. B. Thompson, and R. N. Eisenman.** 1985. c-myc oncogene protein synthesis is independent of the cell cycle in human and avian cells. *Nature* **314**: 366–369.

450. **Hannan, R. D., F. A. Stennard, and A. K. West.** 1994. Localization of c-myc protooncogene expression in the rat heart *in vivo* and in the isolated, perfused heart following treatment with norepinephrine. *Biochim. Biophys. Acta* **1217**: 281–290.

451. **Hansen, L. J., B. C. Tennant, C. Seeger, and D. Ganem.** 1993. Differential activation of myc gene family members in hepatic carcinogenesis by closely related hepatitis B viruses. *Mol. Cell Biol.* **13**: 659–667.

452*. **Hanson, K. D., M. Y. Shichirl, M. R. Follansbee, and J. M. Sedivy.** 1994. Effects of c-myc expression on cell cycle progression. *Mol. Cell Biol.* **14**: 5748–5755.

453. **Hara, E., S. Okamoto, S. Nakada, Y. Taya, S. Sekiya, and K. Oda.** 1993. Protein phosphorylation required for the formation of E2F complexes regulates N-myc transcription during differentiation of human embryonal carcinoma cells. *Oncogene* **8**: 1023–1032.

454. **Hara, E., T. Yamaguchi, H. Nojima, T. Ide, J. Campisi, H. Okayama, and K. Oda.** 1994. Id-related genes encoding helix–loop–helix proteins are required for G1 progression and are repressed in senescent human fibroblasts. *J. Biol. Chem.* **269**: 2139–2145.

455. **Harris, L. L., J. C. Talian, and P. S. Zelenka.** 1992. Contrasting patterns of c-myc and N-myc expression in proliferating, quiescent, and differentiating cells of the embryonic chicken lens. *Development* **115**: 813–820.

456. **Harvey, R. P.** 1990. The *Xenopus* MyoD gene: an unlocalised maternal mRNA predates lineage-restricted expression in the early embryo. *Development* **108**: 669–680.

457. **Harvey, R. P.** 1991. Widespread expression of MyoD genes in *Xenopus* embryos is amplified in presumptive muscle as a delayed response to mesoderm induction. *Proc. Natl Acad. Sci. USA* **88**: 9198–9202.

458. **Harvey, R. P.** 1992. MyoD protein expression in *Xenopus* embryos closely follows a mesoderm induction-dependent amplification of MyoD transcription and is synchronous across the future somite axis. *Mech Dev.* **37**: 141–149.

459. **Hasegawa, T., E. Hara, K. Takehana, S. Nakada, K. Oda, M. Kawata, H. Kimura, and S. Sekiya.** 1991. A transient decrease in N-myc expression and its biological role during differentiation of human embryonal carcinoma cells. *Differentiation* **47**: 107–117.

460. **Hashiro, M., K. Matsumoto, H. Okumura, K. Hashimoto, and K. Yoshikawa.** 1991. Growth inhibition of human keratinocytes by antisense c-myc oligomer is not coupled to induction of differentiation. *Biochem. Biophys. Res. Commun.* **174**: 287–292.

461. **Hasty, P., A. Bradley, J. H. Morris, D. G. Edmondson, J. M. Venuti, E. N. Olson, and W. H. Klein.** 1993. Muscle deficiency and neonatal death in mice with a targeted mutation in the myogenin gene. *Nature* **364**: 501–506.

462. **Haupt, Y., A. W. Harris, and J. M. Adams.** 1992. Retroviral infection accelerates T lymphomagenesis in E mu-N-ras transgenic mice by activating c-myc or N-myc. *Oncogene* **7**: 981–986.

463. **Hay, N., J. M. Bishop, and D. Levens.** 1987. Regulatory elements that modulate expression of human c-myc. *Genes Dev.* **1**: 659–671.

464. **Hay, N., M. Takimoto, and J. M. Bishop.** 1989. A FOS protein is present in a complex that binds a negative regulator of MYC. *Genes Dev.* **3**: 293–303.

465. **Hayashi, Y., T. Sugimoto, Y. Horii, H. Hosoi, J. Inazawa, J. T. Kemshead, T. Inaba, R. Hanada, K. Yamamoto, A. M. Gown** *et al.* 1990. Characterization of an embryonal rhabdomyosarcoma cell line showing amplification and over-expression of the N-myc oncogene. *Int. J. Cancer* **45**: 705–711.

466. **Hayday, A. C., S. D. Gillies, H. Saito, C. Wood, K. Wiman, W. S. Hayward, and S. Tonegawa.** 1984. Activation of a translocated human c-myc gene by an enhancer in the immunoglobulin heavy-chain locus. *Nature* **307**: 334–340.

467. **Hayflick, J., P. H. Seeburg, R. Ohlsson, S. Pfeifer Ohlsson, D. Watson, T. Papas, and P. H. Duesberg.** 1985. Nucleotide sequence of two overlapping myc-related genes in avian carcinoma virus OK10 and their relation to the myc genes of other viruses and the cell. *Proc. Natl Acad. Sci. USA* **82**: 2718–2722.

468. **Heikkila, R., G. Schwab, E. Wickstrom, S. L. Loke, D. H. Pluznik, R. Watt, and L. M. Neckers.** 1987. A c-myc antisense oligodeoxynucleotide inhibits entry into S phase but not progress from G0 to G1. *Nature* **328**: 445–449.

469. **Henriksson, M., M. Classon, H. Axelson, G. Klein, and J. Thyberg.** 1992. Nuclear colocalization of c-myc protein and hsp70 in cells transfected with human wild-type and mutant c-myc genes. *Exp. Cell Res.* **203**: 383–394.

470. **Henthorn, P., M. Kiledjian, and T. Kadesch.** 1990. Two distinct transcription factors that bind the immunoglobulin enhancer microE5/kappa 2 motif. *Science* **247**: 467–470.

471. **Henthorn, P., R. McCarrick Walmsley, and T. Kadesch.** 1990. Sequence of the cDNA encoding ITF-1, a positive-acting transcription factor. *Nucleic Acids Res.* **18**: 677.

472. **Henthorn, P., R. McCarrick Walmsley, and T. Kadesch.** 1990. Sequence of the cDNA encoding ITF-2, a positive-acting transcription factor. *Nucleic Acids Res.* **18**: 678.

473. **Herrick, D. J. and J. Ross.** 1994. The half-life of c-myc mRNA in growing and serum-stimulated cells: influence of the coding and 3′ untranslated regions and role of ribosome translocation. *Mol. Cell Biol.* **14**: 2119–2128.

474. **Hiebert, S. W., M. Lipp, and J. R. Nevins.** 1989. E1A-dependent trans-activation of the human MYC promoter is mediated by the E2F factor. *Proc. Natl Acad. Sci. USA* **86**: 3594–3598.

475*. **Hinz, U., B. Giebel, and J. A. Campos-Ortega.** 1994. The basic-helix-loop-helix domain of *Drosophila* Lethal of Scute protein is sufficient for proneural function and activates neurogenic genes. *Cell* **76**: 77–87.

476. **Hirning, U., P. Schmid, W. A. Schulz, L. P. Kozak, and H. Hameister.** 1989. In developing brown adipose tissue c-myc protooncogene expression is restricted to early differentiation stages. *Cell Differ. Dev.* **27**: 243–248.

477. **Hirning, U., P. Schmid, W. A. Schulz, G. Rettenberger, and H. Hameister.** 1991. A comparative analysis of N-myc and c-myc expression and cellular proliferation in mouse organogenesis. *Mech. Dev.* **33**: 119–125.

478. **Hirvonen, H., V. Hukkanen, T. T. Salmi, T. P. Makela, T. T. Pelliniemi, S. Knuutila, and R. Alitalo.** 1991. Expression of L-myc and N-myc proto-oncogenes in human leukemias and leukemia cell lines. *Blood* **78**: 3012–3020.

479. **Hirvonen, H., T. P. Makela, M. Sandberg, H. Kalimo, E. Vuorio, and K. Alitalo.** 1990. Expression of the myc proto-oncogenes in developing human fetal brain. *Oncogene* **5**: 1787–1797.

480. **Hirvonen, H. E., R. Salonen, M. M. Sandberg, E. Vuorio, I. Vastrik, E. Kotilainen, and H. Kalimo.** 1994. Differential expression of myc, max and RB1 genes in human gliomas and glioma cell lines. *Br. J. Cancer* **69**: 16–25.

481. **Hoang, A. T., K. J. Cohen, J. F. Barrett, D. A. Bergstrom, and C. V. Dang.** 1994. Participation of cyclin A in Myc-induced apoptosis. *Proc. Natl Acad. Sci. USA* **91**: 6875–6879.

482. **Hodgkinson, C. A., K. J. Moore, A. Nakayama, E. Steingrimsson, N. G. Copeland, N. A. Jenkins, and H. Arnheiter.** 1993. Mutations at the mouse microphthalmia locus are associated with defects in a gene encoding a novel basic-helix−loop−helix-zipper protein. *Cell* **74**: 395−404.

483. **Hoffman Liebermann, B. and D. A. Liebermann.** 1991. Interleukin-6- and leukemia inhibitory factor-induced terminal differentiation of myeloid leukemia cells is blocked at an intermediate stage by constitutive c-myc. *Mol. Cell Biol.* **11**: 2375−2381.

484. **Hoffman Liebermann, B. and D. A. Liebermann.** 1991. Suppression of c-myc and c-myb is tightly linked to terminal differentiation induced by IL6 or LIF and not growth inhibition in myeloid leukemia cells. *Oncogene* **6**: 903−909.

485. **Hoffman, E. C., H. Reyes, F. F. Chu, F. Sander, L. H. Conley, B. A. Brooks, and O. Hankinson.** 1991. Cloning of a factor required for activity of the Ah (dioxin) receptor. *Science* **252**: 954−958.

486. **Hollenberg, S. M., P. F. Cheng, and H. Weintraub.** 1993. Use of a conditional MyoD transcription factor in studies of MyoD trans-activation and muscle determination. *Proc. Natl Acad. Sci. USA* **90**: 8028−8032.

487. **Hollis, G. F., K. F. Mitchell, J. Battey, H. Potter, R. Taub, G. M. Lenoir, and P. Leder.** 1984. A variant translocation places the lambda immunoglobulin genes 3′ to the c-myc oncogene in Burkitt's lymphoma. *Nature* **307**: 752−755.

488. **Hopwood, N. D. and J. B. Gurdon.** 1990. Activation of muscle genes without myogenesis by ectopic expression of MyoD in frog embryo cells. *Nature* **347**: 197−200.

489. **Hopwood, N. D., A. Pluck, and J. B. Gurdon.** 1989. MyoD expression in the forming somites is an early response to mesoderm induction in *Xenopus* embryos. *EMBO J.* **8**: 3409−3417.

490. **Hopwood, N. D., A. Pluck, and J. B. Gurdon.** 1991. *Xenopus* Myf-5 marks early muscle cells and can activate muscle genes ectopically in early embryos. *Development* **111**: 551−560.

491. **Hourdry, J., A. Brulfert, M. Gusse, D. Schoevaert, M. V. Taylor, and M. Mechali.** 1988. Localization of c-myc expression during oogenesis and embryonic development in *Xenopus laevis*. *Development* **104**: 631−641.

492. **Hsu, H-L., I. Wadman, J. T. Tsan, and R. Baer.** 1994. Positive and negative transcriptional control by the Tal1 helix−loop−helix protein. *Proc. Natl Acad. Sci. USA* **91**: 5947−5951.

493. **Hsu, T., T. Moroy, J. Etiemble, A. Louise, C. Trepo, P. Tiollais, and M. A. Buendia.** 1988. Activation of c-myc by woodchuck hepatitis virus insertion in hepatocellular carcinoma. *Cell* **55**:\Xi 627−635.

494. **Hu, J. S., E. N. Olson, and R. E. Kingston.** 1992. HEB, a helix−loop−helix protein related to E2A and ITF2 that can modulate the DNA-binding ability of myogenic regulatory factors. *Mol. Cell Biol.* **12**: 1031−1042.

495. **Hua, X., C. Yokoyama, J. Wu, M. R. Briggs, M. S. Brown, J. L. Goldstein, and X. Wang.** 1993. SREBP-2, a second basic-helix−loop−helix-leucine zipper protein that stimulates transcription by binding to a sterol regulatory element. *Proc. Natl Acad. Sci. USA* **90**: 11603−11607.

496. **Hughes, M. J., J. B. Lingrel, J. M. Krakowsky, and K. P. Anderson.** 1993. A helix−loop−helix transcription factor-like gene is located at the mi locus. *J. Biol. Chem.* **268**: 20687−20690.

497. **Hughes, S. M., J. M. Taylor, S. J. Tapscott, C. M. Gurley, W. J. Carter, and C. A. Peterson.** 1993. Selective accumulation of MyoD and myogenin mRNAs in fast and slow adult skeletal muscle is controlled by innervation and hormones. *Development* **118**: 1137−1147.

498. **Hultgardh Nilsson, A., U. Krondahl, W. Q. Jiang, J. Nilsson, and N. R. Ringertz.** 1993. Endogenous activation of c-myc expression and DNA synthesis in serum-starved neonatal rat smooth muscle cells. *Differentiation* **52**: 161−168.

499. **Humphries, E. H. and E. J. Filardo.** 1990. The transforming activity of PP59C-MYC is weaker than that of v-myc. *Curr. Top. Microbiol. Immunol.* **166**: 259−265.

500. **Hunger, S. P. and M. L. Cleary.** 1993. Chimaeric oncoproteins resulting from chromosomal translocations in acute lymphoblastic leukaemia. *Semin. Cancer Biol.* **4**: 387−399.

501. **Hunger, S. P., P. E. Devaraj, L. Foroni, L. M. Secker Walker, and M. L. Cleary.** 1994. Two types of genomic rearrangements create alternative E2A-HLF fusion proteins in t(17;19)-ALL. *Blood* **83**: 2970−2977.

502. **Hunt, J. D., M. Valentine, and A. Tereba.** 1990. Excision of N-myc from chromosome 2 in human neuroblastoma cells containing amplified N-myc sequences. *Mol. Cell Biol.* **10**: 823−829.

503. **Hwang, L. Y., M. Siegelman, L. Davis, N. Oppenheimer Marks, and R. Baer.** 1993. Expression of the TAL1 proto-oncogene in cultured endothelial cells and blood vessels of the spleen. *Oncogene* **8**: 3043−3046.

504. **Iavarone, A., P. Garg, A. Lasorella, J. Hsu, and M. A. Israel.** 1994. The helix−loop−helix protein Id-2 enhances cell proliferation and binds to the retinoblastoma protein. *Genes Dev.* **8**: 1270−1284.

505. **Ibson, J. M. and P. H. Rabbitts.** 1988. Sequence of a germ-line N-myc gene and amplification as a mechanism of activation. *Oncogene* **2**: 399−402.

506. **Iguchi Ariga, S. M., T. Itani, Y. Kiji, and H. Ariga.** 1987. Possible function of the c-myc product: promotion of cellular DNA replication. *EMBO J.* **6**: 2365–2371.

507. **Iguchi Ariga, S. M., T. Itani, M. Yamaguchi, and H. Ariga.** 1987. c-myc protein can be substituted for SV40 T antigen in SV40 DNA replication. *Nucleic Acids Res.* **15**: 4889–4899.

508. **Iguchi Ariga, S. M., T. Okazaki, T. Itani, M. Ogata, Y. Sato, and H. Ariga.** 1988. An initiation site of DNA replication with transcriptional enhancer activity present upstream of the c-myc gene. *EMBO J.* **7**: 3135–3142.

509. **Ikegaki, N., J. Minna, and R. H. Kennett.** 1989. The human L-myc gene is expressed as two forms of protein in small cell lung carcinoma cell lines: detection by monoclonal antibodies specific to two myc homology box sequences. *EMBO J.* **8**: 1793–1799.

510. **Imamura, Y., S. M. Iguchi Ariga, and H. Ariga.** 1992. The upstream region of the mouse N-myc gene: identification of an enhancer element that functions preferentially in neuroblastoma IMR32 cells. *Biochim. Biophys. Acta* **1132**: 177–187.

511. **Imamura, Y., T. Nakagawa, S. M. Iguchi Ariga, and H. Ariga.** 1993. Transcriptional regulation of the N-myc gene: identification of positive regulatory element and its double- and single-stranded DNA binding proteins. *Biochim. Biophys. Acta* **1216**: 273–285.

512. **Inghirami, G., F. Grignani, L. Sternas, L. Lombardi, D. M. Knowles, and R. Dalla Favera.** 1990. Down-regulation of LFA-1 adhesion receptors by C-myc oncogene in human B lymphoblastoid cells. *Science* **250**: 682–686.

513. **Ip, Y. T., R. E. Park, D. Kosman, K. Yazdanbakhsh, and M. Levine.** 1992. dorsal–twist interactions establish snail expression in the presumptive mesoderm of the *Drosophila* embryo. *Genes Dev.* **6**: 1518–1530.

514*. **Ishibashi, M., K. Moriyoshi, Y. Sasai, K. Shiota, S. Nakanishi, and R. Kageyama.** 1994. Persistent expression of helix–loop–helix factor HES-1 prevents mammalian neural differentiation in the central nervous system. *EMBO J.* **13**: 1799–1805.

515. **Ishibashi, M., Y. Sasai, S. Nakanishi, and R. Kageyama.** 1993. Molecular characterization of HES-2, a mammalian helix–loop–helix factor structurally related to *Drosophila* hairy and Enhancer of split. *Eur. J. Biochem.* **215**: 645–652.

516. **Ishida, A., H. Asano, M. Hasegawa, H. Koseki, T. Ono, M. C. Yoshida, M. Taniguchi, and M. Kanno.** 1993. Cloning and chromosome mapping of the human Mel-18 gene which encodes a DNA-binding protein with a new 'RING-finger' motif. *Gene* **129**: 249–255.

517. **Ishiguro, N., T. Matsui, and M. Shinagawa.** 1993. Specific expression of cellular oncogenes c-myc and c-myb in T-cell lines established from three types of bovine lymphosarcomas. *Am. J. Vet. Res.* **54**: 2010–2014.

518. **Jackson, S. M., K. M. Barnhart, P. L. Mellon, A. Gutierrez Hartmann, and J. P. Hoeffler.** 1993. Helix–loop–helix proteins are present and differentially expressed in different cell lines from the anterior pituitary. *Mol. Cell Endocrinol.* **96**: 167–176.

519. **Jackson, T., M. F. Allard, C. M. Sreenan, L. K. Doss, S. P. Bishop, and J. L. Swain.** 1990. The c-myc proto-oncogene regulates cardiac development in transgenic mice. *Mol. Cell Biol.* **10**: 3709–3716.

520. **Jacobs, Y., C. Vierra, and C. Nelson.** 1993. E2A expression, nuclear localization, and *in vivo* formation of DNA- and non-DNA-binding species during B-cell development. *Mol. Cell Biol.* **13**: 7321–7333.

521. **Jacobs, Y., X-Q. Xin, K. Dorshkind, and C. Nelson.** 1994. Pan/E2A expression precedes immunoglobulin heavy-chain expression during B lymphopoiesis in nontransformed cells, and Pan/E2A proteins are not detected in myeloid cells. *Mol. Cell Biol.* **14**: 4087–4096.

522. **Jaffredo, T., B. Vandenbunder, and F. Dieterlen Lievre.** 1989. In situ study of c-myc protein expression during avian development. *Development* **105**: 679–695.

523. **Jain, V. K., J. G. Judde, E. E. Max, and I. T. Magrath.** 1993. Variable IgH chain enhancer activity in Burkitt's lymphomas suggests an additional, direct mechanism of c-myc deregulation. *J. Immunol.* **150**: 5418–5428.

524. **Jakobovits, A., M. Schwab, J. M. Bishop, and G. R. Martin.** 1985. Expression of N-myc in teratocarcinoma stem cells and mouse embryos. *Nature* **318**: 188–191.

525. **Jansen Durr, P., A. Meichle, P. Steiner, M. Pagano, K. Finke, J. Botz, J. Wessbecher, G. Draetta, and M. Eilers.** 1993. Differential modulation of cyclin gene expression by MYC. *Proc. Natl Acad. Sci. USA* **90**: 3685–3689.

526. **Jasoni, C. L., M. B. Walker, M. D. Morris, and T. A. Reh.** 1994. A chicken achaete–scute homolog (CASH-1) is expressed in a temporally and spatially discrete manner in the developing nervous system. *Development* **120**: 769–783.

527. **Javaux, F., A. Donda, G. Vassart, and D. Christophe.** 1991. Cloning and sequence analysis of TFE, a helix–loop–helix transcription factor able to recognize the thyroglobulin gene promoter *in vitro*. *Nucleic Acids Res.* **19**: 1121–1127.

528. **Jayaraman, P. S., K. Hirst, and C. R. Goding.** 1994. The activation domain of a basic helix–loop–helix protein is masked by repressor interaction with domains distinct from that required for transcription regulation. *EMBO J.* **13**: 2192–2199.

529*. **Jen, Y., H. Weintraub, and R. Benezra.** 1992. Overexpression of Id protein inhibits the muscle differentiation program: *in vivo* association of Id with E2A proteins. *Genes Dev.* **6**: 1466–1479.

530. Jernberg Wiklund, H., M. Pettersson, L. G. Larsson, R. Anton, and K. Nilsson. 1992. Expression of myc-family genes in established human multiple myeloma cell lines: L-myc but not c-myc gene expression in the U-266 myeloma cell line. *Int. J. Cancer* **51**: 116–123.

531. Jimenez, F. and J. A. Campos Ortega. 1990. Defective neuroblast commitment in mutants of the achaete–scute complex and adjacent genes of *D. melanogaster*. *Neuron* **5**: 81–89.

532. Johnson, J. E., S. J. Birren, and D. J. Anderson. 1990. Two rat homologues of *Drosophila* achaete–scute specifically expressed in neuronal precursors. *Nature* **346**: 858–861.

533. Johnson, J. E., K. Zimmerman, T. Saito, and D. J. Anderson. 1992. Induction and repression of mammalian achaete–scute homologue (MASH) gene expression during neuronal differentiation of P19 embryonal carcinoma cells. *Development* **114**: 75–87.

534. Jonak, G. J. and E. J. Knight. 1984. Selective reduction of c-myc mRNA in Daudi cells by human beta interferon. *Proc. Natl Acad. Sci. USA* **81**: 1747–1750.

535. Jonsson, O. G., R. L. Kitchens, R. J. Baer, G. R. Buchanan, and R. G. Smith. 1991. Rearrangements of the tal-1 locus as clonal markers for T cell acute lymphoblastic leukemia. *J. Clin. Invest.* **87**: 2029–2035.

536. Kaczmarek, L., J. K. Hyland, R. Watt, M. Rosenberg, and R. Baserga. 1985. Microinjected c-myc as a competence factor. *Science* **228**: 1313–1315.

537. Kaddurah Daouk, R., J. M. Greene, A. S. J. Baldwin, and R. E. Kingston. 1987. Activation and repression of mammalian gene expression by the c-myc protein. *Genes Dev.* **1**: 347–357.

538. Kakkis, E. and K. Calame. 1987. A plasmacytoma-specific factor binds the c-myc promoter region. *Proc. Natl Acad. Sci. USA* **84**: 7031–7035.

539. Kakkis, E., J. Prehn, and K. Calame. 1986. An active chromatin structure acquired by translocated c-myc genes. *Mol. Cell Biol.* **6**: 1357–1361.

540. Kakkis, E., K. J. Riggs, W. Gillespie, and K. Calame. 1989. A transcriptional repressor of c-myc. *Nature* **339**: 718–721.

541. Kalemkerian, G. P., R. K. Jasti, P. Celano, B. D. Nelkin, and M. Mabry. 1994. All-trans-retinoic acid alters myc gene expression and inhibits *in vitro* progression in small cell lung cancer. *Cell Growth Differ.* **5**: 55–60.

542. Kallianpur, A. R., J. E. Jordan, and S. J. Brandt. 1994. The SCL/TAL-1 gene is expressed in progenitors of both the hematopoietic and vascular systems during embryogenesis. *Blood* **83**: 1200–1208.

543. Kaminski, H. J., R. A. Fenstermaker, F. W. Abdul Karim, J. Clayman, and R. L. Ruff. 1993. Myf-4 does not mediate AChR receptor subunit mRNA expression in thymic tissues. *Ann. N. Y. Acad. Sci.* **681**: 103–106.

544. Kaminski, H. J., R. A. Fenstermaker, F. W. Abdul Karim, J. Clayman, and R. L. Ruff. 1993. Acetylcholine receptor subunit gene expression in thymic tissue. *Muscle Nerve* **16**: 1332–1337.

545. Kamps, M. P. and D. Baltimore. 1993. E2A-Pbx1, the t(1;19) translocation protein of human pre-B-cell acute lymphocytic leukemia, causes acute myeloid leukemia in mice. *Mol. Cell Biol.* **13**: 351–357.

546. Kamps, M. P., A. T. Look, and D. Baltimore. 1991. The human t(1;19) translocation in pre-B ALL produces multiple nuclear E2A-Pbx1 fusion proteins with differing transforming potentials. *Genes Dev.* **5**: 358–368.

547. Kamps, M. P., C. Murre, X. H. Sun, and D. Baltimore. 1990. A new homeobox gene contributes the DNA binding domain of the t(1;19) translocation protein in pre-B ALL. *Cell* **60**: 547–555.

548. Kang, S. 1993. Functional domains of the transcriptional activator NUC-1 in *Neurospora crassa*. *Gene* **130**: 259–264.

549. Kang, S. and R. L. Metzenberg. 1990. Molecular analysis of nuc-1 +, a gene controlling phosphorus acquisition in *Neurospora crassa*. *Mol. Cell Biol.* **10**: 5839–5848.

550. Karn, J., J. V. Watson, A. D. Lowe, S. M. Green, and W. Vedeckis. 1989. Regulation of cell cycle duration by c-myc levels. *Oncogene* **4**: 773–787.

551. Kato, G. J., J. Barrett, M. Villa Garcia, and C. V. Dang. 1990. An amino-terminal c-myc domain required for neoplastic transformation activates transcription. *Mol. Cell Biol.* **10**: 5914–5920.

552. Kato, G. J., W. M. Lee, L. L. Chen, and C. V. Dang. 1992. Max: functional domains and interaction with c-Myc. *Genes Dev.* **6**: 81–92.

553. Kato, K., A. Kanamori, and H. Kondoh. 1990. Rapid and transient decrease of N-myc expression in retinoic acid-induced differentiation of OTF9 teratocarcinoma stem cells. *Mol. Cell Biol.* **10**: 486–491.

554. Katzav, S., J. L. Cleveland, H. E. Heslop, and D. Pulido. 1991. Loss of the amino-terminal helix–loop–helix domain of the vav proto-oncogene activates its transforming potential. *Mol. Cell Biol.* **11**: 1912–1920.

555. Katzav, S., D. Martin Zanca, and M. Barbacid. 1989. vav, a novel human oncogene derived from a locus ubiquitously expressed in hematopoietic cells. *EMBO J.* **8**: 2283–2290.

556. Kaulen, H., P. Pognonec, P. D. Gregor, and R. G. Roeder. 1991. The *Xenopus* B1 factor is closely related to the mammalian activator USF and is implicated in the developmental regulation of TFIIIA gene expression. *Mol. Cell Biol.* **11**: 412–424.

557. **Kaye, F., J. Battey, M. Nau, B. Brooks, E. Seifter, J. De Greve, M. Birrer, E. Sausville, and J. Minna.** 1988. Structure and expression of the human L-myc gene reveal a complex pattern of alternative mRNA processing. *Mol. Cell Biol.* **8**: 186–195.

558. **Keath, E. J., P. G. Caimi, and M. D. Cole.** 1984. Fibroblast lines expressing activated c-myc oncogenes are tumorigenic in nude mice and syngeneic animals. *Cell* **39**: 339–348.

559. **Keath, E. J., A. Kelekar, and M. D. Cole.** 1984. Transcriptional activation of the translocated c-myc oncogene in mouse plasmacytomas: similar RNA levels in tumor and proliferating normal cells. *Cell* **37**: 521–528.

560. **Kelekar, A. and M. D. Cole.** 1986. Tumorigenicity of fibroblast lines expressing the adenovirus E1a, cellular p53, or normal c-myc genes. *Mol. Cell Biol.* **6**: 7–14.

561. **Kelly, K., B. Cochran, C. Stiles, and P. Leder.** 1984. The regulation of c-myc by growth signals. *Curr. Top. Microbiol. Immunol.* **113**: 117–126.

562. **Kelly, K., B. H. Cochran, C. D. Stiles, and P. Leder.** 1983. Cell-specific regulation of the c-myc gene by lymphocyte mitogens and platelet-derived growth factor. *Cell* **35**: 603–610.

563. **Kelly, K. and U. Siebenlist.** 1985. The role of c-myc in the proliferation of normal and neoplastic cells. *J. Clin. Immunol.* **5**: 65–77.

564. **Kerkhoff, E. and K. Bister.** 1991. Myc protein structure: localization of DNA-binding and protein dimerization domains. *Oncogene* **6**: 93–102.

565. **Kessler, D. J., M. P. Duyao, D. B. Spicer, and G. E. Sonenshein.** 1992. NF-kappa B-like factors mediate interleukin 1 induction of c-myc gene transcription in fibroblasts. *J. Exp. Med.* **176**: 787–792.

566. **Kim, S. J., K. Y. Kim, S. J. Tapscott, T. S. Winokur, K. Park, H. Fujiki, H. Weintraub, and A. B. Roberts.** 1992. Inhibition of protein phosphatases blocks myogenesis by first altering MyoD binding activity. *J. Biol. Chem.* **267**: 15140–15145.

567. **Kim, Y. H., M. A. Buchholz, F. J. Chrest, and A. A. Nordin.** 1994. Up-regulation of c-myc induces the gene expression of the murine homologues of p34cdc2 and cyclin-dependent kinase-2 in T lymphocytes. *J. Immunol.* **152**: 4328–4335.

568. **Kimchi, A., D. Resnitzky, R. Ber, and G. Gat.** 1988. Recessive genetic deregulation abrogates c-myc suppression by interferon and is implicated in oncogenesis. *Mol. Cell Biol.* **8**: 2828–2836.

569. **King, M. W.** 1991. Developmentally regulated alternative splicing in the *Xenopus laevis* c-Myc gene creates an intron-1 containing c-Myc RNA present only in post-midblastula embryos. *Nucleic Acids Res.* **19**: 5777–5783.

570. **King, M. W., J. M. Roberts, and R. N. Eisenman.** 1986. Expression of the c-myc proto-oncogene during development of *Xenopus laevis. Mol. Cell Biol.* **6**: 4499–4508.

571. **Kingston, R. E., A. S. J. Baldwin, and P. A. Sharp.** 1984. Regulation of heat shock protein 70 gene expression by c-myc. *Nature* **312**: 280–282.

572. **Kirschbaum, B. J., P. Pognonec, and R. G. Roeder.** 1992. Definition of the transcriptional activation domain of recombinant 43-kilodalton USF. *Mol. Cell Biol.* **12**: 5094–5101.

573. **Kitaura, H., I. Galli, T. Taira, S. M. Iguchi Ariga, and H. Ariga.** 1991. Activation of c-myc promoter by c-myc protein in serum starved cells. *FEBS Lett.* **290**: 147–152.

574. **Klambt, C., E. Knust, K. Tietze, and J. A. Campos Ortega.** 1989. Closely related transcripts encoded by the neurogenic gene complex enhancer of split of *Drosophila melanogaster. EMBO J.* **8**: 203–210.

575. **Klein, E. S., D. M. Simmons, L. W. Swanson, and M. G. Rosenfeld.** 1993. Tissue-specific RNA splicing generates an ankyrin-like domain that affects the dimerization and DNA-binding properties of a bHLH protein. *Genes Dev.* **7**: 55–71.

576. **Klempnauer, K. H.** 1989. Association of v-myc protein with chromatin. *Oncogene* **4**: 115–118.

577. **Knight, E. J., E. D. Anton, D. Fahey, B. K. Friedland, and G. J. Jonak.** 1985. Interferon regulates c-myc gene expression in Daudi cells at the post-transcriptional level. *Proc. Natl Acad. Sci. USA* **82**: 1151–1154.

578. **Knust, E., H. Schrons, F. Grawe, and J. A. Campos Ortega.** 1992. Seven genes of the Enhancer of split complex of *Drosophila melanogaster* encode helix–loop–helix proteins. *Genetics* **132**: 505–518.

579. **Kohl, N. E., C. E. Gee, and F. W. Alt.** 1984. Activated expression of the N-myc gene in human neuroblastomas and related tumors. *Science* **226**: 1335–1337.

580. **Kohl, N. E., E. Legouy, R. A. DePinho, P. D. Nisen, R. K. Smith, C. E. Gee, and F. W. Alt.** 1986. Human N-myc is closely related in organization and nucleotide sequence to c-myc. *Nature* **319**: 73–77.

581. **Kohlhuber, F., L. J. Strobl, and D. Eick.** 1993. Early down-regulation of c-myc in dimethylsulfoxide-induced mouse erythroleukemia (MEL) cells is mediated at the P1/P2 promoters. *Oncogene* **8**: 1099–1102.

582. **Kokontis, J., K. Takakura, N. Hay, and S. Liao.** 1994. Increased androgen receptor activity and altered c-myc expression in prostate cancer cells after long-term androgen deprivation. *Cancer Res.* **54**: 1566–1573.

583. **Kopan, R., J. S. Nye, and H. Weintraub.** 1994. The intracellular domain of mouse Notch: a constitutively activated repressor of myogenesis directed at the basic helix–loop–helix region of MyoD. *Development* **120**: 2385–2396.

584. **Korkolopoulou, P., J. Oates, C. Kittas, and J. Crocker.** 1994. p53, c-myc p62 and proliferating cell nuclear antigen (PCNA) expression in non-Hodgkin's lymphomas. *J. Clin. Pathol.* **47**: 9–14.

585. **Koskinen, P. J., L. Sistonen, G. Evan, R. Morimoto, and K. Alitalo.** 1991. Nuclear colocalization of cellular and viral myc proteins with HSP70 in myc-overexpressing cells. *J. Virol.* **65**: 842–851.

586. **Kozlowski, M. T., L. Gan, J. M. Venuti, M. Sawadogo, and W. H. Klein.** 1991. Sea urchin USF: a helix–loop–helix protein active in embryonic ectoderm cells. *Dev. Biol.* **148**: 625–630.

587. **Kramatschek, B. and J. A. Campos-Ortega.** 1994. Neuroectodermal transcription of the *Drosophila* neurogenic genes E(spl) and HLH-m5 is regulated by proneural genes. *Development* **120**: 815–826.

588. **Krause, M., A. Fire, S. White Harrison, H. Weintraub, and S. Tapscott.** 1992. Functional conservation of nematode and vertebrate myogenic regulatory factors. *J. Cell Sci. Suppl.* **16**: 111–115.

589. **Krause, M. and H. Weintraub.** 1992. CeMyoD expression and myogenesis in *C. elegans. Semin. Dev. Biol.* **3**: 277–285.

590*. **Kreider, B. L., R. Benezra, G. Rovera, and T. Kadesch.** 1992. Inhibition of myeloid differentiation by the helix–loop–helix protein Id. *Science* **255**: 1700–1702.

591. **Kretzner, L., E. M. Blackwood, and R. N. Eisenman.** 1992. Transcriptional activities of the Myc and Max proteins in mammalian cells. *Curr. Top. Microbiol. Immunol.* **182**: 435–443.

592*. **Kretzner, L., E. M. Blackwood, and R. N. Eisenman.** 1992. Myc and Max proteins possess distinct transcriptional activities. *Nature* **359**: 426–429.

593. **Krumm, A., T. Meulia, M. Brunvand, and M. Groudine.** 1992. The block to transcriptional elongation within the human c-myc gene is determined in the promoter–proximal region. *Genes Dev.* **6**: 2201–2213.

594. **Krystal, G., M. Birrer, J. Way, M. Nau, E. Sausville, C. Thompson, J. Minna, and J. Battey.** 1988. Multiple mechanisms for transcriptional regulation of the myc gene family in small-cell lung cancer. *Mol. Cell Biol.* **8**: 3373–3381.

595. **Krystal, G., J. Way, and J. Battey.** 1988. Comparison of c-, N-, and L-myc transcriptional regulation. *Curr. Top. Microbiol. Immunol.* **141**: 274–281.

596. **Krystal, G. W., B. C. Armstrong, and J. F. Battey.** 1990. N-myc mRNA forms an RNA–RNA duplex with endogenous antisense transcripts. *Mol. Cell Biol.* **10**: 4180–4191.

597. **Kubota, Y., S. H. Kim, S. M. Iguchi Ariga, and H. Ariga.** 1989. Transrepression of the N-myc expression by c-myc protein. *Biochem. Biophys. Res. Commun.* **162**: 991–997.

598. **Kugler, W., M. Kaling, K. Ross, U. Wagner, and G. U. Ryffel.** 1990. BAP, a rat liver protein that activates transcription through a promoter element with similarity to the USF/MLTF binding site. *Nucleic Acids Res.* **18**: 6943–6951.

599. **Kumar, S. and M. Leffak.** 1989. DNA topology of the ordered chromatin domain 5$'$ to the human c-myc gene. *Nucleic Acids Res.* **17**: 2819–2833.

600. **Kume, T. U., S. Takada, and M. Obinata.** 1988. Probability that the commitment of murine erythroleukemia cell differentiation is determined by the c-myc level. *J. Mol. Biol.* **202**: 779–786.

601. **Kuo, S. S., J. D. Mellentin, N. G. Copeland, D. J. Gilbert, N. A. Jenkins, and M. L. Cleary.** 1991. Structure, chromosome mapping, and expression of the mouse Lyl-1 gene. *Oncogene* **6**: 961–968.

602. **Kurabayashi, M., R. Jeyaseelan, and L. Kedes.** 1993. Two distinct cDNA sequences encoding the human helix–loop–helix protein Id2. *Gene* **133**: 305–306.

603. **Kurabayashi, M., R. Jeyaseelan, and L. Kedes.** 1994. Doxorubicin represses the function of the myogenic helix–loop–helix transcription factor MyoD. Involvement of Id gene induction. *J. Biol. Chem.* **269**: 6031–6039.

604. **La Rocca, S. A., M. Grossi, G. Falcone, S. Alema, and F. Tato.** 1989. Interaction with normal cells suppresses the transformed phenotype of v-myc-transformed quail muscle cells. *Cell* **58**: 123–131.

605. **La Rosa, F. A., J. W. Pierce, and G. E. Sonenshein.** 1994. Differential regulation of the c-myc oncogene promoter by the NF-kappa B rel family of transcription factors. *Mol. Cell Biol.* **14**: 1039–1044.

606. **Lachman, H. M., G. H. Cheng, and A. I. Skoultchi.** 1986. Transfection of mouse erythroleukemia cells with myc sequences changes the rate of induced commitment to differentiate. *Proc. Natl Acad. Sci. USA* **83**: 6480–6484.

607. **Lachman, H. M., K. S. Hatton, A. I. Skoultchi, and C. L. Schildkraut.** 1985. c-myc mRNA levels in the cell cycle change in mouse erythroleukemia cells following inducer treatment. *Proc. Natl Acad. Sci. USA* **82**: 5323–5327.

608. **Lachman, H. M. and A. I. Skoultchi.** 1984. Expression of c-myc changes during differentiation of mouse erythroleukaemia cells. *Nature* **310**: 592–594.

609. **Lacy, J., W. P. Summers, and W. C. Summers.** 1989. Post-transcriptional mechanisms of deregulation of MYC following conversion of a human B cell line by Epstein–Barr virus. *EMBO J.* **8**: 1973–1980.

610*. **Lahoz, E. G., L. Xu, N. Schreiber-Agus, and R. A. DePinho.** 1994. Suppression of Myc, but not E1a, transformation activity by Max-associated proteins, Mad and Mxi1. *Proc. Natl Acad. Sci. USA* **91**: 5503–5507.

611. **Laird Offringa, I. A., C. L. de Wit, P. Elfferich, and A. J. van der Eb.** 1990. Poly(A) tail shortening is the translation-dependent step in c-myc mRNA degradation. *Mol. Cell Biol.* **10**: 6132–6140.

612. **Laird Offringa, I. A., P. Elfferich, H. J. Knaken, J. de Ruiter, and A. J. van der Eb.** 1989. Analysis of polyadenylation site usage of the c-myc oncogene. *Nucleic Acids Res.* **17**: 6499–6514.

613. **Laird Offringa, I. A., P. Elfferich, and A. J. van der Eb.** 1991. Rapid c-myc mRNA degradation does not require (A + U)-rich sequences or complete translation of the mRNA. *Nucleic Acids Res.* **19**: 2387–2394.

614. **Land, H., A. C. Chen, J. P. Morgenstern, L. F. Parada, and R. A. Weinberg.** 1986. Behavior of myc and ras oncogenes in transformation of rat embryo fibroblasts. *Mol. Cell Biol.* **6**: 1917–1925.

615. **Langer, S. J., D. M. Bortner, M. F. Roussel, C. J. Sherr, and M. C. Ostrowski.** 1992. Mitogenic signaling by colony-stimulating factor 1 and ras is suppressed by the ets-2 DNA-binding domain and restored by myc overexpression. *Mol. Cell Biol.* **12**: 5355–5362.

616. **Larcher, J. C., J. L. Vayssiere, L. Lossouarn, F. Gros, and B. Croizat.** 1991. Regulation of c- and N-myc expression during induced differentiation of murine neuroblastoma cells. *Oncogene* **6**: 633–638.

617. **Largaespada, D. A., D. A. Kaehler, H. Mishak, E. Weissinger, M. Potter, J. F. Mushinski, and R. Risser.** 1992. A retrovirus that expresses v-abl and c-myc oncogenes rapidly induces plasmacytomas. *Oncogene* **7**: 811–819.

618*. **Larsson, L. -G., M. Pettersson, F. Oberg, K. Nilsson, and B. Luscher.** 1994. Expression of mad, mxi1, max and c-myc during induced differentiation of hematopoietic cells: opposite regulation of mad and c-myc. *Oncogene* **9**: 1247–1252.

619. **Larsson, L. G., H. E. Gray, T. Totterman, U. Pettersson, and K. Nilsson.** 1987. Drastically increased expression of MYC and FOS protooncogenes during *in vitro* differentiation of chronic lymphocytic leukemia cells. *Proc. Natl Acad. Sci. USA* **84**: 223–227.

620. **Larsson, L. G., M. Pettersson, F. Oberg, K. Nilsson, and B. Luscher.** 1994. Expression of mad, mxi1, max and c-myc during induced differentiation of hematopoietic cells: opposite regulation of mad and c-myc. *Oncogene* **9**: 1247–1252.

621. **Larsson, L. G., M. Schena, M. Carlsson, J. Sallstrom, and K. Nilsson.** 1991. Expression of the c-myc protein is down-regulated at the terminal stages during *in vitro* differentiation of B-type chronic lymphocytic leukemia cells. *Blood* **77**: 1025–1032.

622. **Lassar, A. B., J. N. Buskin, D. Lockshon, R. L. Davis, S. Apone, S. D. Hauschka, and H. Weintraub.** 1989. MyoD is a sequence-specific DNA binding protein requiring a region of myc homology to bind to the muscle creatine kinase enhancer. *Cell* **58**: 823–831.

623. **Lau, L. F. and D. Nathans.** 1987. Expression of a set of growth-related immediate early genes in BALB/c 3T3 cells: coordinate regulation with c-fos or c-myc. *Proc. Natl Acad. Sci. USA* **84**: 1182–1186.

624. **Lavenu, A., S. Pournin, C. Babinet, and D. Morello.** 1994. The cis-acting elements known to regulate c-myc expression ex vivo are not sufficient for correct transcription *in vivo*. *Oncogene* **9**: 527–536.

625. **Lazarus, P.** 1992. The regulation of translation by the 5′ untranslated region of *Xenopus* c-myc I mRNA during early development. *Oncogene* **7**: 1037–1041.

626. **LeBrun, D. P. and M. L. Cleary.** 1994. Fusion with E2A alters the transcriptional properties of the homeodomain protein PBX1 in t(1;19) leukemias. *Oncogene* **9**: 1641–1647.

627. **Leder, A., P. K. Pattengale, A. Kuo, T. A. Stewart, and P. Leder.** 1986. Consequences of widespread deregulation of the c-myc gene in transgenic mice: multiple neoplasms and normal development. *Cell* **45**: 485–495.

628. **Lee, N. G., J. Yamaguchi, and K. N. Subramanian.** 1991. Efficient replication of plasmids containing the SV40 origin in N-myc overexpressing human neuroblastoma cells. *Oncogene* **6**: 1161–1169.

629. **Lee, S. Y., A. Sugiyama, N. Sueoka, and Y. Kuchino.** 1990. Point mutation of the neu gene in rat neural tumor RT4-AC cells: suppression of tumorigenicity by s-Myc. *Jpn. J. Cancer Res.* **81**: 1085–1088.

630. **Lee, T. C., Y. Zhang, and R. J. Schwartz.** 1994. Bifunctional transcriptional properties of YY1 in regulating muscle actin and c-myc gene expression during myogenesis. *Oncogene* **9**: 1047–1052.

631. **Lee, W. H., A. L. Murphree, and W. F. Benedict.** 1984. Expression and amplification of the N-myc gene in primary retinoblastoma. *Nature* **309**: 458–460.

632. **Lee, W. M., M. Schwab, D. Westaway, and H. E. Varmus.** 1985. Augmented expression of normal c-myc is sufficient for cotransformation of rat embryo cells with a mutant ras gene. *Mol. Cell Biol.* **5**: 3345–3356.

633. **Legouy, E., R. DePinho, K. Zimmerman, R. Collum, G. Yancopoulos, L. Mitsock, R. Kriz, and F. W. Alt.** 1987. Structure and expression of the murine L-myc gene. *EMBO J.* **6**: 3359–3366.

634. **Legrain, M., M. De Wilde, and F. Hilger.** 1986. Isolation, physical characterization and expression analysis of the *Saccharomyces cerevisiae* positive regulatory gene PHO4. *Nucleic Acids Res.* **14**: 3059–3073.

635. **Lenardo, M., A. K. Rustgi, A. R. Schievella, and R. Bernards.** 1989. Suppression of MHC class I gene expression by N-myc through enhancer inactivation. *EMBO J.* **8**: 3351–3355.

636. **Leptin, M.** 1991. twist and snail as positive and negative regulators during *Drosophila* mesoderm development. *Genes Dev.* **5**: 1568–1576.

637. **Levine, R. A., J. E. McCormack, A. Buckler, and G. E. Sonenshein.** 1986. Complex regulation of c-myc gene expression in a murine B cell lymphoma. *Curr. Top. Microbiol. Immunol.* **132**: 305–312.

638. **Levine, R. A., J. E. McCormack, A. Buckler, and G. E. Sonenshein.** 1986. Transcriptional and posttranscriptional control of c-myc gene expression in WEHI 231 cells. *Mol. Cell Biol.* **6**: 4112–4116.

639. **Levy, L. S., M. B. Gardner, and J. W. Casey.** 1984. Isolation of a feline leukaemia provirus containing the oncogene myc from a feline lymphosarcoma. *Nature* **308**: 853–856.

640. **Levy, N., E. Yonish Rouach, M. Oren, and A. Kimchi.** 1993. Complementation by wild-type p53 of interleukin-6 effects on M1 cells: induction of cell cycle exit and cooperativity with c-myc suppression. *Mol. Cell Biol.* **13**: 7942–7952.

641. **Li, H. and Y. Capetanaki.** 1993. Regulation of the mouse desmin gene: transactivated by MyoD, myogenin, MRF4 and Myf5. *Nucleic Acids Res.* **21**: 335–343.

642. **Li, H. and Y. Capetanaki.** 1994. An E box in the desmin promoter cooperates with the E box and MEF-2 sites of a distal enhancer to direct muscle-specific transcription. *EMBO J.* **13**: 3580–3589.

643. **Li, H. and Y. Capetanaki.** 1991. Regulation and transactivation of the mouse desmin gene by different members of the MyoD families. *J. Cell Biol.* **115**: 395a.

644. **Li, H., S. K. Choudhary, D. J. Milner, M. I. Munir, I. R. Kuisk, and Y. Capetanaki.** 1994. Inhibition of desmin expression blocks myoblast fusion and interferes with the myogenic regulators MyoD and myogenin. *J. Cell Biol.* **124**: 827–841.

645. **Li, J. M., R. A. Parsons, and W. F. Marzluff.** 1994. Transcription of the sea urchin U6 gene *in vitro* requires a TATA-like box, a proximal sequence element, and sea urchin USF, which binds an essential E box. *Mol. Cell Biol.* **14**: 2191–2200.

646. **Li, L-H., C. Nerlov, G. Prendergast, D. MacGregor, and E. B. Ziff.** 1994. c-Myc represses transcription *in vivo* by a novel mechanism dependent on the initiator element and Myc box II. *EMBO J.* **13**: 4070–4079.

647. **Li, L., J. C. Chambard, M. Karin, and E. N. Olson.** 1992. Fos and Jun repress transcriptional activation by myogenin and MyoD: the amino terminus of Jun can mediate repression. *Genes Dev.* **6**: 676–689.

648. **Lin, H. H., W. Y. Li, and D. K. Ann.** 1993. The helix–loop–helix proteins (salivary-specific cAMP response element-binding proteins) can modulate cAMP-inducible RP4 gene expression in salivary cells. *J. Biol. Chem.* **268**: 10214–10220.

649. **Lin, Z. Y., C. A. Dechesne, J. Eldridge, and B. M. Paterson.** 1989. An avian muscle factor related to MyoD1 activates muscle-specific promoters in nonmuscle cells of different germ-layer origin and in BrdU-treated myoblasts. *Genes Dev.* **3**: 986–996.

650. **Lipkowitz, S., V. Gobel, M. L. Varterasian, K. Nakahara, K. Tchorz, and I. R. Kirsch.** 1992. A comparative structural characterization of the human NSCL-1 and NSCL-2 genes. Two basic helix–loop–helix genes expressed in the developing nervous system. *J. Biol. Chem.* **267**: 21065–21071.

651. **Lipp, M., R. Schilling, and G. Bernhardt.** 1989. Trans-activation of human MYC: the second promoter is target for the stimulation by adenovirus E1a proteins. *Oncogene* **4**: 535–541.

652. **Liu, E., G. Santos, W. M. Lee, C. K. Osborne, and C. C. Benz.** 1989. Effects of c-myc overexpression on the growth characteristics of MCF-7 human breast cancer cells. *Oncogene* **4**: 979–984.

653. **Liu, J., C. H. Clegg, and M. Shoyab.** 1992. Regulation of EGR-1, c-jun, and c-myc gene expression by oncostatin M. *Cell Growth Differ.* **3**: 307–313.

654. **Lo, L. C., J. E. Johnson, C. W. Wuenschell, T. Saito, and D. J. Anderson.** 1991. Mammalian achaete–scute homolog 1 is transiently expressed by spatially restricted subsets of early neuroepithelial and neural crest cells. *Genes Dev.* **5**: 1524–1537.

655. **Lombardi, L., F. Grignani, L. Sternas, K. Cechova, G. Inghirami, and R. Dalla Favera.** 1990. Mechanism of negative feed-back regulation of c-myc gene expression in B-cells and its inactivation in tumor cells. *Curr. Top. Microbiol. Immunol.* **166**: 293–301.

656. **Lombardi, L., E. W. Newcomb, and R. Dalla Favera.** 1987. Pathogenesis of Burkitt lymphoma: expression of an activated c-myc oncogene causes the tumorigenic conversion of EBV-infected human B lymphoblasts. *Cell* **49**: 161–170.

657. **London, L., R. G. Keene, and R. Landick.** 1991. Analysis of premature termination in c-myc during transcription by RNA polymerase II in a HeLa nuclear extract. *Mol. Cell Biol.* **11**: 4599–4615.

658. **Lotem, J. and L. Sachs.** 1993. Regulation by bcl-2, c-myc, and p53 of susceptibility to induction of apoptosis by heat shock and cancer chemotherapy compounds in differentiation-competent and -defective myeloid leukemic cells. *Cell Growth Differ.* **4**: 41–47.

659. **Lu, L. and C. D. Logsdon.** 1992. CCK, bombesin, and carbachol stimulate c-fos, c-jun, and c-myc oncogene expression in rat pancreatic acini. *Am. J. Physiol.* **263**: G327-G332.

660. **Lu, Q., D. D. Wright, and M. P. Kamps.** 1994. Fusion with E2A converts the Pbx1 homeodomain protein into a constitutive transcriptional activator in human leukemias carrying the t(1;19) translocation. *Mol. Cell Biol.* **14**: 3938–3948.

661. **Lucas, J. M., N. M. Wilkie, and J. C. Lang.** 1993. c-MYC repression of promoter activity through core promoter elements. *Biochem. Biophys. Res. Commun.* **194**: 1446–1452.

662. **Ludwig, S. R., L. F. Habera, S. L. Dellaporta, and S. R. Wessler.** 1989. Lc, a member of the maize R gene family responsible for tissue-specific anthocyanin production, encodes a protein similar to transcriptional activators and contains the myc-homology region. *Proc. Natl Acad. Sci. USA* **86**: 7092–7096.

663*. **Ludwig, S. R. and S. R. Wessler.** 1990. Maize R gene family: tissue-specific helix–loop–helix proteins. *Cell* **62**: 849–851.

664. **Luscher, B. and R. N. Eisenman.** 1988. c-myc and c-myb protein degradation: effect of metabolic inhibitors and heat shock. *Mol. Cell Biol.* **8**: 2504–2512.

665. **Ma, A., R. K. Smith, A. Tesfaye, P. Achacoso, R. Dildrop, N. Rosenberg, and F. W. Alt.** 1991. Mechanism of endogenous myc gene down-regulation in E mu-N-myc tumors. *Mol. Cell Biol.* **11**: 440–444.

666. **Mackay, T. F. and C. H. Langley.** 1990. Molecular and phenotypic variation in the achaete–scute region of *Drosophila melanogaster*. Nature **348**: 64–66.

667. **Macpherson, J. N., B. S. Weir, and A. J. Leigh Brown.** 1990. Extensive linkage disequilibrium in the achaete–scute complex of *Drosophila melanogaster*. *Genetics* **126**: 121–129.

668. **Maekawa, T., T. Sudo, M. Kurimoto, and S. Ishii.** 1991. USF-related transcription factor, HIV-TF1, stimulates transcription of human immunodeficiency virus-1. *Nucleic Acids Res.* **19**: 4689–4694.

669. **Mai, S. and A. Jalava.** 1994. C-Myc binds to the $5'$ flanking sequence motifs of the dihydrofolate reductase gene in cellular extracts: role in proliferation. *Nucleic Acids Res.* **22**: 2264–2273.

670. **Mak, K. L., R. Q. To, Y. Kong, and S. F. Konieczny.** 1992. The MRF4 activation domain is required to induce muscle-specific gene expression. *Mol. Cell Biol.* **12**: 4334–4346.

671. **Makela, T. P., J. Kere, R. Winqvist, and K. Alitalo.** 1991. Intrachromosomal rearrangements fusing L-myc and rlf in small-cell lung cancer. *Mol. Cell Biol.* **11**: 4015–4021.

672. **Makela, T. P., P. J. Koskinen, I. Vastrik, and K. Alitalo.** 1992. Alternative forms of Max as enhancers or suppressors of Myc-ras cotransformation. *Science* **256**: 373–377.

673. **Makela, T. P., K. Saksela, and K. Alitalo.** 1989. Two N-myc polypeptides with distinct amino termini encoded by the second and third exons of the gene. *Mol. Cell Biol.* **9**: 1545–1552.

674. **Makela, T. P., K. Saksela, and K. Alitalo.** 1992. Amplification and rearrangement of L-myc in human small-cell lung cancer. *Mutat. Res.* **276**: 307–315.

675. **Makela, T. P., K. Saksela, G. Evan, and K. Alitalo.** 1991. A fusion protein formed by L-myc and a novel gene in SCLC. *EMBO J.* **10**: 1331–1335.

676. **Makela, T. P., M. Shiraishi, M. G. Borrello, T. Sekiya, and K. Alitalo.** 1992. Rearrangement and co-amplification of L-myc and rlf in primary lung cancer. *Oncogene* **7**: 405–409.

677. **Maley, M. A., Y. Fan, M. W. Beilharz, and M. D. Grounds.** 1994. Intrinsic differences in MyoD and myogenin expression between primary cultures of SJL/J and BALB/C skeletal muscle. *Exp. Cell Res.* **211**: 99–107.

678. **Mangasarian, K. and W. S. Mellon.** 1993. 1,25-Dihydroxyvitamin D-3 destabilizes c-myc mRNA in HL-60 leukemic cells. *Biochim. Biophys. Acta* 1172: 55–63.

679. **Mangiacapra, F. J., S. L. Roof, D. Z. Ewton, and J. R. Florini.** 1992. Paradoxical decrease in myf-5 messenger RNA levels during induction of myogenic differentiation by insulin-like growth factors. *Mol. Endocrinol.* **6**: 2038–2044.

680. **Mango, S. E., G. D. Schuler, M. E. Steele, and M. D. Cole.** 1989. Germ line c-myc is not down-regulated by loss or exclusion of activating factors in myc-induced macrophage tumors. *Mol. Cell Biol.* **9**: 3482–3490.

681. **Marck, C., O. Lefebvre, C. Carles, M. Riva, N. Chaussivert, A. Ruet, and A. Sentenac.** 1993. The TFIIIB-assembling subunit of yeast transcription factor TFIIIC has both tetratricopeptide repeats and basic helix–loop–helix motifs. *Proc. Natl Acad. Sci. USA* **90**: 4027–4031.

682. **Marcu, K. B.** 1987. Regulation of expression of the c-myc proto-oncogene. *Bioessays* **6**: 28–32.

683. **Marcu, K. B., C. Asselin, A. Nepveu, S. Weisinger, and J. Q. Yang.** 1988. Negative control elements within and near the murine c-myc gene. *Curr. Top. Microbiol. Immunol.* **141**: 253–263.

684. **Marcu, K. B., P. D. Fahrlander, M. A. Julius, A. Nepveu, E. F. Remmers, and J. Q. Yang.** 1986. Studies on c-myc regulation in normal and transformed cells. *Curr. Top. Microbiol. Immunol.* **132**: 345–354.

685. **Martin, J. F., L. Li, and E. N. Olson.** 1992. Repression of myogenin function by TGF-beta 1 is targeted at the basic helix–loop–helix motif and is independent of E2A products. *J. Biol. Chem.* **267**: 10956–10960.

686. **Martinez, C., J. Modolell, and J. Garrell.** 1993. Regulation of the proneural gene achaete by helix–loop–helix proteins. *Mol. Cell Biol.* **13**: 3514–3521.

687. **Martinotti, S., A. Richman, and A. Hayday.** 1988. Disruption of the putative c-myc auto-regulation mechanism in a human B cell line. *Curr. Top. Microbiol. Immunol.* **141**: 264–268.

688. Marui, N., T. Sakai, N. Hosokawa, M. Yoshida, A. Aoike, K. Kawai, H. Nishino, and M. Fukushima. 1990. N-myc suppression and cell cycle arrest at G1 phase by prostaglandins. *FEBS Lett.* **270**: 15–18.

689. Maruyama, K., S. C. Schiavi, W. Huse, G. L. Johnson, and H. E. Ruley. 1987. myc and E1A oncogenes alter the responses of PC12 cells to nerve growth factor and block differentiation. *Oncogene* **1**: 361–367.

690. Masison, D. C., K. F. O'Connell, and R. E. Baker. 1993. Mutational analysis of the *Saccharomyces cerevisiae* general regulatory factor CP1. *Nucleic Acids Res.* **21**: 4133–4141.

691. Mason, G. G., A. M. Witte, M. L. Whitelaw, C. Antonsson, J. McGuire, A. Wilhelmsson, L. Poellinger, and J. A. Gustafsson. 1994. Purification of the DNA binding form of dioxin receptor. Role of the Arnt cofactor in regulation of dioxin receptor function. *J. Biol. Chem.* **269**: 4438–4449.

692. Matsushita, N., K. Sogawa, M. Ema, A. Yoshida, and Y. Fujii Kuriyama. 1993. A factor binding to the xenobiotic responsive element (XRE) of P-4501A1 gene consists of at least two helix–loop–helix proteins, Ah receptor and Arnt. *J. Biol. Chem.* **268**: 21002–21006.

693. Mattei, M. G., C. Stoetzel, and F. Perrin Schmitt. 1993. The B-HLH protein encoding the M-twist gene is located by in situ hybridization on murine chromosome 12. *Mamm. Genome* **4**: 127–128.

694. McGuire, J., M. L. Whitelaw, I. Pongratz, J. A. Gustafsson, and L. Poellinger. 1994. A cellular factor stimulates ligand-dependent release of hsp90 from the basic helix–loop–helix dioxin receptor. *Mol. Cell Biol.* **14**: 2438–2446.

695. McLachlan, A. D. and D. R. Boswell. 1985. Confidence limits for homology in protein or gene sequences. The c-myc oncogene and adenovirus E1a protein. *J. Mol. Biol.* **185**: 39–49.

696. Mechti, N., M. Piechaczyk, J. M. Blanchard, L. Marty, A. Bonnieu, P. Jeanteur, and B. Lebleu. 1986. Transcriptional and post-transcriptional regulation of c-myc expression during the differentiation of murine erythroleukemia Friend cells. *Nucleic Acids Res.* **14**: 9653–9666.

697. Mehmet, H., J. Taylor Papadimitriou, and E. Rozengurt. 1989. Interferon inhibition of bombesin-stimulated mitogenesis in Swiss 3T3 cells occurs without blocking c-fos and c-myc expression. *J. Interferon Res.* **9**: 205–213.

698. Meier, J. L., X. Luo, M. Sawadogo, and S. E. Straus. 1994. The cellular transcription factor USF cooperates with Varicella–Zoster virus immediate-early protein 62 to symmetrically activate a bidirectional viral promoter. *Mol. Cell Biol.* **14**: 6896–6906.

699. Meisterernst, M., M. Horikoshi, and R. G. Roeder. 1990. Recombinant yeast TFIID, a general transcription factor, mediates activation by the gene-specific factor USF in a chromatin assembly assay. *Proc. Natl Acad. Sci. USA* **87**: 9153–9157.

700. Mellentin, J. D., C. Murre, T. A. Donlon, P. S. McCaw, S. D. Smith, A. J. Carroll, M. E. McDonald, D. Baltimore, and M. L. Cleary. 1989. The gene for enhancer binding proteins E12/E47 lies at the t(1;19) breakpoint in acute leukemias. *Science* **246**: 379–382.

701. Mellentin, J. D., S. D. Smith, and M. L. Cleary. 1989. lyl-1, a novel gene altered by chromosomal translocation in T cell leukemia, codes for a protein with a helix–loop–helix DNA binding motif. *Cell* **58**: 77–83.

702. Mellor, J., W. Jiang, M. Funk, J. Rathjen, C. A. Barnes, T. Hinz, J. H. Hegemann, and P. Philippsen. 1990. CPF1, a yeast protein which functions in centromeres and promoters. *EMBO J.* **9**: 4017–4026.

703. Messina, J. L. 1991. Inhibition and stimulation of c-myc gene transcription by insulin in rat hepatoma cells. Insulin alters the intragenic pausing of c-myc transcription. *J. Biol. Chem.* **266**: 17995–18001.

704. Meulia, T., A. Krumm, C. Spencer, and M. Groudine. 1992. Sequences in the human c-myc P2 promoter affect the elongation and premature termination of transcripts initiated from the upstream P1 promoter. *Mol. Cell Biol.* **12**: 4590–4600.

705. Michelson, A. M., S. M. Abmayr, M. Bate, A. M. Arias, and T. Maniatis. 1990. Expression of a MyoD family member prefigures muscle pattern in *Drosophila* embryos. *Genes Dev.* **4**: 2086–2097.

706. Michitsch, R. W. and P. W. Melera. 1985. Nucleotide sequence of the 3′ exon of the human N-myc gene. *Nucleic Acids Res.* **13**: 2545–2558.

707. Miller, H., C. Asselin, D. Dufort, J. Q. Yang, K. Gupta, K. B. Marcu, and A. Nepveu. 1989. A cis-acting element in the promoter region of the murine c-myc gene is necessary for transcriptional block. *Mol. Cell Biol.* **9**: 5340–5349.

708. Milner, A. E., R. J. Grand, C. M. Waters, and C. D. Gregory. 1993. Apoptosis in Burkitt lymphoma cells is driven by c-myc. *Oncogene* **8**: 3385–3391.

709. Min, S., S. J. Crider-Miller, and E. J. Taparowshy. 1994. The transcription activation domains of v-Myc and VP16 interact with common factors required for cellular transformation and proliferation. *Cell Growth Differ.* **5**: 563–573.

710. Min, S. and E. J. Taparowsky. 1992. v-Myc, but not Max, possesses domains that function in both transcription activation and cellular transformation. *Oncogene* **7**: 1531–1540.

711. **Miner, J. H., J. B. Miller, and B. J. Wold.** 1992. Skeletal muscle phenotypes initiated by ectopic MyoD in transgenic mouse heart. *Development* **114**: 853−860.

712. **Miner, J. H. and B. Wold.** 1990. Herculin, a fourth member of the MyoD family of myogenic regulatory genes. *Proc. Natl Acad. Sci. USA* **87**: 1089−1093.

713. **Miner, J. H. and B. J. Wold.** 1991. c-myc inhibition of MyoD and myogenin-initiated myogenic differentiation. *Mol. Cell Biol.* **11**: 2842−2851.

714. **Mitchell, L. S., R. A. Neill, and G. D. Birnie.** 1992. Temporal relationships between induced changes in c-myc mRNA abundance, proliferation, and differentiation in HL60 cells. *Differentiation* **49**: 119−125.

715. **Miyamoto, N. G., V. Moncollin, J. M. Egly, and P. Chambon.** 1985. Specific interaction between a transcription factor and the upstream element of the adenovirus-2 major late promoter. *EMBO J.* **4**: 3563−3570.

716. **Miyazawa, T., M. Kohmoto, Y. Kawaguchi, K. Tomonaga, T. Toyosaki, K. Ikuta, A. Adachi, and T. Mikami.** 1993. The AP-1 binding site in the feline immunodeficiency virus long terminal repeat is not required for virus replication in feline T lymphocytes. *J. Gen. Virol.* **74**: 1573−1580.

717. **Moberg, K. H., T. J. Logan, W. A. Tyndall, and D. J. Hall.** 1992. Three distinct elements within the murine c-myc promoter are required for transcription. *Oncogene* **7**: 411−421.

718. **Moberg, K. H., W. A. Tyndall, J. Pyrc, and D. J. Hall.** 1991. Analysis of the c-myc P2 promoter. *J. Cell Physiol.* **148**: 75−84.

719. **Modak, S. P., E. Principaud, and G. Spohr.** 1993. Regulation of *Xenopus* c-myc promoter activity in oocytes and embryos. *Oncogene* **8**: 645−654.

720. **Moelling, K., T. Benter, T. Bunte, E. Pfaff, W. Deppert, J. M. Egly, and N. B. Miyamoto.** 1984. Properties of the myc-gene product: nuclear association, inhibition of transcription and activation in stimulated lymphocytes. *Curr. Top. Microbiol. Immunol.* **113**: 198−207.

721. **Montarras, D., J. Chelly, E. Bober, H. Arnold, M. O. Ott, F. Gros, and C. Pinset.** 1991. Developmental patterns in the expression of Myf5, MyoD, myogenin, and MRF4 during myogenesis. *New Biol.* **3**: 592−600.

722. **Mori, M., G. F. Barnard, R. J. Staniunas, J. M. Jessup, G. D. J. Steele, and L. B. Chen.** 1993. Prothymosin-alpha mRNA expression correlates with that of c-myc in human colon cancer. *Oncogene* **8**: 2821−2826.

723. **Moroy, T., P. Fisher, C. Guidos, A. Ma, K. Zimmerman, A. Tesfaye, R. DePinho, I. Weissman, and F. W. Alt.** 1990. IgH enhancer deregulated expression of L-myc: abnormal T lymphocyte development and T cell lymphomagenesis. *EMBO J.* **9**: 3659−3666.

724. **Moroy, T., S. Verbeek, A. Ma, P. Achacoso, A. Berns, and F. Alt.** 1991. E mu N- and E mu L-myc cooperate with E mu pim-1 to generate lymphoid tumors at high frequency in double-transgenic mice. *Oncogene* **6**: 1941−1948.

725. **Morrow, M. A., G. Lee, S. Gillis, G. D. Yancopoulos, and F. W. Alt.** 1992. Interleukin-7 induces N-myc and c-myc expression in normal precursor B lymphocytes. *Genes Dev.* **6**: 61−70.

726. **Morse, B., V. J. South, P. G. Rothberg, and S. M. Astrin.** 1989. Somatic mutation and transcriptional deregulation of myc in endemic Burkitt's lymphoma disease: heptamer−nonamer recognition mistakes? *Mol. Cell Biol.* **9**: 74−82.

727. **Mothersill, C., J. Harney, and C. B. Seymour.** 1994. Induction of stable p53 oncoprotein and of c-myc overexpression in cultured normal human uroepithelium by radiation and *N*-nitrosodiethanolamine. *Radiat. Res.* **138**: 93−98.

728. **Mothersill, C., C. B. Seymour, J. Harney, and T. P. Hennessy.** 1994. High levels of stable p53 protein and the expression of c-myc in cultured human epithelial tissue after cobalt-60 irradiation. *Radiat. Res.* **137**: 317−322.

729. **Motoyama, J. and K. Eto.** 1994. Antisense c-myc oligonucleotide promotes chondrogenesis and enhances RA responsiveness of mouse limb mesenchymal cells *in vitro*. *FEBS Lett.* **338**: 323−325.

730. **Mougneau, E., L. Lemieux, M. Rassoulzadegan, and F. Cuzin.** 1984. Biological activities of v-myc and rearranged c-myc oncogenes in rat fibroblast cells in culture. *Proc. Natl Acad. Sci. USA* **81**: 5758−5762.

731. **Mouthon, M. A., O. Bernard, M. T. Mitjavila, P. H. Romeo, W. Vainchenker, and D. Mathieu Mahul.** 1993. Expression of tal-1 and GATA-binding proteins during human hematopoiesis. *Blood* **81**: 647−655.

732. **Mugrauer, G., F. W. Alt, and P. Ekblom.** 1988. N-myc proto-oncogene expression during organogenesis in the developing mouse as revealed by in situ hybridization. *J. Cell Biol.* **107**: 1325−1335.

733. **Mugrauer, G. and P. Ekblom.** 1991. Contrasting expression patterns of three members of the myc family of protooncogenes in the developing and adult mouse kidney. *J. Cell Biol.* **112**: 13−25.

734. **Muir, W. M. and A. E. Bell.** 1987. Multiple vital functions of the daughterless (da) gene in *Drosophila melanogaster* and factors influencing its expression. *Genetica* **72**: 43−54.

735. **Mukherjee, B., S. D. Morgenbesser, and R. A. DePinho.** 1992. Myc family oncoproteins function through a common pathway to transform normal cells in culture: cross-interference by Max and trans-acting dominant mutants. *Genes Dev.* **6**: 1480−1492.

736. **Mullins, J. I., D. S. Brody, R. C. J. Binari, and S. M. Cotter.** 1984. Viral transduction of c-myc gene in naturally occurring feline leukaemias. *Nature* **308**: 856–858.

737. **Munger, K., J. A. Pietenpol, M. R. Pittelkow, J. T. Holt, and H. L. Moses.** 1992. Transforming growth factor beta 1 regulation of c-myc expression, pRB phosphorylation, and cell cycle progression in keratinocytes. *Cell Growth Differ.* **3**: 291–298.

738. **Murphy, C. S., J. A. Pietenpol, K. Munger, P. M. Howley, and H. L. Moses.** 1991. c-myc and pRB: role in TGF-beta 1 inhibition of keratinocyte proliferation. *Cold Spring Harb. Symp. Quant. Biol.* **56**: 129–135.

739. **Murray, S. S., C. A. Glackin, K. A. Winters, D. Gazit, A. J. Kahn, and E. J. Murray.** 1992. Expression of helix–loop–helix regulatory genes during differentiation of mouse osteoblastic cells. *J. Bone. Miner. Res.* **7**: 1131–1138.

740. **Murray, S. S., E. J. Murray, C. A. Glackin, and M. R. Urist.** 1993. Bone morphogenetic protein inhibits differentiation and affects expression of helix–loop–helix regulatory molecules in myoblastic cells. *J. Cell Biochem.* **53**: 51–60.

741*. **Murre, C., P. S. McCaw, and D. Baltimore.** 1989. A new DNA binding and dimerization motif in immunoglobulin enhancer binding, daughterless, MyoD, and myc proteins. *Cell* **56**: 777–783.

742. **Murre, C., A. Voronova, and D. Baltimore.** 1991. B-cell- and myocyte-specific E2-box-binding factors contain E12/E47-like subunits. *Mol. Cell Biol.* **11**: 1156–1160.

743. **Muscat, G. E., L. Mynett Johnson, D. Dowhan, M. Downes, and R. Griggs.** 1994. Activation of myoD gene transcription by 3,5,3'-triiodo-L-thyronine: a direct role for the thyroid hormone and retinoid X receptors. *Nucleic Acids Res.* **22**: 583–591.

744. **Nabeshima, Y., K. Hanaoka, M. Hayasaka, E. Esumi, S. Li, and I. Nonaka.** 1993. Myogenin gene disruption results in perinatal lethality because of severe muscle defect. *Nature* **364**: 532–535.

745. **Nagata, Y. and K. Todokoro.** 1994. Activation of helix–loop–helix proteins Id1, Id2 and Id3 during neural differentiation. *Biochem. Biophys. Res. Commun.* **199**: 1355–1362.

746. **Nakagoshi, H., C. Kanei Ishii, T. Sawazaki, G. Mizuguchi, and S. Ishii.** 1992. Transcriptional activation of the c-myc gene by the c-myb and B-myb gene products. *Oncogene* **7**: 1233–1240.

747. **Nakajima, H., M. Ikeda, N. Tsuchida, S. Nishimura, and Y. Taya.** 1989. Inactivation of the N-myc gene product by single amino acid substitution of leucine residues located in the leucine-zipper region. *Oncogene* **4**: 999–1002.

748. **Nambu, J. R., J. O. Lewis, K. A. J. Wharton, and S. T. Crews.** 1991. The *Drosophila* single-minded gene encodes a helix–loop–helix protein that acts as a master regulator of CNS midline development. *Cell* **67**: 1157–1167.

749. **Nau, M. M., B. J. Brooks, J. Battey, E. Sausville, A. F. Gazdar, I. R. Kirsch, O. W. McBride, V. Bertness, G. F. Hollis, and J. D. Minna.** 1985. L-myc, a new myc-related gene amplified and expressed in human small cell lung cancer. *Nature* **318**: 69–73.

750. **Nau, M. M., B. J. J. Brooks, D. N. Carney, A. F. Gazdar, J. F. Battey, E. A. Sausville, and J. D. Minna.** 1986. Human small-cell lung cancers show amplification and expression of the N-myc gene. *Proc. Natl Acad. Sci. USA* **83**: 1092–1096.

751. **Nau, M. M., D. N. Carney, J. Battey, B. Johnson, C. Little, A. Gazdar, and J. D. Minna.** 1984. Amplification, expression and rearrangement of c-myc and N-myc oncogenes in human lung cancer. *Curr. Top. Microbiol. Immunol.* **113**: 172–177.

752. **Negishi, Y., Y. Nishita, Y. Saegusa, I. Kakizaki, I. Galli, F. Kihara, K. Tamai, N. Miyajima, S. M. Iguchi Ariga, and H. Ariga.** 1994. Identification and cDNA cloning of single-stranded DNA binding proteins that interact with the region upstream of the human c-myc gene. *Oncogene* **9**: 1133–1143.

753. **Nelson, C., L. P. Shen, A. Meister, E. Fodor, and W. J. Rutter.** 1990. Pan: a transcriptional regulator that binds chymotrypsin, insulin, and AP-4 enhancer motifs. *Genes Dev.* **4**: 1035–1043.

754. **Nepveu, A., P. D. Fahrlander, J. Q. Yang, and K. B. Marcu.** 1985. Amplification and altered expression of the c-myc oncogene in A-MuLV-transformed fibroblasts. *Nature* **317**: 440–443.

755. **Nepveu, A., R. A. Levine, J. Campisi, M. E. Greenberg, E. B. Ziff, and K. B. Marcu.** 1987. Alternative modes of c-myc regulation in growth factor-stimulated and differentiating cells. *Oncogene* **1**: 243–250.

756. **Nepveu, A. and K. B. Marcu.** 1986. Intragenic pausing and anti-sense transcription within the murine c-myc locus. *EMBO J.* **5**: 2859–2865.

757. **Nepveu, A., K. B. Marcu, A. I. Skoultchi, and H. M. Lachman.** 1987. Contributions of transcriptional and post-transcriptional mechanisms to the regulation of c-myc expression in mouse erythroleukemia cells. *Genes Dev.* **1**: 938–945.

758. **Neuman, T., A. Keen, E. Knapik, D. Shain, M. Ross, H. O. Nornes, and M. X. Zuber.** 1993. ME1 and GE1:basic helix–loop–helix transcription factors expressed at high levels in the developing nervous system and in morphogenetically active regions. *Eur. J. Neurosci.* **5**: 311–318.

759. **Neuman, T., A. Keen, M. X. Zuber, G. I. Kristjansson, P. Gruss, and H. O. Nornes.** 1993. Neuronal expression of regulatory helix—loop—helix factor Id2 gene in mouse. *Dev. Biol.* **160**: 186—195.

760. **Neuveut, C., R. Vigne, J. E. Clements, and J. Sire.** 1993. The visna transcriptional activator Tat: effects on the viral LTR and on cellular genes. *Virology* **197**: 236—244.

761. **Ninomiya Tsuji, J., F. M. Torti, and G. M. Ringold.** 1993. Tumor necrosis factor-induced c-myc expression in the absence of mitogenesis is associated with inhibition of adipocyte differentiation. *Proc. Natl Acad. Sci. USA* **90**: 9611—9615.

762. **Nishi, Y., K. Akiyama, and B. R. Korf.** 1992. Characterization of N-myc amplification in a human neuroblastoma cell line by clones isolated following the phenol emulsion reassociation technique and by hexagonal field gel electrophoresis. *Mamm. Genome* **2**: 11—20.

763. **Nishikura, K.** 1987. Expression of c-myc proto-oncogene during the early development of *Xenopus* laevis. *Oncogene Res.* **1**: 179—191.

764. **Nishikura, K., A. ar Rushdi, J. Erikson, R. Watt, G. Rovera, and C. M. Croce.** 1983. Differential expression of the normal and of the translocated human c-myc oncogenes in B cells. *Proc. Natl Acad. Sci. USA* **80**: 4822—4826.

765. **Nishikura, K., S. Goldflam, and G. A. Vuocolo.** 1985. Accurate and efficient transcription of human c-myc genes injected into *Xenopus* laevis oocytes. *Mol. Cell Biol.* **5**: 1434—1441.

766. **Nishikura, K., U. Kim, and J. M. Murray.** 1990. Differentiation of F9 cells is independent of c-myc expression. *Oncogene* **5**: 981—988.

767. **Ogata, T. and M. Noda.** 1991. Expression of Id, a negative regulator of helix—loop—helix DNA binding proteins, is down-regulated at confluence and enhanced by dexamethasone in a mouse osteoblastic cell line, MC3T3E1. *Biochem. Biophys. Res. Commun.* **180**: 1194—1199.

768. **Ogata, T., J. M. Wozney, R. Benezra, and M. Noda.** 1993. Bone morphogenetic protein 2 transiently enhances expression of a gene, Id (inhibitor of differentiation), encoding a helix—loop—helix molecule in osteoblast-like cells. *Proc. Natl Acad. Sci. USA* **90**: 9219—9222.

769. **Ogawa, N. and Y. Oshima.** 1990. Functional domains of a positive regulatory protein, PHO4, for transcriptional control of the phosphatase regulon in *Saccharomyces cerevisiae*. *Mol. Cell Biol.* **10**: 2224—2236.

770. **Ohlsson, R. I. and S. Pfeifer Ohlsson.** 1986. myc expression *in vivo* during human embryogenesis. *Curr. Top. Microbiol. Immunol.* **132**: 272—279.

771. **Ohmori, Y., J. Tanabe, S. Takada, W. M. Lee, and M. Obinata.** 1993. Functional domains of c-Myc involved in the commitment and differentiation of murine erythroleukemia cells. *Oncogene* **8**: 379—386.

772. **Olson, E.** 1992. Activation of muscle-specific transcription by myogenic helix—loop—helix proteins. *Symp. Soc. Exp. Biol.* **46**: 331—341.

773. **Olson, E. N., T. J. Brennan, T. Chakraborty, T. C. Cheng, P. Cserjesi, D. Edmondson, G. James, and L. Li.** 1991. Molecular control of myogenesis: antagonism between growth and differentiation. *Mol. Cell Biochem.* **104**: 7—13.

774. **Onclercq, R., C. Babinet, and C. Cremisi.** 1989. Exogenous c-myc gene overexpression interferes with early events in F9 cell differentiation. *Oncogene Res.* **4**: 293—302.

775. **Onclercq, R., A. Lavenu, and C. Cremisi.** 1989. Pleiotropic derepression of developmentally regulated cellular and viral genes by c-myc protooncogene products in undifferentiated embryonal carcinoma cells. *Nucleic Acids Res.* **17**: 735—753.

776. **Osanto, S., R. Jansen, and M. Vloemans.** 1992. Downmodulation of c-myc expression by interferon gamma and tumour necrosis factor alpha precedes growth arrest in human melanoma cells. *Eur. J. Cancer* **28A**: 1622—1627.

777. **Ott, M. O., E. Bober, G. Lyons, H. Arnold, and M. Buckingham.** 1991. Early expression of the myogenic regulatory gene, myf-5, in precursor cells of skeletal muscle in the mouse embryo. *Development* **111**: 1097—1107.

778. **Packham, G. and J. L. Cleveland.** 1994. Ornithine decarboxylase is a mediator of c-Myc-induced apoptosis. *Mol. Cell Biol.* **14**: 5741—5747.

779. **Pallavicini, M. G., C. Rosette, M. Reitsma, P. S. DeTeresa, and J. W. Gray.** 1990. Relationship of c-myc gene copy number and gene expression: cellular effects of elevated c-myc protein. *J. Cell Physiol.* **143**: 372—380.

780. **Panno, J. P. and B. A. McKeown.** 1993. Expression of the myc proto-oncogene in the rainbow trout *Oncorhynchus mykiss*. *Comp. Biochem. Physiol. B.* **104**: 649—652.

781. **Parkhurst, S. M., D. Bopp, and D. Ish Horowicz.** 1990. X:A ratio, the primary sex-determining signal in *Drosophila*, is transduced by helix—loop—helix proteins [published erratum appears in *Cell* 1991 Mar. 8; 64(5): following 1046]. *Cell* **63**: 1179—1191.

782. **Parkhurst, S. M., H. D. Lipshitz, and D. Ish Horowicz.** 1993. achaete—scute feminizing activities and *Drosophila* sex determination. *Development* **117**: 737—749.

783. **Patapoutian, A., J. H. Miner, G. E. Lyons, and B. Wold.** 1993. Isolated sequences from the linked Myf-5 and MRF4 genes drive distinct patterns of muscle-specific expression in transgenic mice. *Development* **118**: 61−69.

784. **Paterson, B. M., M. Shirakata, S. Nakamura, C. Dechesne, U. Walldorf, J. Eldridge, A. Dubendorfer, M. Frasch, and W. J. Gehring.** 1992. Isolation and functional comparison of Dmyd, the *Drosophila* homologue of the vertebrate myogenic determination genes, with CMD1. *Symp. Soc. Exp. Biol.* **46**: 89−109.

785. **Paterson, B. M., U. Walldorf, J. Eldridge, A. Dubendorfer, M. Frasch, and W. J. Gehring.** 1991. The *Drosophila* homologue of vertebrate myogenic-determination genes encodes a transiently expressed nuclear protein marking primary myogenic cells. *Proc. Natl Acad. Sci. USA* **88**: 3782−3786.

786. **Pearson White, S. H.** 1991. Human MyoD: cDNA and deduced amino acid sequence. *Nucleic Acids Res.* **19**: 1148.

787. **Pedrazzoli, P., M. A. Bains, R. Watson, J. Fisher, T. G. Hoy, and A. Jacobs.** 1989. c-myc and c-myb oncoproteins during induced maturation of myeloid and erythroid human leukemic cell lines. *Cancer Res.* **49**: 6911−6916.

788. **Pei, R. and K. Calame.** 1988. Differential stability of c-myc mRNAS in a cell-free system. *Mol. Cell Biol.* **8**: 2860−2868.

789. **Pellegrini, S. and C. Basilico.** 1986. Rat fibroblasts expressing high levels of human c-myc transcripts are anchorage-independent and tumorigenic. *J. Cell Physiol.* **126**: 107−114.

790. **Peltenburg, L. T., R. Dee, and P. I. Schrier.** 1993. Downregulation of HLA class I expression by c-myc in human melanoma is independent of enhancer A. *Nucleic Acids Res.* **21**: 1179−1185.

791*. **Pena, A.** 1993. A switch from Myc:Max to Mad:Max heterocomplexes accompanies monocyte/macrophage differentiation. *Genes Dev.* **7**: 2110−2119.

792. **Pena, A., C. D. Reddy, S. Wu, N. J. Hickok, E. P. Reddy, G. Yumet, D. R. Soprano, and K. J. Soprano.** 1993. Regulation of human ornithine decarboxylase expression by the c-Myc.Max protein complex. *J. Biol. Chem.* **268**: 27277−27285.

793. **Penn, L. J., M. W. Brooks, E. M. Laufer, and H. Land.** 1990. Negative autoregulation of c-myc transcription. *EMBO J.* **9**: 1113−1121.

794. **Penn, L. J., M. W. Brooks, E. M. Laufer, T. D. Littlewood, J. P. Morgenstern, G. I. Evan, W. M. Lee, and H. Land.** 1990. Domains of human c-myc protein required for autosuppression and cooperation with ras oncogenes are overlapping. *Mol. Cell Biol.* **10**: 4961−4966.

795. **Perrot, G. H. and K. C. Cone.** 1989. Nucleotide sequence of the maize R-S gene. *Nucleic Acids Res.* **17**: 8003.

796. **Persson, H., H. E. Gray, and F. Godeau.** 1985. Growth-dependent synthesis of c-myc-encoded proteins: early stimulation by serum factors in synchronized mouse 3T3 cells. *Mol. Cell Biol.* **5**: 2903−2912.

797. **Persson, H., H. E. Gray, F. Godeau, S. Braunhut, and A. R. Bellve.** 1986. Multiple growth-associated nuclear proteins immunoprecipitated by antisera raised against human c-myc peptide antigens. *Mol. Cell Biol.* **6**: 942−949.

798. **Persson, H., L. Hennighausen, R. Taub, W. DeGrado, and P. Leder.** 1984. Antibodies to human c-myc oncogene product: evidence of an evolutionarily conserved protein induced during cell proliferation. *Science* **225**: 687−693.

799. **Persson, H. and P. Leder.** 1984. Nuclear localization and DNA binding properties of a protein expressed by human c-myc oncogene. *Science* **225**: 718−721.

800. **Pesce, S. and R. Benezra.** 1993. The loop region of the helix−loop−helix protein Id1 is critical for its dominant negative activity. *Mol. Cell Biol.* **13**: 7874−7880.

801. **Peterson, C. A., H. Gordon, Z. W. Hall, B. M. Paterson, and H. M. Blau.** 1990. Negative control of the helix−loop−helix family of myogenic regulators in the NFB mutant. *Cell* **62**: 493−502.

802. **Pfeifer Ohlsson, S., A. S. Goustin, J. Rydnert, T. Wahlstrom, L. Bjersing, D. Stehelin, and R. Ohlsson.** 1984. Spatial and temporal pattern of cellular myc oncogene expression in developing human placenta:implications for embryonic cell proliferation. *Cell* **38**: 585−596.

803. **Pfeifer Ohlsson, S., J. Rydnert, A. S. Goustin, E. Larsson, C. Betsholtz, and R. Ohlsson.** 1985. Cell-type-specific pattern of myc protooncogene expression in developing human embryos. *Proc. Natl Acad. Sci. USA* **82**: 5050−5054.

804. **Pfeifer, S., J. Zabielski, R. Ohlsson, L. Frykberg, J. Knowles, R. Pettersson, N. Oker Blom, L. Philipson, A. Vaheri, and B. Vennstrom.** 1983. Avian acute leukemia virus OK 10: analysis of its myc oncogene by molecular cloning. *J. Virol.* **46**: 347−354.

805. **Philipp, A., A. Schneider, I. Vasrik, K. Finke, Y. Xiong, D. Beach, K. Alitalo, and M. Eilers.** 1994. Repression of cyclin D1:a novel function of MYC. *Mol. Cell Biol.* **14**: 4032−4043.

806. **Piechaczyk, M., A. Bonnieu, D. Eick, E. Remmers, J. Q. Yang, K. Marcu, P. Jeanteur, and J. M. Blanchard.** 1986. Altered c-myc RNA metabolism in Burkitt's lymphomas and mouse plasmacytomas. *Curr. Top. Microbiol. Immunol.* **132**: 331−338.

807. **Pietenpol, J. A., J. T. Holt, R. W. Stein, and H. L. Moses.** 1990. Transforming growth factor beta 1 suppression of c-myc gene transcription: role in inhibition of keratinocyte proliferation. *Proc. Natl Acad. Sci. USA* **87**: 3758–3762.

808. **Pietenpol, J. A., K. Munger, P. M. Howley, R. W. Stein, and H. L. Moses.** 1991. Factor-binding element in the human c-myc promoter involved in transcriptional regulation by transforming growth factor beta 1 and by the retinoblastoma gene product. *Proc. Natl Acad. Sci. USA* **88**: 10227–10231.

809. **Pietenpol, J. A., R. W. Stein, E. Moran, P. Yaciuk, R. Schlegel, R. M. Lyons, M. R. Pittelkow, K. Munger, P. M. Howley, and H. L. Moses.** 1990. TGF-beta 1 inhibition of c-myc transcription and growth in keratinocytes is abrogated by viral transforming proteins with pRB binding domains. *Cell* **61**: 777–785.

810. **Pognonec, P. and R. G. Roeder.** 1991. Recombinant 43-kDa USF binds to DNA and activates transcription in a manner indistinguishable from that of natural 43/44-kDa USF. *Mol. Cell Biol.* **11**: 5125–5136.

811. **Pohjanpelto, P. and E. Holtta.** 1990. Deprivation of a single amino acid induces protein synthesis-dependent increases in c-jun, c-myc, and ornithine decarboxylase mRNAs in Chinese hamster ovary cells. *Mol. Cell Biol.* **10**: 5814–5821.

812. **Polack, A., R. Feederle, G. Klobeck, and K. Hortnagel.** 1993. Regulatory elements in the immunoglobulin kappa locus induce c-myc activation and the promoter shift in Burkitt's lymphoma cells. *EMBO J.* **12**: 3913–3920.

813. **Pollack, P. S., S. R. Houser, R. Budjak, and B. Goldman.** 1994. c-myc gene expression is localized to the myocyte following hemodynamic overload *in vivo*. *J. Cell Biochem.* **54**: 78–84.

814. **Pongubala, J. M. and M. L. Atchison.** 1991. Functional characterization of the developmentally controlled immunoglobulin kappa 3' enhancer: regulation by Id, a repressor of helix–loop–helix transcription factors. *Mol. Cell Biol.* **11**: 1040–1047.

815. **Postel, E. H., S. E. Mango, and S. J. Flint.** 1989. A nuclease-hypersensitive element of the human c-myc promoter interacts with a transcription initiation factor. *Mol. Cell Biol.* **9**: 5123–5133.

816. **Prendergast, G. C. and M. D. Cole.** 1989. Posttranscriptional regulation of cellular gene expression by the c-myc oncogene. *Mol. Cell Biol.* **9**: 124–134.

817. **Prendergast, G. C., L. E. Diamond, D. Dahl, and M. D. Cole.** 1990. The c-myc-regulated gene mr1 encodes plasminogen activator inhibitor 1. *Mol. Cell Biol.* **10**: 1265–1269.

818. **Prendergast, G. C., R. Hopewell, B. J. Gorham, and E. B. Ziff.** 1992. Biphasic effect of Max on Myc cotransformation activity and dependence on amino- and carboxy-terminal Max functions. *Genes Dev.* **6**: 2429–2439.

819. **Principaud, E. and G. Spohr.** 1991. *Xenopus laevis* c-myc I and II genes: molecular structure and developmental expression. *Nucleic Acids Res.* **19**: 3081–3088.

820. **Privitera, E., M. P. Kamps, Y. Hayashi, T. Inaba, L. H. Shapiro, S. C. Raimondi, F. Behm, L. Hendershot, A. J. Carroll, D. Baltimore** *et al*. 1992. Different molecular consequences of the 1;19 chromosomal translocation in childhood B-cell precursor acute lymphoblastic leukemia. *Blood* **79**: 1781–1788.

821. **Prochownik, E. V. and J. Kukowska.** 1986. Deregulated expression of c-myc by murine erythroleukaemia cells prevents differentiation. *Nature* **322**: 848–850.

822. **Prochownik, E. V., J. Kukowska, and C. Rodgers.** 1988. c-myc antisense transcripts accelerate differentiation and inhibit G1 progression in murine erythroleukemia cells. *Mol. Cell Biol.* **8**: 3683–3695.

823. **Prody, C. A. and J. P. Merlie.** 1992. The 5′-flanking region of the mouse muscle nicotinic acetylcholine receptor beta subunit gene promotes expression in cultured muscle cells and is activated by MRF4, myogenin and myoD. *Nucleic Acids Res.* **20**: 2367–2372.

824. **Quertermous, E. A., H. Hidai, M. A. Blanar, and T. Quertermous.** 1994. Cloning and characterization of a basic helix–loop–helix protein expressed in early mesoderm and the developing somites. *Proc. Natl Acad. Sci. USA* **91**: 7066–7070.

825. **Quik, M., R. Odeh, J. Philie, and M. Szyf.** 1993. Functional nicotinic receptor expression in mesodermal cells transfected with MyoD cDNA. *Neuroscience* **57**: 787–795.

826*. **Quong, M. W., M. E. Massari, R. Zwart, and C. Murre.** 1993. A new transcriptional-activation motif restricted to a class of helix–loop–helix proteins is functionally conserved in both yeast and mammalian cells. *Mol. Cell Biol.* **13**: 792–800.

827. **Rabbits, P. H., A. Forster, M. A. Stinson, and T. H. Rabbitts.** 1985. Truncation of exon 1 from the c-myc gene results in prolonged c-myc mRNa stability. *EMBO J.* **4**: 3727–3733.

828. **Rabbitts, P. H., J. V. Watson, A. Lamond, A. Forster, M. A. Stinson, G. Evan, W. Fischer, E. Atherton, R. Sheppard, and T. H. Rabbitts.** 1985. Metabolism of c-myc gene products: c-myc mRNA and protein expression in the cell cycle. *EMBO J.* **4**: 2009–2015.

829. **Rabbitts, T. H., A. Forster, P. Hamlyn, and R. Baer.** 1984. Effect of somatic mutation within translocated c-myc genes in Burkitt's lymphoma. *Nature* **309**: 592–597.

830. **Rabbitts, T. H., P. H. Hamlyn, and R. Baer.** 1983. Altered nucleotide sequences of a translocated c-myc gene in Burkitt lymphoma. *Nature* **306**: 760–765.

831. **Radicella, J. P., D. Brown, L. A. Tolar, and V. L. Chandler.** 1992. Allelic diversity of the maize B regulatory gene: different leader and promoter sequences of two B alleles determine distinct tissue specificities of anthocyanin production. *Genes Dev.* **6**: 2152–2164.

832. **Radicella, J. P., D. Turks, and V. L. Chandler.** 1991. Cloning and nucleotide sequence of a cDNA encoding B-Peru, a regulatory protein of the anthocyanin pathway in maize. *Plant Mol. Biol.* **17**: 127–130.

833. **Ralston, R.** 1991. Complementation of transforming domains in E1a/myc chimaeras. *Nature* **353**: 866–868.

834. **Ralston, R. and J. M. Bishop.** 1983. The protein products of the myc and myb oncogenes and adenovirus E1a are structurally related. *Nature* **306**: 803–806.

835. **Ramain, P., P. Heitzler, M. Haenlin, and P. Simpson.** 1993. pannier, a negative regulator of achaete and scute in *Drosophila*, encodes a zinc finger protein with homology to the vertebrate transcription factor GATA-1. *Development* **119**: 1277–1291.

836. **Ramos-Morales, F., B. Druker, and S. Fischer.** 1994. Vav binds to sereral SH2/SH3 containing proteins in activated lymphocytes. *Oncogene* **9**: 1917–1923.

837. **Ramsay, G., G. I. Evan, and J. M. Bishop.** 1984. The protein encoded by the human proto-oncogene c-myc. *Proc. Natl Acad. Sci. USA* **81**: 7742–7746.

838. **Ramsay, G. M., P. J. Enrietto, T. Graf, and M. J. Hayman.** 1982. Recovery of myc-specific sequences by a partially transformation-defective mutant of avian myelocytomatosis virus, MC29, correlates with the restoration of transforming activity. *Proc. Natl Acad. Sci. USA* **79**: 6885–6889.

839. **Ramsay, G. M. and M. J. Hayman.** 1982. Isolation and biochemical characterization of partially transformation-defective mutants of avian myelocytomatosis virus strain MC29:localization of the mutation to the myc domain of the 110,000-dalton gag–myc polyprotein. *J. Virol.* **41**: 745–753.

840. **Ramsay, G. M., G. Moscovici, C. Moscovici, and J. M. Bishop.** 1990. Neoplastic transformation and tumorigenesis by the human protooncogene MYC. *Proc. Natl Acad. Sci. USA* **87**: 2102–2106.

841. **Rao, G. N. and R. L. Church.** 1989. Regulation of expression of c-myc protoocogene in a clonal line of mouse lens epithelial cells by serum growth factors. *Exp. Cell Res.* **183**: 140–148.

842*. **Rao, S. S., C. Chu, and D. S. Kohtz.** 1994. Ectopic expression of cyclin D1 prevents activation of gene transcription by myogenic basic helix–loop–helix regulators. *Mol. Cell Biol.* **14**: 5259–5267.

843. **Rao, V. N., T. Ohno, D. D. Prasad, G. Bhattacharya, and E. S. Reddy.** 1993. Analysis of the DNA-binding and transcriptional activation functions of human Fli-1 protein. *Oncogene* **8**: 2167–2173.

844. **Ray, R. and D. M. Miller.** 1991. Cloning and characterization of a human c-myc promoter-binding protein. *Mol. Cell Biol.* **11**: 2154–2161.

845. **Read, M. L., A. R. Clark, and K. Docherty.** 1993. The helix–loop–helix transcription factor USF (upstream stimulating factor) binds to a regulatory sequence of the human insulin gene enhancer. *Biochem. J.* **295**: 233–237.

846*. **Reddy, C. D., P. Dasgupta, P. Saikumar, H. Dudek, F. J. Rauscher, and E. P. Reddy.** 1992. Mutational analysis of Max: role of basic, helix–loop–helix/leucine zipper domains in DNA binding, dimerization and regulation of Myc-mediated transcriptional activation. *Oncogene* **7**: 2085–2092.

847. **Reddy, E. P., R. K. Reynolds, D. K. Watson, R. A. Schultz, J. Lautenberger, and T. S. Papas.** 1983. Nucleotide sequence analysis of the proviral genome of avian myelocytomatosis virus (MC29). *Proc. Natl Acad. Sci. USA* **80**: 2500–2504.

848. **Reed, J. C., M. Cuddy, S. Haldar, C. Croce, P. Nowell, D. Makover, and K. Bradley.** 1990. BCL2-mediated tumorigenicity of a human T-lymphoid cell line: synergy with MYC and inhibition by BCL2 antisense. *Proc. Natl Acad. Sci. USA* **87**: 3660–3664.

849. **Reed, J. C., P. C. Nowell, and R. G. Hoover.** 1985. Regulation of c-myc mRNA levels in normal human lymphocytes by modulators of cell proliferation. *Proc. Natl Acad. Sci. USA* **82**: 4221–4224.

850. **Reick, M., R. W. Robertson, D. S. Pasco, and J. B. Fagan.** 1994. Down-regulation of nuclear aryl hydrocarbon receptor DNA-binding and transactivation functions: requirement for a labile or inducible factor. *Mol. Cell Biol.* **14**: 5653–5660.

851. **Reisman, D., N. B. Elkind, B. Roy, J. Beamon, and V. Rotter.** 1993. c-Myc trans-activates the p53 promoter through a required downstream CACGTG motif. *Cell Growth Differ.* **4**: 57–65.

852. **Reisman, D. and V. Rotter.** 1993. The helix–loop–helix containing transcription factor USF binds to and transactivates the promoter of the p53 tumor suppressor gene. *Nucleic Acids Res.* **21**: 345–350.

853. **Reisz-Porszasz, S., M. R. Probst, B. N. Fukunaga, and O. Hankinson.** 1994. Identification of functional domains of the aryl hydrocarbon receptor nuclear translocator protein (ARNT). *Mol. Cell Biol.* **14**: 6075–6086.

854. **Reitsma, P. H., P. G. Rothberg, S. M. Astrin, J. Trial, Z. Bar Shavit, A. Hall, S. L. Teitelbaum, and A. J. Kahn.** 1983. Regulation of myc gene expression in HL-60 leukacmia cells by a vitamin D metabolite. *Nature* **306**: 492–494.

855. **Remmers, E. F., J. Q. Yang, and K. B. Marcu.** 1986. A negative transcriptional control element located upstream of the murine c-myc gene. *EMBO J.* **5**: 899−904.

856. **Resar, L. M., C. Dolde, J. F. Barrett, and C. V. Dang.** 1993. B-myc inhibits neoplastic transformation and transcriptional activation by c-myc. *Mol. Cell Biol.* **13**: 1130−1136.

857. **Resnitzky, D. and A. Kimchi.** 1991. Deregulated c-myc expression abrogates the interferon- and interleukin 6-mediated G0/G1 cell cycle arrest but not other inhibitory responses in M1 myeloblastic cells. *Cell Growth Differ.* **2**: 33−41.

858. **Resnitzky, D., A. Yarden, D. Zipori, and A. Kimchi.** 1986. Autocrine beta-related interferon controls c-myc suppression and growth arrest during hematopoietic cell differentiation. *Cell* **46**: 31−40.

859. **Reuter, R. and M. Leptin.** 1994. Interacting functions of snail, twist and huckebein during the early development of germ layers in *Drosophila*. *Development* **120**: 1137−1150.

860. **Reyes, H., S. Reisz Porszasz, and O. Hankinson.** 1992. Identification of the Ah receptor nuclear translocator protein (Arnt) as a component of the DNA binding form of the Ah receptor. *Science* **256**: 1193−1195.

861. **Rhodes, S. J. and S. F. Konieczny.** 1989. Identification of MRF4:a new member of the muscle regulatory factor gene family. *Genes Dev.* **3**: 2050−2061.

862. **Riccio, A., P. V. Pedone, L. R. Lund, T. Olesen, H. S. Olsen, and P. A. Andreasen.** 1992. Transforming growth factor beta 1-responsive element: closely associated binding sites for USF and CCAAT-binding transcription factor−nuclear factor I in the type 1 plasminogen activator inhibitor gene. *Mol. Cell Biol.* **12**: 1846−1855.

863. **Richman, A. and A. Hayday.** 1989. Serum-inducible expression of transfected human c-myc genes. *Mol. Cell Biol.* **9**: 4962−4969.

864. **Richman, A. and A. Hayday.** 1989. Normal expression of a rearranged and mutated c-myc oncogene after transfection into fibroblasts. *Science* **246**: 494−497.

865. **Richon, V. M., R. G. Ramsay, R. A. Rifkind, and P. A. Marks.** 1989. Modulation of the c-myb, c-myc and p53 mRNA and protein levels during induced murine erythroleukemia cell differentiation. *Oncogene* **4**: 165−173.

866. **Riechmann, V., I. van Cruchten, and F. Sablitzky.** 1994. The expression pattern of Id4, a novel dominant negative helix−loop−helix protein, is distinct from Id1, Id2 and Id3. *Nucleic Acids Res.* **22(5)**: 749−755.

867. **Riggs, K. J., K. T. Merrell, G. Wilson, and K. Calame.** 1991. Common factor 1 is a transcriptional activator which binds in the c-myc promoter, the skeletal alpha-actin promoter, and the immunoglobulin heavy-chain enhancer. *Mol. Cell Biol.* **11**: 1765−1769.

868. **Riggs, K. J., S. Saleque, K. K. Wong, K. T. Merrell, J. S. Lee, Y. Shi, and K. Calame.** 1993. Yin-yang 1 activates the c-myc promoter. *Mol. Cell Biol.* **13**: 7487−7495.

869. **Rivera, R. R., M. H. Stuiver, R. Steenbergen, and C. Murre.** 1993. Ets proteins: new factors that regulate immunoglobulin heavy-chain gene expression. *Mol. Cell Biol.* **13**: 7163−7169.

870. **Roberts, S., T. Purton, and D. L. Bentley.** 1992. A protein-binding site in the c-myc promoter functions as a terminator of RNA polymerase II transcription. *Genes Dev.* **6**: 1562−1574.

871. **Robins, T., K. Bister, C. Garon, T. Papas, and P. Duesberg.** 1982. Structural relationship between a normal chicken DNA locus and the transforming gene of the avian acute leukemia virus MC29. *Virology* **41(2)**: 635−642.

872. **Robinson Benion, C., K. E. Salhany, S. R. Hann, and J. T. Holt.** 1991. Antisense inhibition of c-myc expression reveals common and distinct mechanisms of growth inhibition by TGF beta and TNF alpha. *J. Cell Biochem.* **45**: 188−195.

873. **Roland, J. and D. Morello.** 1993. H-2/myc, E mu/myc, and c-myc transgenic mice: potent sources of early hematopoietic cell lines. *Cell Growth Differ.* **4**: 891−900.

874. **Roman, C., A. G. Matera, C. Cooper, S. Artandi, S. Blain, D. C. Ward, and K. Calame.** 1992. mTFE3, an X-linked transcriptional activator containing basic helix−loop−helix and zipper domains, utilizes the zipper to stabilize both DNA binding and multimerization. *Mol. Cell Biol.* **12**: 817−827.

875. **Rosolen, A., L. Whitesell, N. Ikegaki, R. H. Kennett, and L. M. Neckers.** 1990. Antisense inhibition of single copy N-myc expression results in decreased cell growth without reduction of c-myc protein in a neuroepithelioma cell line. *Cancer Res.* **50**: 6316−6322.

876. **Rothberg, P. G., M. D. Erisman, R. E. Diehl, U. G. Rovigatti, and S. M. Astrin.** 1984. Structure and expression of the oncogene c-myc in fresh tumor material from patients with hematopoietic malignancies. *Mol. Cell Biol.* **4**: 1096−1103.

877. **Roussel, M. F., J. L. Cleveland, S. A. Shurtleff, and C. J. Sherr.** 1991. Myc rescue of a mutant CSF-1 receptor impaired in mitogenic signalling. *Nature* **353**: 361−363.

878. **Roussel, M. F., J. N. Davis, J. L. Cleveland, J. Ghysdael, and S. W. Hiebert.** 1994. Dual control of myc expression through a single DNA binding site targeted by ets family proteins and E2F-1. *Oncogene* **9**: 405−415.

879*. **Roy, A. L., C. Carruthers, T. Gutjahr, and R. G. Roeder.** 1993. Direct role for Myc in transcription initiation mediated by interactions with TFII-I. *Nature* **365**: 359−361.

880. **Rudduck, C., R. E. Lukeis, T. L. McRobert, C. W. Chow, and O. M. Garson.** 1992. Chromosomal localization of amplified N-myc in neuroblastoma cells using a biotinylated probe. *Cancer Genet. Cytogenet.* **58**: 55−59.

881. **Rudnicki, M. A., T. Braun, S. Hinuma, and R. Jaenisch.** 1992. Inactivation of MyoD in mice leads to up-regulation of the myogenic HLH gene Myf-5 and results in apparently normal muscle development. *Cell* **71**: 383−390.

882. **Rudnicki, M. A., P. N. Schnegelsberg, R. H. Stead, T. Braun, H. H. Arnold, and R. Jaenisch.** 1993. MyoD or Myf-5 is required for the formation of skeletal muscle. *Cell* **75**: 1351−1359.

883. **Ruezinsky, D., H. Beckmann, and T. Kadesch.** 1991. Modulation of the IgH enhancer's cell type specificity through a genetic switch. *Genes Dev.* **5**: 29−37.

884. **Ruiz Gomez, M. and A. Ghysen.** 1993. The expression and role of a proneural gene, achaete, in the development of the larval nervous system of *Drosophila*. *EMBO J.* **12**: 1121−1130.

885. **Ruiz Gomez, M. and J. Modolell.** 1987. Deletion analysis of the achaete−scute locus of *Drosophila melanogaster*. *Genes Dev.* **1**: 1238−1246.

886. **Rupp, R. A. and H. Weintraub.** 1991. Ubiquitous MyoD transcription at the midblastula transition precedes induction-dependent MyoD expression in presumptive mesoderm of *X. laevis*. *Cell* **65**: 927−937.

887. **Rupp, R. A. W., L. Snider, and H. Weintraub.** 1994. *Xenopus* embryos regulate the nuclear localization of XMyoD. *Genes Dev.* **8**: 1311−1323.

888. **Rushlow, C. A., A. Hogan, S. M. Pinchin, K. M. Howe, M. Lardelli, and D. Ish Horowicz.** 1989. The *Drosophila* hairy protein acts in both segmentation and bristle patterning and shows homology to N-myc. *EMBO J.* **8**: 3095−3103.

889. **Ryan, J. J., E. Prochownik, C. A. Gottlieb, I. J. Apel, R. Merino, G. Nunez, and M. F. Clarke.** 1994. c-*myc* and *bcl-2* modulate p53 function by altering p53 subcellular trafficking during the cell cycle. *Proc. Natl Acad. Sci. USA* **91**: 5878−5882.

890. **Sacca, R. and B. H. Cochran.** 1990. Identification of a PDGF-responsive element in the murine c-myc gene. *Oncogene* **5**: 1499−1505.

891. **Saito, H., A. C. Hayday, K. Wiman, W. S. Hayward, and S. Tonegawa.** 1983. Activation of the c-myc gene by translocation: a model for translational control. *Proc. Natl Acad. Sci. USA* **80**: 7476−7480.

892. **Saksela, K., J. Bergh, V. P. Lehto, K. Nilsson, and K. Alitalo.** 1985. Amplification of the c-myc oncogene in a subpopulation of human small cell lung cancer. *Cancer Res.* **45**: 1823−1827.

893. **Saksela, K., P. J. Koskinen, and K. Alitalo.** 1991. Binding of a nuclear factor to the upstream region of the c-myc gene. *Oncogene Res.* **6**: 73−76.

894. **Salminen, A., T. Braun, A. Buchberger, S. Jurs, B. Winter, and H. H. Arnold.** 1991. Transcription of the muscle regulatory gene Myf4 is regulated by serum components, peptide growth factors and signaling pathways involving G proteins. *J. Cell Biol.* **115**: 905−917.

895. **Sanchez-Garcia, I. and T. H. Rabbitts.** 1994. Transcriptional activation by Tal1 and FUS-CHOP proteins expressed in acute malignancies as a result of chromosomal abnormalities. *Proc. Natl Acad. Sci. USA* **91**: 7869−7873.

896. **Sarid, J., T. D. Halazonetis, W. Murphy, and P. Leder.** 1987. Evolutionarily conserved regions of the human c-myc protein can be uncoupled from transforming activity. *Proc. Natl Acad. Sci. USA* **84**: 170−173.

897. **Sartorelli, V., N. A. Hong, N. H. Bishopric, and L. Kedes.** 1992. Myocardial activation of the human cardiac alpha-actin promoter by helix−loop−helix proteins. *Proc. Natl Acad. Sci. USA* **89**: 4047−4051.

898. **Sasai, Y., R. Kageyama, Y. Tagawa, R. Shigemoto, and S. Nakanishi.** 1992. Two mammalian helix−loop−helix factors structurally related to *Drosophila* hairy and Enhancer of split. *Genes Dev.* **6**: 2620−2634.

899. **Sawada, S. and D. R. Littman.** 1993. A heterodimer of HEB and an E12-related protein interacts with the CD4 enhancer and regulates its activity in T-cell lines. *Mol. Cell Biol.* **13**: 5620−5628.

900. **Sawadogo, M.** 1988. Multiple forms of the human gene-specific transcription factor USF. II. DNA binding properties and transcriptional activity of the purified HeLa USF. *J. Biol. Chem.* **263**: 11994−12001.

901. **Sawadogo, M. and R. G. Roeder.** 1985. Interaction of a gene-specific transcription factor with the adenovirus major late promoter upstream of the TATA box region. *Cell* **43**: 165−175.

902. **Sawadogo, M., M. W. Van Dyke, P. D. Gregor, and R. G. Roeder.** 1987. Multiple forms of the human gene-specific transcription factor USF. I. Complete purification and identification of USF from HeLa cell nuclei. *J. Biol. Chem.* **263**: 11985−11993.

903. **Sawai, S., K. Kato, Y. Wakamatsu, and H. Kondoh.** 1990. Organization and expression of the chicken N-myc gene. *Mol. Cell Biol.* **10**: 2017−2026.

904. **Sawai, S., A. Shimono, K. Hanaoka, and H. Kondoh.** 1991. Embryonic lethality resulting from disruption of both N-myc alleles in mouse zygotes. *New Biol.* **3**: 861−869.

905. **Sawai, S., A. Shimono, Y. Wakamatsu, C. Palmes, K. Hanaoka, and H. Kondoh.** 1993. Defects of embryonic organogenesis resulting from targeted disruption of the N-myc gene in the mouse. *Development* **117**: 1445−1455.

906. **Sawyers, C. L., W. Callahan, and O. N. Witte.** 1992. Dominant negative MYC blocks transformation by ABL oncogenes. *Cell* **70**: 901−910.

907. **Scales, J. B., E. N. Olson, and M. Perry.** 1991. Differential expression of two distinct MyoD genes in *Xenopus*. *Cell Growth Differ.* **2**: 619−629.

908. **Schafer, B. W., B. T. Blakely, G. J. Darlington, and H. M. Blau.** 1990. Effect of cell history on response to helix−loop−helix family of myogenic regulators. *Nature* **344**: 454−458.

909. **Scheuermann, R. H. and S. R. Bauer.** 1990. Tumorigenesis in transgenic mice expressing the c-myc oncogene with various lymphoid enhancer elements. *Curr. Top. Microbiol. Immunol.* **166**: 221−231.

910. **Schlissel, M., A. Voronova, and D. Baltimore.** 1991. Helix−loop−helix transcription factor E47 activates germ-line immunoglobulin heavy-chain gene transcription and rearrangement in a pre-T-cell line. *Genes Dev.* **5**: 1367−1376.

911. **Schmid, P., W. A. Schulz, and H. Hameister.** 1989. Dynamic expression pattern of the myc protooncogene in midgestation mouse embryos. *Science* **243**: 226−229.

912. **Schofield, P. N., W. Engstrom, A. J. Lee, C. Biddle, and C. F. Graham.** 1987. Expression of c-myc during differentiation of the human teratocarcinoma cell line Tera-2. *J. Cell Sci.* **88**: 57−64.

913. **Schreiber Agus, N., J. Horner, R. Torres, F. C. Chiu, and R. A. DePinho.** 1993. Zebra fish myc family and max genes: differential expression and oncogenic activity throughout vertebrate evolution. *Mol. Cell Biol.* **13**: 2765−2775.

914. **Schreiber Agus, N., R. Torres, J. Horner, A. Lau, M. Jamrich, and R. A. DePinho.** 1993. Comparative analysis of the expression and oncogenic activities of *Xenopus* c-, N-, and L-myc homologs. *Mol. Cell Biol.* **13**: 2456−2468.

915. **Schrier, P. I. and L. T. Peltenburg.** 1993. Relationship between myc oncogene activation and MHC class I expression. *Adv. Cancer Res.* **60**: 181−246.

916. **Schubach, W. and M. Groudine.** 1984. Alteration of c-myc chromatin structure by avian leukosis virus integration. *Nature* **307**: 702−708.

917. **Schulz, W. A. and G. Gais.** 1989. Constitutive c-myc expression enhances proliferation of differentiating F9 teratocarcinoma cells. *Biochim. Biophys. Acta* **1013**: 125−132.

918. **Schwab, M.** 1993. Amplification of N-myc as a prognostic marker for patients with neuroblastoma. *Semin. Cancer Biol.* **4**: 13−18.

919. **Schwab, M., K. Alitalo, K. H. Klempnauer, H. E. Varmus, J. M. Bishop, F. Gilbert, G. Brodeur, M. Goldstein, and J. Trent.** 1983. Amplified DNA with limited homology to myc cellular oncogene is shared by human neuroblastoma cell lines and a neuroblastoma tumour. *Nature* **305**: 245−248.

920. **Schwab, M., J. Ellison, M. Busch, W. Rosenau, H. E. Varmus, and J. M. Bishop.** 1984. Enhanced expression of the human gene N-myc consequent to amplification of DNA may contribute to malignant progression of neuroblastoma. *Proc. Natl Acad. Sci. USA* **81**: 4940−4944.

921. **Schwab, M., K. H. Klempnauer, K. Alitalo, H. Varmus, and M. Bishop.** 1986. Rearrangement at the 5′ end of amplified c-myc in human COLO 320 cells is associated with abnormal transcription. *Mol. Cell Biol.* **6**: 2752−2755.

922. **Schwab, M., G. Ramsay, K. Alitalo, H. E. Varmus, J. M. Bishop, T. Martinsson, G. Levan, and A. Levan.** 1985. Amplification and enhanced expression of the c-myc oncogene in mouse SEWA tumour cells. *Nature* **315**: 345−347.

923. **Schwab, M., H. E. Varmus, and J. M. Bishop.** 1985. Human N-myc gene contributes to neoplastic transformation of mammalian cells in culture. *Nature* **316**: 160−162.

924. **Schwab, M., H. E. Varmus, J. M. Bishop, K. H. Grzeschik, S. L. Naylor, A. Y. Sakaguchi, G. Brodeur, and J. Trent.** 1984. Chromosome localization in normal human cells and neuroblastomas of a gene related to c-myc. *Nature* **308**: 288−291.

925. **Schweinfest, C. W., S. Fujiwara, L. F. Lau, and T. S. Papas.** 1988. c-myc can induce expression of G0/G1 transition genes. *Mol. Cell Biol.* **8**: 3080−3087.

926. **Seeger, R. C., G. M. Brodeur, H. Sather, A. Dalton, S. E. Siegel, K. Y. Wong, and D. Hammond.** 1985. Association of multiple copies of the N-myc oncogene with rapid progression of neuroblastomas. *N. Engl. J. Med.* **313**: 1111−1116.

927. **Seipel, K., O. Georgiev, and W. Schaffner.** 1992. Different activation domains stimulate transcrip- tion from remote ('enhancer') and proximal ('promoter') positions. *EMBO J.* **11**: 4961−4968.

928. **Sejersen, T., H. Bjorklund, J. Sumegi, and N. R. Ringertz.** 1986. N-myc and c-src genes are differentially regulated in PCC7 embryonal carcinoma cells undergoing neuronal differentiation. *J. Cell Physiol.* **127**: 274−280.

929. **Sejersen, T., M. Rahm, G. Szabo, S. Ingvarsson, and J. Sumegi.** 1987. Similarities and differences in the regulation of N-myc and c-myc genes in murine embryonal carcinoma cells. *Exp. Cell Res.* **172**: 304−317.

930. **Sekido, Y., T. Takahashi, T. P. Makela, Y. Obata, R. Ueda, T. Hida, K. Hibi, K. Shimokata, and K. Alitalo.** 1992. Complex intrachromosomal rearrangement in the process of amplification of the L-myc gene in small-cell lung cancer. *Mol. Cell Biol.* **12**: 1747–1754.

931. **Selten, G., H. T. Cuypers, M. Zijlstra, C. Melief, and A. Berns.** 1984. Involvement of c-myc in MuLV-induced T cell lymphomas in mice: frequency and mechanisms of activation. *EMBO J.* **3**: 3215–3222.

932. **Selvakumaran, M., D. Liebermann, and B. Hoffman Liebermann.** 1993. Myeloblastic leukemia cells conditionally blocked by myc-estrogen receptor chimeric transgenes for terminal differentiation coupled to growth arrest and apoptosis. *Blood* **81**: 2257–2262.

933. **Selvakumaran, M., H. K. Lin, R. T. Sjin, J. C. Reed, D. A. Liebermann, and B. Hoffman.** 1994. The novel primary response gene MyD118 and the proto-oncogenes myb, myc, and bcl-2 modulate transforming growth factor beta 1-induced apoptosis of myeloid leukemia cells. *Mol. Cell Biol.* **14**: 2352–2360.

934. **Semsei, I., S. Y. Ma, and R. G. Cutler.** 1989. Tissue and age specific expression of the myc proto-oncogene family throughout the life span of the C57BL/6J mouse strain. *Oncogene* **4**: 465–471.

935. **Shaknovich, R., G. Shue, and D. S. Kohtz.** 1992. Conformational activation of a basic helix–loop–helix protein (MyoD1) by the C-terminal region of murine HSP90 (HSP84). *Mol. Cell Biol.* **12**: 5059–5068.

936. **Shaughnessy, J., F. Wiener, K. Huppi, J. F. Mushinski, and M. Potter.** 1994. A novel c-myc-activating reciprocal T(12;15) chromosomal translocation juxtaposes S alpha to Pvt-1 in a mouse plasmacytoma. *Oncogene* **9**: 247–253.

937. **Shi, Y., J. M. Glynn, L. J. Guilbert, T. G. Cotter, R. P. Bissonnette, and D. R. Green.** 1992. Role for c-myc in activation-induced apoptotic cell death in T cell hybridomas. *Science* **257**: 212–214.

938. **Shi, Y., H. G. Hutchinson, D. J. Hall, and A. Zalewski.** 1993. Downregulation of c-myc expression by antisense oligonucleotides inhibits proliferation of human smooth muscle cells. *Circulation* **88**: 1190–1195.

939. **Shibasaki, Y., H. Sakura, F. Takaku, and M. Kasuga.** 1990. Insulin enhancer binding protein has helix–loop–helix structure. *Biochem. Biophys. Res. Commun.* **170**: 314–321.

940. **Shichiri, M., K. D. Hanson, and J. M. Sedivy.** 1993. Effects of c-myc expression on proliferation, quiescence, and the G0 to G1 transition in nontransformed cells. *Cell Growth Differ.* **4**: 93–104.

941. **Shieh, B. H., R. S. Sparkes, R. B. Gaynor, and A. J. Lusis.** 1993. Localization of the gene-encoding upstream stimulatory factor (USF) to human chromosome 1q22–q23. *Genomics* **16**: 266–268.

942. **Shieh, S. Y. and M. J. Tsai.** 1991. Cell-specific and ubiquitous factors are responsible for the enhancer activity of the rat insulin II gene. *J. Biol. Chem.* **266**: 16708–16714.

943. **Shih, C. K., M. Linial, M. M. Goodenow, and W. S. Hayward.** 1984. Nucleotide sequence 5' of the chicken c-myc coding region: localization of a noncoding exon that is absent from myc transcripts in most avian leukosis virus-induced lymphomas. *Proc. Natl Acad. Sci. USA* **81**: 4697–4701.

944. **Shoji, W., T. Yamamoto, and M. Obinata.** 1994. The helix–loop–helix protein Id inhibits differentiation of murine erythroleukemia cells. *J. Biol. Chem.* **269**: 5078–5084.

945. **Shue, G. and D. S. Kohtz.** 1994. Structural and functional aspects of basic helix–loop–helix protein folding by heat-shock protein 90. *J. Biol. Chem.* **269**: 2707–2711.

946. **Sidman, C. L., T. M. Denial, J. D. Marshall, and J. B. Roths.** 1993. Multiple mechanisms of tumorigenesis in E mu-myc transgenic mice. *Cancer Res.* **53**: 1665–1669.

947. **Siebenlist, U., P. Bressler, and K. Kelly.** 1988. Two distinct mechanisms of transcriptional control operate on c-myc during differentiation of HL60 cells. *Mol. Cell Biol.* **8**: 867–874.

948. **Siebenlist, U., L. Hennighausen, J. Battey, and P. Leder.** 1984. Chromatin structure and protein binding in the putative regulatory region of the c-myc gene in Burkitt lymphoma. *Cell* **37**: 381–391.

949. **Simonson, M. S., A. Rooney, and W. H. Herman.** 1993. Expression and differential regulation of Id1, a dominant negative regulator of basic helix–loop–helix transcription factors, in glomerular mesangial cells. *Nucleic Acids Res.* **21**: 5767–5774.

950. **Sirito, M., Q. Lin, T. Maity, and M. Sawadogo.** 1994. Ubiquitous expression of the 43- and 44-kDa forms of transcription factor USF in mammalian cells. *Nucleic Acids Res.* **22**: 427–433.

951. **Skeath, J. B. and S. B. Carroll.** 1991. Regulation of achaete–scute gene expression and sensory organ pattern formation in the *Drosophila* wing. *Genes Dev.* **5**: 984–995.

952. **Skeath, J. B., G. Panganiban, J. Selegue, and S. B. Carroll.** 1992. Gene regulation in two dimensions: the proneural achaete and scute genes are controlled by combinations of axis-patterning genes through a common intergenic control region. *Genes Dev.* **6**: 2606–2619.

953. **Skerka, C., P. F. Zipfel, and U. Siebenlist.** 1993. Two regulatory domains are required for downregulation of c-myc transcription in differentiating U937 cells. *Oncogene* **8**: 2135–2143.

954. Sklar, M. D., E. Thompson, M. J. Welsh, M. Liebert, J. Harney, H. B. Grossman, M. Smith, and E. V. Prochownik. 1991. Depletion of c-myc with specific antisense sequences reverses the transformed phenotype in ras oncogene-transformed NIH 3T3 cells. *Mol. Cell Biol.* **11**: 3699–3710.

955. Slamon, D. J., T. C. Boone, R. C. Seeger, D. E. Keith, V. Chazin, H. C. Lee, and L. M. Souza. 1986. Identification and characterization of the protein encoded by the human N-myc oncogene. *Science* **232**: 768–772.

956. Slavc, I., R. Ellenbogen, W. H. Jung, G. F. Vawter, C. Kretschmar, H. Grier, and B. R. Korf. 1990. myc gene amplification and expression in primary human neuroblastoma. *Cancer Res.* **50**: 1459–1463.

957. Small, M. B., N. Hay, M. Schwab, and J. M. Bishop. 1987. Neoplastic transformation by the human gene N-myc. *Mol. Cell Biol.* **7**: 1638–1645.

958. Smeland, E. B., K. Beiske, B. Ek, R. Watt, S. Pfeifer Ohlsson, H. K. Blomhoff, T. Godal, and R. Ohlsson. 1987. Regulation of c-myc transcription and protein expression during activation of normal human B cells. *Exp. Cell Res.* **172**: 101–109.

959. Smeland, E. B., T. Godal, K. Beiske, R. Watt, S. Pfeifer Ohlsson, and R. Ohlsson. 1986. Regulation of c-myc mRNA and protein levels during activation of normal human B cells. *Curr. Top. Microbiol. Immunol.* **132**: 290–296.

960. Smith, C. K., M. J. Janney, and R. E. Allen. 1994. Temporal expression of myogenic regulatory genes during activation, proliferation, and differentiation of rat skeletal muscle satellite cells. *J. Cell Physiol.* **159**: 379–385.

961. Smith, M. J., D. C. Charron Prochownik, and E. V. Prochownik. 1990. The leucine zipper of c-Myc is required for full inhibition of erythroleukemia differentiation. *Mol. Cell Biol.* **10**: 5333–5339.

962. Smith, R. K., K. Zimmerman, G. D. Yancopoulos, A. Ma, and F. W. Alt. 1992. Transcriptional down-regulation of N-myc expression during B-cell development. *Mol. Cell Biol.* **12**: 1578–1584.

963. Sorrentino, V., V. Drozdoff, M. D. McKinney, L. Zeitz, and E. Fleissner. 1986. Potentiation of growth factor activity by exogenous c-myc expression. *Proc. Natl Acad. Sci. USA* **83**: 8167–8171.

964. Spector, D. L., R. A. Watt, and N. F. Sullivan. 1987. The v- and c-myc oncogene proteins colocalize in situ with small nuclear ribonucleoprotein particles. *Oncogene* **1**: 5–12.

965. Spencer, C. A. and M. A. Kilvert. 1993. Transcription elongation in the human c-myc gene is governed by overall transcription initiation levels in *Xenopus* oocytes. *Mol. Cell Biol.* **13**: 1296–1305.

966. Spencer, C. A., R. C. LeStrange, U. Novak, W. S. Hayward, and M. Groudine. 1990. The block to transcription elongation is promoter dependent in normal and Burkitt's lymphoma c-myc alleles. *Genes Dev.* **4**: 75–88.

967. Spicer, D. B. and G. E. Sonenshein. 1992. An antisense promoter of the murine c-myc gene is localized within intron 2. *Mol. Cell Biol.* **12**: 1324–1329.

968. Spotts, G. D. and S. R. Hann. 1990. Enhanced translation and increased turnover of c-myc proteins occur during differentiation of murine erythroleukemia cells. *Mol. Cell Biol.* **10**: 3952–3964.

969. Stanton, B. R., A. S. Perkins, L. Tessarollo, D. A. Sassoon, and L. F. Parada. 1992. Loss of N-myc function results in embryonic lethality and failure of the epithelial component of the embryo to develop. *Genes Dev.* **6**: 2235–2247.

970. Stanton, L. W., P. D. Fahrlander, P. M. Tesser, and K. B. Marcu. 1984. Nucleotide sequence comparison of normal and translocated murine c-myc genes. *Nature* **310**: 423–425.

971. Stanton, L. W., M. Schwab, and J. M. Bishop. 1986. Nucleotide sequence of the human N-myc gene. *Proc. Natl Acad. Sci. USA* **83**: 1772–1776.

972. Stern, D. F., A. B. Roberts, N. S. Roche, M. B. Sporn, and R. A. Weinberg. 1986. Differential responsiveness of myc- and ras-transfected cells to growth factors: selective stimulation of myc-transfected cells by epidermal growth factor. *Mol. Cell Biol.* **6**: 870–877.

973. Stewart, M. A., D. Forrest, R. McFarlane, D. Onions, N. Wilkie, and J. C. Neil. 1986. Conservation of the c-myc coding sequence in transduced feline v-myc genes. *Virology* **154**: 121–134.

974. Stone, J., T. de Lange, G. Ramsay, E. Jakobovits, J. M. Bishop, H. Varmus, and W. Lee. 1987. Definition of regions in human c-myc that are involved in transformation and nuclear localization. *Mol. Cell Biol.* **7**: 1697–1709.

975. Strasser, A., A. W. Harris, M. L. Bath, and S. Cory. 1990. Novel primitive lymphoid tumours induced in transgenic mice by cooperation between myc and bcl-2. *Nature* **348**: 331–333.

976. Strobl, L. J. and D. Eick. 1992. Hold back of RNA polymerase II at the transcription start site mediates down-regulation of c-myc *in vivo*. *EMBO J.* **11**: 3307–3314.

977. Studzinski, G. P., Z. S. Brelvi, S. C. Feldman, and R. A. Watt. 1986. Participation of c-myc protein in DNA synthesis of human cells. *Science* **234**: 467–470.

978. Suen, T. C. and M. C. Hung. 1991. c-myc reverses neu-induced transformed morphology by transcriptional repression. *Mol. Cell Biol.* **11**: 354–362.

979. Sugiyama, A., A. Kume, K. Nemoto, S. Y. Lee, Y. Asami, F. Nemoto, S. Nishimura, and Y. Kuchino. 1989. Isolation and characterization of s-myc, a member of the rat myc gene family. *Proc. Natl Acad. Sci. USA* **86**: 9144–9148.

980. **Sullivan, K. F. and C. A. Glass.** 1991. CENP-B is a highly conserved mammalian centromere protein with homology to the helix−loop−helix family of proteins. *Chromosoma* **100**: 360−370.

981. **Sullivan, N., C. Green, M. Pasdar, and R. Watt.** 1986. Characterization and nuclear localization of the v- and c-myc proteins. *Curr. Top. Microbiol. Immunol.* **132**: 355−361.

982. **Sullivan, N. F., R. A. Watt, M. R. Delannoy, C. L. Green, and D. L. Spector.** 1986. Colocalization of the myc oncogene protein and small nuclear ribonucleoprotein particles. *Cold Spring Harb. Symp. Quant. Biol.* 51 Pt **2**: 943−947.

983. **Sumegi, J., T. Sejersen, H. Bjorklund, G. Klein, and N. R. Ringertz.** 1986. Differential expression of N-myc, c-myc and c-src proto-oncogenes during the course of induced differentiation of murine embryonal carcinoma cells. *Curr. Top. Microbiol. Immunol.* **132**: 297−304.

984. **Sun, X. H. and D. Baltimore.** 1991. An inhibitory domain of E12 transcription factor prevents DNA binding in E12 homodimers but not in E12 heterodimers [published erratum appears in *Cell* 1991 Aug 9; 66(3): 423]. *Cell* **64**: 459−470.

985. **Sussman, D. J., J. Chung, and P. Leder.** 1991. *In vitro* and *in vivo* analysis of the c-myc RNA polymerase III promoter. *Nucleic Acids Res.* **19**: 5045−5052.

986. **Swartwout, S. G. and A. J. Kinniburgh.** 1989. c-myc RNA degradation in growing and differentiating cells: possible alternate pathways. *Mol. Cell Biol.* **9**: 288−295.

987. **Symonds, G., A. Hartshorn, A. Kennewell, M. A. O'Mara, A. Bruskin, and J. M. Bishop.** 1989. Transformation of murine myelomonocytic cells by myc: point mutations in v-myc contribute synergistically to transforming potential. *Oncogene* **4**: 285−294.

988. **Szabo, G. J., L. Szekely, M. Schablik, G. Klein, J. Sumegi, and G. Szabo.** 1991. Inositol derivatives down-regulate c-myc inducing growth arrest without differentiation. *Exp. Cell Res.* **193**: 420−424.

989. **Tachibana, K., N. Takayama, K. Matsuo, S. Kato, K. Yamamoto, K. Ohyama, A. Umezawa, and T. Takano.** 1993. Allele-specific activation of the c-myc gene in an atypical Burkitt's lymphoma carrying the t(2;8) chromosomal translocation 250 kb downstream from c-myc. *Gene* **124**: 231−237.

990. **Tajbakhsh, S. and M. E. Buckingham.** 1994. Mouse limb muscle is determined in the absence of the earliest myogenic factor myf-5. *Proc. Natl Acad. Sci. USA* **91**: 747−751.

991. **Takada, S., T. Yamamoto, Y. Ohmori, Y. Matsui, and M. Obinata.** 1992. c-Myc interferes with the commitment to differentiation of murine erythroleukemia cells at a reversible point. *Jpn. J. Cancer Res.* **83**: 61−65.

992. **Takebayashi, K., Y. Sasai, Y. Sakai, T. Watanabe, S. Nakanishi, and R. Kageyama.** 1994. Structure, chromosomal locus, and promoter analysis of the gene encoding the mouse helix−loop−helix factor HES-1. Negative autoregulation through the multiple N box elements. *J. Biol. Chem.* **269**: 5150−5156.

993. **Takimoto, M., J. P. Quinn, A. R. Farina, L. M. Staudt, and D. Levens.** 1989. fos/jun and octamer-binding protein interact with a common site in a negative element of the human c-myc gene. *J. Biol. Chem.* **264**: 8992−8999.

994. **Tanigawa, T., L. Robb, A. R. Green, and C. G. Begley.** 1994. Constitutive expression of the putative transcription factor *SCL* associated with proviral insertion in the myeloid leukemia cell line WEHI-3BD[-1]. *Cell Growth Differ.* **5**: 557−561.

995*. **Tapscott, S. J., R. L. Davis, M. J. Thayer, P. F. Cheng, H. Weintraub, and A. B. Lassar.** 1988. MyoD1:a nuclear phosphoprotein requiring a Myc homology region to convert fibroblasts to myoblasts. *Science* **242**: 405−411.

996. **Tapscott, S. J., A. B. Lassar, and H. Weintraub.** 1992. A novel myoblast enhancer element mediates MyoD transcription. *Mol. Cell Biol.* **12**: 4994−5003.

997. **Tapscott, S. J., M. J. Thayer, and H. Weintraub.** 1993. Deficiency in rhabdomyosarcomas of a factor required for MyoD activity and myogenesis. *Science* **259**: 1450−1453.

998. **Taya, Y., S. Mizusawa, and S. Nishimura.** 1986. Nucleotide sequence of the coding region of the mouse N-myc gene. *EMBO J.* **5**: 1215−1219.

999. **Taylor, M. V., J. B. Gurdon, N. D. Hopwood, N. Towers, and T. J. Mohun.** 1991. *Xenopus* embryos contain a somite-specific, MyoD-like protein that binds to a promoter site required for muscle actin expression. *Genes Dev.* **5**: 1149−1160.

1000. **Taylor, M. V., M. Gusse, G. I. Evan, N. Dathan, and M. Mechali.** 1986. *Xenopus* myc proto-oncogene during development: expression as a stable maternal mRNA uncoupled from cell division. *EMBO J.* **5**: 3563−3570.

1001. **Taylor, W. R., S. E. Egan, M. Mowat, A. H. Greenberg, and J. A. Wright.** 1992. Evidence for synergistic interactions between ras, myc and a mutant form of p53 in cellular transformation and tumor dissemination. *Oncogene* **7**: 1383−1390.

1002. **Tchang, F., S. Vriz, and M. Mechali.** 1991. Posttranscriptional regulation of c-myc RNA during early development of *Xenopus laevis*. *FEBS Lett.* **291**: 177−180.

1003. **Thalmeier, K., H. Synovzik, R. Mertz, E. L. Winnacker, and M. Lipp.** 1989. Nuclear factor E2F mediates basic transcription and trans activation by E1a of the human MYC promoter. *Genes Dev.* **3**: 527−536.

1004. **Therrien, M. and J. Drouin.** 1993. Cell-specific helix—loop—helix factor required for pituitary expression of the pro-opiomelanocortin gene. *Mol. Cell Biol.* **13**: 2342–2353.

1005. **Thisse, B., C. Stoetzel, C. Gorostiza Thisse, and F. Perrin Schmitt.** 1988. Sequence of the twist gene and nuclear localization of its protein in endomesodermal cells of early *Drosophila* embryos. *EMBO J.* **7**: 2175–2183.

1006. **Thomas, D., I. Jacquemin, and Y. Surdin Kerjan.** 1992. MET4, a leucine zipper protein, and centromere-binding factor 1 are both required for transcriptional activation of sulfur metabolism in *Saccharomyces cerevisiae*. *Mol. Cell Biol.* **12**: 1719–1727.

1007. **Thomas, J. B., S. T. Crews, and C. S. Goodman.** 1988. Molecular genetics of the single-minded locus: a gene involved in the development of the *Drosophila* nervous system. *Cell* **52**: 133–141.

1008. **Thompson, C. B., P. B. Challoner, P. E. Neiman, and M. Groudine.** 1985. Levels of c-myc oncogene mRNA are invariant throughout the cell cycle. *Nature* **314**: 363–366.

1009. **Thompson, T. C., J. Southgate, G. Kitchener, and H. Land.** 1989. Multistage carcinogenesis induced by ras and myc oncogenes in a reconstituted organ. *Cell* **56**: 917–930.

1010. **Thorburn, A. M., P. A. Walton, and J. R. Feramisco.** 1993. MyoD induced cell cycle arrest is associated with increased nuclear affinity of the Rb protein. *Mol. Biol. Cell* **4**: 705–713.

1011. **Tietze, K., N. Oellers, and E. Knust.** 1992. Enhancer of splitD, a dominant mutation of *Drosophila*, and its use in the study of functional domains of a helix—loop—helix protein. *Proc. Natl Acad. Sci. USA* **89**: 6152–6156.

1012. **Tomlinson, C. R., M. T. Kozlowski, and W. H. Klein.** 1990. Ectoderm nuclei from sea urchin embryos contain a Spec-DNA binding protein similar to the vertebrate transcription factor USF. *Development* **110**: 259–272.

1013. **Tonelli, C., G. Consonni, S. F. Dolfini, S. L. Dellaporta, A. Viotti, and G. Gavazzi.** 1991. Genetic and molecular analysis of Sn, a light-inducible, tissue specific regulatory gene in maize. *Mol. Gen. Genet.* **225**: 401–410.

1014. **Tonissen, K. F. and P. A. Krieg.** 1994. Analysis of a variant Max sequence expressed in *Xenopus laevis*. *Oncogene* **9**: 33–38.

1015. **Tontonoz, P., J. B. Kim, R. A. Graves, and B. M. Spiegelman.** 1993. ADD1:a novel helix—loop—helix transcription factor associated with adipocyte determination and differentiation. *Mol. Cell Biol.* **13**: 4753–4759.

1016. **Toth, E. C., L. Marusic, A. Ochem, A. Patthy, S. Pongor, M. Giacca, and A. Falaschi.** 1993. Interactions of USF and Ku antigen with a human DNA region containing a replication origin. *Nucleic Acids Res.* **21**: 3257–3263.

1017. **Toth, M., W. Doerfler, and T. Shenk.** 1992. Adenovirus DNA replication facilitates binding of the MLTF/USF transcription factor to the viral major late promoter within infected cells. *Nucleic Acids Res.* **20**: 5143–5148.

1018. **Trouche, D., M. Grigoriev, J. L. Lenormand, P. Robin, S. A. Leibovitch, P. Sassone Corsi, and A. Harel Bellan.** 1993. Repression of c-fos promoter by MyoD on muscle cell differentiation. *Nature* **363**: 79–82.

1019. **Tsay, H. J., Y. H. Choe, C. M. Neville, and J. Schmidt.** 1992. CTF4, a chicken transcription factor of the helix—loop—helix class A family. *Nucleic Acids Res.* **20**: 1805.

1020. **Tsay, H. J., Y. H. Choe, C. M. Neville, and J. Schmidt.** 1992. CTF4, a chicken transcription factor of the helix—loop—helix class A family. *Nucleic Acids Res.* **20**: 2624.

1021. **Tulchin, N., L. Ornstein, J. Guillem, K. O'Toole, M. E. Lambert, and I. B. Weinstein.** 1988. Distribution of the c-myc oncoprotein in normal and neoplastic tissues of the rat colon. *Oncogene* **3**: 697–701.

1022. **Turner, D. L. and H. Weintraub.** 1994. Expression of achaete—scute homolog 3 in *Xenopus* embryos converts ectodermal cells to a neural fate. *Genes Dev.* **8**: 1434–1447.

1023. **Tverberg, L. A. and A. F. Russo.** 1993. Regulation of the calcitonin/calcitonin gene-related peptide gene by cell-specific synergy between helix—loop—helix and octamer-binding transcription factors. *J. Biol. Chem.* **268**: 15965–15973.

1024. **Vaessin, H., M. Brand, L. Y. Jan, and Y. N. Jan.** 1994. daughterless is essential for neuronal precursor differentiation but not for initiation of neuronal precursor formation in *Drosophila* embryo. *Development* **120**: 935–945.

1025. **Vaidya, T. B., S. J. Rhodes, J. L. Moore, D. A. Sherman, S. F. Konieczny, and E. J. Taparowsky.** 1992. Isolation and structural analysis of the rat MyoD gene. *Gene* **116**: 223–230.

1026. **Van Beneden, R. J., D. K. Watson, T. T. Chen, J. A. Lautenberger, and T. S. Papas.** 1986. Cellular myc (c-myc) in fish (rainbow trout): its relationship to other vertebrate myc genes and to the transforming genes of the MC29 family of viruses. *Proc. Natl Acad. Sci. USA* **83**: 3698–3702.

1027. **Van Doren, M., P. A. Powell, D. Pasternak, A. Singson, and J. W. Posakony.** 1992. Spatial regulation of proneural gene activity: auto- and cross-activation of achaete is antagonized by extramacrochaetae. *Genes Dev.* **6**: 2592–2605.

1028. **van Lohuizen, M., M. Breuer, and A. Berns.** 1989. N-myc is frequently activated by proviral insertion in MuLV-induced T cell lymphomas. *EMBO J.* **8**: 133–136.

1029. **van't Veer, L. J., R. L. Beijersbergen, and R. Bernards.** 1993. N-myc suppresses major histocompatibility complex class I gene expression through down-regulation of the p50 subunit of NF-kappa B. *EMBO J.* **12**: 195–200.

1030. **Vass, J. K., R. Neill, T. Jamieson, and G. D. Birnie.** 1990. Regulation of the relative abundances of c-myc mRNAs in human promyelocytic HL60 cells. *Differentiation* **45**: 49–54.

1031. **Vassilev, L. and E. M. Johnson.** 1990. An initiation zone of chromosomal DNA replication located upstream of the c-myc gene in proliferating HeLa cells. *Mol. Cell Biol.* **10**: 4899–4904.

1032. **Vaux, D. L. and I. L. Weissman.** 1993. Neither macromolecular synthesis nor myc is required for cell death via the mechanism that can be controlled by Bcl-2. *Mol. Cell Biol.* **13**: 7000–7005.

1033. **Vennstrom, B., P. Kahn, B. Adkins, P. Enrietto, M. J. Hayman, T. Graf, and P. Luciw.** 1984. Transformation of mammalian fibroblasts and macrophages *in vitro* by a murine retrovirus encoding an avian v-myc oncogene. *EMBO J.* **3**: 3223–3229.

1034. **Vennstrom, B., D. Sheiness, J. Zabielski, and J. M. Bishop.** 1982. Isolation and characterization of c-myc, a cellular homolog of the oncogene (v-myc) of avian myelocytomatosis virus strain 29. *J. Virol.* **42**: 773–779.

1035. **Venuti, J. M., L. Goldberg, T. Chakraborty, E. N. Olson, and W. H. Klein.** 1991. A myogenic factor from sea urchin embryos capable of programming muscle differentiation in mammalian cells. *Proc. Natl Acad. Sci. USA* **88**: 6219–6223.

1036. **Versteeg, R., I. A. Noordermeer, M. Kruse Wolters, D. J. Ruiter, and P. I. Schrier.** 1988. c-myc down-regulates class I HLA expression in human melanomas. *EMBO J.* **7**: 1023–1029.

1037. **Vidal, M., R. Strich, R. E. Esposito, and R. F. Gaber.** 1991. RPD1 (SIN3/UME4) is required for maximal activation and repression of diverse yeast genes. *Mol. Cell Biol.* **11**: 6306–6316.

1038. **Vierra, C. A., Y. Jacobs, L. Ly, and C. Nelson.** 1994. Patterns of Pan expression and role of Pan proteins in endocrine cell type-specific complex formation. *Mol. Endocrinol.* **8**: 197–209.

1039. **Villares, R. and C. V. Cabrera.** 1987. The achaete–scute gene complex of D. *melanogaster*: conserved domains in a subset of genes required for neurogenesis and their homology to myc. *Cell* **50**: 415–424.

1040. **Visvader, J., C. G. Begley, and J. M. Adams.** 1991. Differential expression of the LYL, SCL and E2A helix–loop–helix genes within the hemopoietic system. *Oncogene* **6**: 187–194.

1041. **Vize, P. D., A. Vaughan, and P. Krieg.** 1990. Expression of the N-myc proto-oncogene during the early development of *Xenopus laevis*. *Development* **110**: 885–896.

1042. **Vogt, M., J. Lesley, J. M. Bogenberger, C. Haggblom, S. Swift, and M. Haas.** 1987. The induction of growth factor-independence in murine myelocytes by oncogenes results in monoclonal cell lines and is correlated with cell crisis and karyotypic instability. *Oncogene Res.* **2**: 49–63.

1043. **Voliva, C. F., A. Aronheim, M. D. Walker, and B. M. Peterlin.** 1992. B-cell factor 1 is required for optimal expression of the DRA promoter in B cells. *Mol. Cell Biol.* **12**: 2383–2390.

1044. **Voronova, A. and D. Baltimore.** 1990. Mutations that disrupt DNA binding and dimer formation in the E47 helix–loop–helix protein map to distinct domains. *Proc. Natl Acad. Sci. USA* **87**: 4722–4726.

1045. **Voytik, S. L., M. Przyborski, S. F. Badylak, and S. F. Konieczny.** 1993. Differential expression of muscle regulatory factor genes in normal and denervated adult rat hindlimb muscles. *Dev. Dyn.* **198**: 214–224.

1046. **Vriz, S., J. M. Lemaitre, M. Leibovici, N. Thierry, and M. Mechali.** 1992. Comparative analysis of the intracellular localization of c-Myc, c-Fos, and replicative proteins during cell cycle progression. *Mol. Cell Biol.* **12**: 3548–3555.

1047. **Vriz, S. and M. Mechali.** 1989. Analysis of 3'-untranslated regions of seven c-myc genes reveals conserved elements prevalent in post-transcriptionally regulated genes. *FEBS Lett.* **251**: 201–206.

1048. **Vriz, S., M. Taylor, and M. Mechali.** 1989. Differential expression of two *Xenopus* c-myc proto-oncogenes during development. *EMBO J.* **8**: 4091–4097.

1049. **Wagner, A. J., M. M. Le Beau, M. O. Diaz, and N. Hay.** 1992. Expression, regulation, and chromosomal localization of the Max gene. *Proc. Natl Acad. Sci. USA* **89**: 3111–3115.

1050. **Wagner, A. J., C. Meyers, L. A. Laimins, and N. Hay.** 1993. c-Myc induces the expression and activity of ornithine decarboxylase. *Cell Growth Differ.* **4**: 879–883.

1051. **Wagner, A. J., M. B. Small, and N. Hay.** 1993. Myc-mediated apoptosis is blocked by ectopic expression of Bcl-2. *Mol. Cell Biol.* **13**: 2432–2440.

1052. **Wainwright, S. M. and D. Ish Horowicz.** 1992. Point mutations in the *Drosophila* hairy gene demonstrate *in vivo* requirements for basic, helix–loop–helix, and WRPW domains. *Mol. Cell Biol.* **12**: 2475–2483.

1053. **Waitz, W. and P. Loidl.** 1991. Cell cycle dependent association of c-myc protein with the nuclear matrix. *Oncogene* **6**: 29—35.

1054. **Wakamatsu, Y., Y. Watanabe, A. Shimono, and H. Kondoh.** 1993. Transition of localization of the N-Myc protein from nucleus to cytoplasm in differentiating neurons. *Neuron* **10**: 1—9.

1055. **Walker, C. W., J. D. Boom, and A. G. Marsh.** 1992. First non-vertebrate member of the myc gene family is seasonally expressed in an invertebrate testis. *Oncogene* **7**: 2007—2012.

1056. **Walker, M. D., C. W. Park, A. Rosen, and A. Aronheim.** 1990. A cDNA from a mouse pancreatic beta cell encoding a putative transcription factor of the insulin gene. *Nucleic Acids Res.* **18**: 1159—1166.

1057. **Walther, N., H. W. Jansen, C. Trachmann, and K. Bister.** 1986. Nucleotide sequence of the CMII v-myc allele. *Virology* **154**: 219—223.

1058. **Walther, N., R. Lurz, T. Patschinsky, H. W. Jansen, and K. Bister.** 1985. Molecular cloning of proviral DNA and structural analysis of the transduced myc oncogene of avian oncovirus CMII. *J. Virol.* **54**: 576—585.

1059. **Wang, H., I. Clark, P. R. Nicholson, I. Herskowitz, and D. J. Stillman.** 1990. The *Saccharomyces cerevisiae* SIN3 gene, a negative regulator of HO, contains four paired amphipathic helix motifs. *Mol. Cell Biol.* **10**: 5927—5936.

1060. **Wang, H. and D. J. Stillman.** 1993. Transcriptional repression in *Saccharomyces cerevisiae* by a SIN3-LexA fusion protein. *Mol. Cell Biol.* **13**: 1805—1814.

1061. **Wang, X., M. R. Briggs, X. Hua, C. Yokoyama, J. L. Goldstein, and M. S. Brown.** 1993. Nuclear protein that binds sterol regulatory element of low density lipoprotein receptor promoter. II. Purification and characterization. *J. Biol. Chem.* **268**: 14497—14504.

1062. **Wang, X., R. Sato, M. S. Brown, X. Hua, and J. L. Goldstein.** 1994. SREBP-1, a membrane-bound transcription factor released by sterol-regulated proteolysis. *Cell* **77**: 53—62.

1063. **Wang, Y., H. Sugiyama, H. Axelson, C. K. Panda, M. Babonits, A. Ma, J. M. Steinberg, F. W. Alt, G. Klein, and F. Wiener.** 1992. Functional homology between N-myc and c-myc in murine plasmacytomagenesis: plasmacytoma development in N-myc transgenic mice. *Oncogene* **7**: 1241—1247.

1064. **Watanabe, T., E. Sariban, T. Mitchell, and D. Kufe.** 1985. Human c-myc and N-ras expression during induction of HL-60 cellular differentiation. *Biochem. Biophys. Res. Commun.* **126**: 999—1005.

1065. **Waters, C. M., T. D. Littlewood, D. C. Hancock, J. P. Moore, and G. I. Evan.** 1991. c-myc protein expression in untransformed fibroblasts. *Oncogene* **6**: 797—805.

1066. **Watson, D. K., M. C. Psallidopoulos, K. P. Samuel, R. Dalla Favera, and T. S. Papas.** 1983. Nucleotide sequence analysis of human c-myc locus, chicken homologue, and myelocytomatosis virus MC29 transforming gene reveals a highly conserved gene product. *Proc. Natl Acad. Sci. USA* **80**: 3642—3645.

1067. **Watson, D. K., E. P. Reddy, P. H. Duesberg, and T. S. Papas.** 1983. Nucleotide sequence analysis of the chicken c-myc gene reveals homologous and unique coding regions by comparison with the transforming gene of avian myelocytomatosis virus MC29, delta gag—myc. *Proc. Natl Acad. Sci. USA* **80**: 2146—2150.

1068. **Watson, P. H., R. T. Pon, and R. P. Shiu.** 1991. Inhibition of c-myc expression by phosphorothioate antisense oligonucleotide identifies a critical role for c-myc in the growth of human breast cancer. *Cancer Res.* **51**: 3996—4000.

1069. **Watson, R. J.** 1988. Expression of the c-myb and c-myc genes is regulated independently in differentiating mouse erythroleukemia cells by common processes of premature transcription arrest and increased mRNA turnover. *Mol. Cell Biol.* **8**: 3938—3942.

1070. **Watt, R., K. Nishikura, J. Sorrentino, A. ar Rushdi, C. M. Croce, and G. Rovera.** 1983. The structure and nucleotide sequence of the 5′ end of the human c-myc oncogene. *Proc. Natl Acad. Sci. USA* **80**: 6307—6311.

1071. **Watt, R., L. W. Stanton, K. B. Marcu, R. C. Gallo, C. M. Croce, and G. Rovera.** 1983. Nucleotide sequence of cloned cDNA of human c-myc oncogene. *Nature* **303**: 725—728.

1072. **Wei, Y., T. Y. Hsu, P. Tiollais, M. A. Buendia, and J. Etiemble.** 1990. Evolutionary conservation of target sequences for cis-acting regulation in c-myc exon 1 and its upstream region. *Gene* **93**: 301—305.

1073*. **Weintraub, H., V. J. Dwarki, I. Verma, R. Davis, S. Hollenberg, L. Snider, A. Lassar, and S. J. Tapscott.** 1991. Muscle-specific transcriptional activation by MyoD. *Genes Dev.* **5**: 1377—1386.

1074. **Weintraub, H., S. J. Tapscott, R. L. Davis, M. J. Thayer, M. A. Adam, A. B. Lassar, and A. D. Miller.** 1989. Activation of muscle-specific genes in pigment, nerve, fat, liver, and fibroblast cell lines by forced expression of MyoD. *Proc. Natl Acad. Sci. USA* **86**: 5434—5438.

1075. **Weisinger, G., E. F. Remmers, P. Hearing, and K. B. Marcu.** 1988. Multiple negative elements upstream of the murine c-myc gene share nuclear factor binding sites with SV40 and polyoma enhancers. *Oncogene* **3**: 635—646.

1076. **Weissinger, E. M., H. Mischak, J. Goodnight, W. F. Davidson, and J. F. Mushinski.** 1993. Addition of constitutive c-myc expression to Abelson murine leukemia virus changes the phenotype of the cells transformed by the virus from pre-B-cell lymphomas to plasmacytomas. *Mol. Cell Biol.* **13**: 2578—2585.

1077. Whitelaw, M., I. Pongratz, A. Wilhelmsson, J. A. Gustafsson, and L. Poellinger. 1993. Ligand-dependent recruitment of the Arnt coregulator determines DNA recognition by the dioxin receptor. *Mol. Cell Biol.* **13**: 2504–2514.

1078. Whitelaw, M. L., M. Gottlicher, J. A. Gustafsson, and L. Poellinger. 1993. Definition of a novel ligand binding domain of a nuclear bHLH receptor: co-localization of ligand and hsp90 binding activities within the regulable inactivation domain of the dioxin receptor. *EMBO J.* **12**: 4169–4179.

1079. Wilhelmsson, A., M. L. Whitelaw, J-A. Gustafsson, and L. Poellinger. 1994. Agonistic and antagonistic effects of a-naphthoflavone on dioxin receptor function. *J. Biol. Chem.* **269**: 19028–19033.

1080*. Wilson, R. B., M. Kiledjian, C. P. Shen, R. Benezra, P. Zwollo, S. M. Dymecki, S. V. Desiderio, and T. Kadesch. 1991. Repression of immunoglobulin enhancers by the helix–loop–helix protein Id: implications for B-lymphoid-cell development. *Mol. Cell Biol.* **11**: 6185–6191.

1081. Wingrove, T. G., R. Watt, P. Keng, and I. G. Macara. 1988. Stabilization of myc proto-oncogene proteins during Friend murine erythroleukemia cell differentiation. *J. Biol. Chem.* **263**: 8918–8924.

1082. Winqvist, R., K. Saksela, and K. Alitalo. 1984. The myc proteins are not associated with chromatin in mitotic cells. *EMBO J.* **3**: 2947–2950.

1083. Winter, B., T. Braun, and H. H. Arnold. 1992. Co-operativity of functional domains in the muscle-specific transcription factor Myf-5. *EMBO J.* **11**: 1843–1855.

1084. Wisdom, R. and W. Lee. 1991. The protein-coding region of c-myc mRNA contains a sequence that specifies rapid mRNA turnover and induction by protein synthesis inhibitors. *Genes Dev.* **5**: 232–243.

1085. Wittig, B., S. Wolfl, T. Dorbic, W. Vahrson, and A. Rich. 1992. Transcription of human c-myc in permeabilized nuclei is associated with formation of Z-DNA in three discrete regions of the gene. *EMBO J.* **11**: 4653–4663.

1086. Witzemann, V. and B. Sakmann. 1991. Differential regulation of MyoD and myogenin mRNA levels by nerve induced muscle activity. *FEBS Lett.* **282**: 259–264.

1087. Wolf, C., C. Thisse, C. Stoetzel, B. Thisse, P. Gerlinger, and F. Perrin Schmitt. 1991. The M-twist gene of Mus is expressed in subsets of mesodermal cells and is closely related to the *Xenopus* X-twi and the *Drosophila* twist genes. *Dev. Biol.* **143**: 363–373.

1088. Wolf, J. R., R. R. Hirschhorn, and S. M. Steiner. 1992. Growth factor responsiveness: role of MyoD and myogenin. *Exp. Cell Res.* **202**: 105–112.

1089. Wolf, J. R., Y. Hu, R. R. Hirschhorn, and S. M. Steiner. 1993. MyoD and regulation of prostaglandin H synthase. *Exp. Cell Res.* **207**: 439–441.

1090. Wood, A. C., C. M. Waters, A. Garner, and J. A. Hickman. 1994. Changes in c-myc expression and the kinetics of dexamethasone-induced programmed cell death (apoptosis) in human lymphoid leukaemia cells. *Br. J. Cancer* **69**: 663–669.

1091. Workman, J. L., R. G. Roeder, and R. E. Kingston. 1990. An upstream transcription factor, USF (MLTF), facilitates the formation of preinitiation complexes during *in vitro* chromatin assembly. *EMBO J.* **9**: 1299–1308.

1092. Wright, S. and J. M. Bishop. 1989. DNA sequences that mediate attenuation of transcription from the mouse protooncogene myc. *Proc. Natl Acad. Sci. USA* **86**: 505–509.

1093. Wright, S., L. F. Mirels, M. C. Calayag, and J. M. Bishop. 1991. Premature termination of transcription from the P1 promoter of the mouse c-myc gene. *Proc. Natl Acad. Sci. USA* **88**: 11383–11387.

1094. Wright, W. E., D. A. Sassoon, and V. K. Lin. 1989. Myogenin, a factor regulating myogenesis, has a domain homologous to MyoD. *Cell* **56**: 607–617.

1095. Wu, F. Y., N. T. Chang, W. J. Chen, and C. C. Juan. 1993. Vitamin K3-induced cell cycle arrest and apoptotic cell death are accompanied by altered expression of c-fos and c-myc in nasopharyngeal carcinoma cells. *Oncogene* **8**: 2237–2244.

1096. Wu, L. and J. P. J. Whitlock. 1993. Mechanism of dioxin action: receptor–enhancer interactions in intact cells. *Nucleic Acids Res.* **21**: 119–125.

1097. Wyllie, A. H., K. A. Rose, R. G. Morris, C. M. Steel, E. Foster, and D. A. Spandidos. 1987. Rodent fibroblast tumours expressing human myc and ras genes: growth, metastasis and endogenous oncogene expression. *Br. J. Cancer* **56**: 251–259.

1098. Xia, Y., L. Brown, C. Y. Yang, J. T. Tsan, M. J. Siciliano, R. I. I. Espinosa, M. M. Le Beau, and R. J. Baer. 1991. TAL2, a helix–loop–helix gene activated by the (7;9)(q34;q32) translocation in human T-cell leukemia. *Proc. Natl Acad. Sci. USA* **88**: 11416–11420.

1099. Xu, L., S. D. Morgenbesser, and R. A. DePinho. 1991. Complex transcriptional regulation of myc family gene expression in the developing mouse brain and liver. *Mol. Cell Biol.* **11**: 6007–6015.

1100. Xu, L., R. Wallen, V. Patel, and R. A. DePinho. 1993. Role of first exon/intron sequences in the regulation of myc family oncogenic potency. *Oncogene* **8**: 2547–2553.

1101. Yancopoulos, G. D., P. D. Nisen, A. Tesfaye, N. E. Kohl, M. P. Goldfarb, and F. W. Alt. 1985. N-myc can cooperate with ras to transform normal cells in culture. *Proc. Natl Acad. Sci. USA* **82**: 5455–5459.

1102. **Yang, B. S., T. J. Geddes, R. J. Pogulis, B. de Crombrugghe, and S. O. Freytag.** 1991. Transcriptional suppression of cellular gene expression by c-Myc. *Mol. Cell Biol.* **11**: 2291–2295.

1103. **Yang, B. S., J. D. Gilbert, and S. O. Freytag.** 1993. Overexpression of Myc suppresses CCAAT transcription factor/nuclear factor 1-dependent promoters *in vivo*. *Mol. Cell Biol.* **13**: 3093–3102.

1104. **Yang, J., R. Sato, J. L. Golstein, and M. S. Brown.** 1994. Sterol-resistant transcription in CHO cells caused by gene rearrangement that truncates SREBP-2. *Genes Dev.* **8**: 1910–1919.

1105. **Yang, J. Q., S. R. Bauer, J. F. Mushinski, and K. B. Marcu.** 1985. Chromosome translocations clustered 5′ of the murine c-myc gene qualitatively affect promoter usage: implications for the site of normal c-myc regulation. *EMBO J.* **4**: 1441–1447.

1106. **Yano, T., C. A. Sander, H. M. Clark, M. V. Dolezal, E. S. Jaffe, and M. Raffeld.** 1993. Clustered mutations in the second exon of the MYC gene in sporadic Burkitt's lymphoma. *Oncogene* **8**: 2741–2748.

1107. **Yarden, A. and A. Kimchi.** 1986. Tumor necrosis factor reduces c-myc expression and cooperates with interferon-gamma in HeLa cells. *Science* **234**: 1419–1421.

1108. **Yokota, J., Y. Tsunetsugu Yokota, H. Battifora, C. Le Fevre, and M. J. Cline.** 1986. Alterations of myc, myb, and rasHa proto-oncogenes in cancers are frequent and show clinical correlation. *Science* **231**: 261–265.

1109. **Yokoyama, C., X. Wang, M. R. Briggs, A. Admon, J. Wu, X. Hua, J. L. Goldstein, and M. S. Brown.** 1993. SREBP-1, a basic-helix–loop–helix-leucine zipper protein that controls transcription of the low density lipoprotein receptor gene. *Cell* **75**: 187–197.

1110. **Yoon, H. and D. Boettiger.** 1994. Expression of v-src alters the expression of myogenic regulatory factor genes. *Oncogene* **9**: 801–807.

1111. **Yoshida, K., Z. Kuromitsu, N. Ogawa, and Y. Oshima.** 1989. Mode of expression of the positive regulatory genes PHO2 and PHO4 of the phosphatase regulon in *Saccharomyces cerevisiae*. *Mol. Gen. Genet.* **217**: 31–39.

1112. **Yoshida, K., N. Ogawa, and Y. Oshima.** 1989. Function of the PHO regulatory genes for repressible acid phosphatase synthesis in *Saccharomyces cerevisiae*. *Mol. Gen. Genet.* **217**: 40–46.

1113. **Younger Shepherd, S., H. Vaessin, E. Bier, L. Y. Jan, and Y. N. Jan.** 1992. deadpan, an essential pan-neural gene encoding an HLH protein, acts as a denominator in *Drosophila* sex determination. *Cell* **70**: 911–922.

1114. **Yu, Y. T., R. E. Breitbart, L. B. Smoot, Y. Lee, V. Mahdavi, and B. Nadal Ginard.** 1992. Human myocyte-specific enhancer factor 2 comprises a group of tissue-restricted MADS box transcription factors. *Genes Dev.* **6**: 1783–1798.

1115. **Yuh, Y. S. and E. B. Thompson.** 1989. Glucocorticoid effect on oncogene/growth gene expression in human T lymphoblastic leukemic cell line CCRF-CEM. Specific c-myc mRNA suppression by dexamethasone. *J. Biol. Chem.* **264**: 10904–10910.

1116. **Zajac Kaye, M., E. P. Gelmann, and D. Levens.** 1988. A point mutation in the c-myc locus of a Burkitt lymphoma abolishes binding of a nuclear protein. *Science* **240**: 1776–1780.

1117. **Zajac Kaye, M. and D. Levens.** 1990. Phosphorylation-dependent binding of a 138-kDa myc intron factor to a regulatory element in the first intron of the c-myc gene. *J. Biol. Chem.* **265**: 4547–4551.

1118. **Zajac Kaye, M., B. Yu, and N. Ben Baruch.** 1990. Downstream regulatory elements in the c-myc gene. *Curr. Top. Microbiol. Immunol.* **166**: 279–284.

1119. **Zerlin, M., M. A. Julius, C. Cerni, and K. B. Marcu.** 1986. Biological effects of high level c-myc expression in FR3T3 fibroblasts. *Curr. Top. Microbiol. Immunol.* **132**: 320–326.

1120. **Zhang, Y., J. Babin, A. L. Feldhaus, H. Singh, P. A. Sharp, and M. Bina.** 1991. HTF4:a new human helix–loop–helix protein. *Nucleic Acids Res.* **19**: 4555.

1121. **Zhang, Y. and M. Bina.** 1991. Sequence of a HeLa cDNA provides the DNA binding domain and carboxy terminus of HE47:a human helix–loop–helix protein related to the enhancer binding factor E47. *DNA Seq.* **2**: 197–202.

1122. **Zhang, Y., K. Doyle, and M. Bina.** 1992. Interactions of HTF4 with E-box motifs in the long terminal repeat of human immunodeficiency virus type 1. *J. Virol.* **66**: 5631–5634.

1123. **Zhao, G. Q., Q. Zhao, X. Zhou, M. G. Mattei, and B. de Crombrugghe.** 1993. TFEC, a basic helix–loop–helix protein, forms heterodimers with TFE3 and inhibits TFE3-dependent transcription activation. *Mol. Cell Biol.* **13**: 4505–4512.

1124. **Zhuang, Y., C. G. Kim, S. Bartelmez, P. Cheng, M. Groudine, and H. Weintraub.** 1992. Helix–loop–helix transcription factors E12 and E47 are not essential for skeletal or cardiac myogenesis, erythropoiesis, chondrogenesis, or neurogenesis. *Proc. Natl Acad. Sci. USA* **89**: 12132–12136.

1125. **Zimmerman, K., E. Legouy, V. Stewart, R. DePinho, and F. W. Alt.** 1990. Differential regulation of the N-myc gene in transfected cells and transgenic mice. *Mol. Cell Biol.* **10**: 2096–2103.

1126. **Zimmerman, K., J. Shih, J. Bars, A. Collazo, and D. J. Anderson.** 1993. XASH-3, a novel *Xenopus* achaete–scute homolog, provides an early marker of planar neural induction and position along the mediolateral axis of the neural plate. *Development* **119**: 221–232.

1127. **Zimmerman, K. A., G. D. Yancopoulos, R. G. Collum, R. K. Smith, N. E. Kohl, K. A. Denis, M. M. Nau, O. N. Witte, D. Toran Allerand, C. E. Gee** *et al.* 1986. Differential expression of myc family genes during murine development. *Nature* **319**: 780–783.

1128. **Zingg, J-M., G. Pedraza-Alva, and J-P. Jost.** 1994. MyoD1 promoter autoregulation is mediated by two proximal E-boxes. *Nucleic Acids Res.* **22**: 2234–2241.

1129. **Zobel, A., F. Kalkbrenner, S. Guehmann, M. Nawrath, G. Vorbrueggen, and K. Moelling.** 1991. Interaction of the v- and c-Myb proteins with regulatory sequences of the human c-myc gene. *Oncogene* **6**: 1397–1407.

1130. **Zobel, A., F. Kalkbrenner, G. Vorbrueggen, and K. Moelling.** 1992. Transactivation of the human c-myc gene by c-Myb. *Biochem. Biophys. Res. Commun.* **186**: 715–722.

1131. **Zoidl, G., D. Brockmann, and H. Esche.** 1993. Deletion of the beta-turn/alpha-helix motif at the exon 2/3 boundary of human c-Myc leads to the loss of its immortalizing function. *Gene* **131**: 269–274.

1132. **Zwartkruis, F., T. Hoeijmakers, J. Deschamps, and F. Meijlink.** 1991. Characterization of the murine Hox-2.3 promoter: involvement of the transcription factor USF (MLTF). *Mech. Dev.* **33**: 179–190.

Structure/function relationships of HLH proteins

1133. **Anthony Cahill, S. J., P. A. Benfield, R. Fairman, Z. R. Wasserman, S. L. Brenner, W. F. Stafford, C. Altenbach, W. L. Hubbell, and W. F. DeGrado.** 1992. Molecular characterization of helix–loop–helix peptides. *Science* **255**: 979–983.

1134. **Armstrong, K. M. and R. L. Baldwin.** 1993. Charged histidine affects alpha-helix stability at all positions in the helix by interacting with the backbone charges. *Proc. Natl Acad. Sci. USA* **90**: 11337–11340.

1135. **Auer, M., H. U. Gremlich, J. M. Seifert, T. J. Daly, T. G. Parslow, G. Casari, and H. Gstach.** 1994. Helix–loop–helix motif in HIV-1 Rev. *Biochemistry* **33**: 2988–2996.

1136. **Brandt Rauf, P. W., M. R. Pincus, J. M. Chen, and G. Lee.** 1989. Conformational energy analysis of the leucine repeat regions of C/EBP, GCN4, and the proteins of the myc, jun, and fos oncogenes. *J. Protein Chem.* **8**: 679–688.

1137*. **Burley, S. K.** 1994. DNA-binding motifs from eukaryotic transcription factors. *Curr. Opin. Cell Biol.* **4**: 3–11.

1138. **Chakrabartty, A., A. J. Doig, and R. L. Baldwin.** 1993. Helix capping propensities in peptides parallel those in proteins. *Proc. Natl Acad. Sci. USA* **90**: 11332–11336.

1139. **Dong, Q., E. E. Blatter, Y. W. Ebright, K. Bister, and R. H. Ebright.** 1994. Identification of amino acid-base contacts in the Myc-DNA complex by site-specific bromouracil mediated photocrosslinking. *EMBO J.* **13**: 200–204.

1140. **Draeger, L. J. and G. P. Mullen.** 1994. Interaction of the bHLH-zip domain of c-Myc with H1-type peptides. Characterization of helicity in the H1 peptides by NMR. *J. Biol. Chem.* **269**: 1785–1793.

1141*. **Ellenberger, T.** 1994. Getting a grip on DNA recognition: structures of the basic region leucine zipper, and the basic region helix–loop–helix DNA-binding domains. *Curr. Opin. Cell Biol.* **4**: 12–21.

1142*. **Ellenberger, T., D. Fass, M. Arnaud, and S. C. Harrison.** 1994. Crystal structure of transcription factor E**47**:E-box recognition by a basic region helix–loop–helix dimer. *Genes Dev.* **8**: 970–980.

1143*. **Ferre, D. A., P. Pognonec, R. G. Roeder, and S. K. Burley.** 1994. Structure and function of the b/HLH/Z domain of USF. *EMBO J.* **13**: 180–189.

1144*. **Ferre, D. A., G. C. Prendergast, E. B. Ziff, and S. K. Burley.** 1993. Recognition by Max of its cognate DNA through a dimeric b/HLH/Z domain. *Nature* **363**: 38–45.

1145. **Gibson, T. J., J. D. Thompson, and R. A. Abagyan.** 1993. Proposed structure for the DNA-binding domain of the helix–loop–helix family of eukaryotic gene regulatory proteins. *Protein Eng.* **6**: 41–50.

1146. **Halazonetis, T. D. and A. N. Kandil.** 1992. Predicted structural similarities of the DNA binding domains of c-Myc and endonuclease *Eco* RI. *Science* **255**: 464–466.

1147. **Hu, J. C., N. E. Newell, B. Tidor, and R. T. Sauer.** 1993. Probing the roles of residues at the e and g positions of the GCN4 leucine zipper by combinatorial mutagenesis. *Protein Sci.* **2**: 1072–1084.

1148. **Landschulz, W. H., P. F. Johnson, and S. L. McKnight.** 1988. The leucine zipper: a hypothetical structure common to a new class of DNA binding proteins. *Science* **240**: 1759–1764.

1149*. **Ma, P. C. M., M. A. Rould, H. Weintraub, and C. O. Pabo.** 1994. Crystal structure of MyoD bLHL domain-DNA complex: perspectives on DNA recognition and implications for transcriptional activation. *Cell* **77**: 451–459.

1150. **O'Shea, E. K., J. D. Klemm, P. S. Kim, and T. Alber.** 1991. X-ray structure of the GCN4 leucine zipper, a two-stranded, parallel coiled coil. *Science* **254**: 539–544.

1151. **O'Shea, E. K., R. Rutkowski, and P. S. Kim.** 1992. Mechanism of specificity in the Fos–Jun oncoprotein heterodimer. *Cell* **68**: 699–708.

1152. **Phillips, S. E. V.** 1994. Built by association: structure and function of helix–loop–helix DNA binding proteins. *Curr. Opin. Cell Biol.* **2**: 1–4.

1153. **Presta, L. G. and G. D. Rose.** 1988. Helix signals in proteins. *Science* **240**: 1632−1641.

1154*. **Regan, L.** 1993. What determines where alpha-helices begin and end? comment. *Proc. Natl Acad. Sci. USA* **90**: 10907−10908.

1155. **Richardson, J. S. and D. C. Richardson.** 1988. Amino acid preferences for specific locations at the ends of alpha helices [published erratum appears in *Science* 1988 Dec 23; 242(4886): 1624]. *Science* **240**: 1648−1652.

1156. **Starovasnik, M. A., T. K. Blackwell, T. M. Laue, H. Weintraub, and R. E. Klevit.** 1992. Folding topology of the disulfide-bonded dimeric DNA-binding domain of the myogenic determination factor MyoD. *Biochemistry* **31**: 9891−9903.

1157. **Suzuki, M.** 1993. Common features in DNA recognition helices of eukaryotic transcription factors. *EMBO J.* **12**: 3221−3226.

Sequence-specific DNA binding by HLH proteins

1158. **Alex, R., O. Sozeri, S. Meyer, and R. Dildrop.** 1992. Determination of the DNA sequence recognized by the bHLH−zip domain of the N-Myc protein. *Nucleic Acids Res.* **20**: 2257−2263.

1159. **Ariga, H., Y. Imamura, and S. M. Iguchi Ariga.** 1989. DNA replication origin and transcriptional enhancer in c-myc gene share the c-myc protein binding sequences. *EMBO J.* **8**: 4273−4279.

1160. **Bendall, A. J. and P. L. Molloy.** 1994. Base preferences for DNA binding by the bHLH-Zip protein USF: effects of $MgCl_2$ on specificity and comparison with binding of Myc family members. *Nucleic Acids Res.* **22**: 2801−2810.

1161. **Billaud, M., K. J. Isselbacher, and R. Bernards.** 1993. A dominant-negative mutant of Max that inhibits sequence-specific DNA binding by Myc proteins. *Proc. Natl Acad. Sci. USA* **90**: 2739−2743.

1162. **Blackwell, T. K., J. Huang, A. Ma, L. Kretzner, F. W. Alt, R. N. Eisenman, and H. Weintraub.** 1993. Binding of myc proteins to canonical and noncanonical DNA sequences. *Mol. Cell Biol.* **13**: 5216−5224.

1163. **Blackwell, T. K., L. Kretzner, E. M. Blackwood, R. N. Eisenman, and H. Weintraub.** 1990. Sequence-specific DNA binding by the c-Myc protein. *Science* **250**: 1149−1151.

1164*. **Blackwell, T. K. and H. Weintraub.** 1990. Differences and similarities in DNA-binding preferences of MyoD and E2A protein complexes revealed by binding site selection. *Science* **250**: 1104−1110.

1165. **Brown, L. and R. Baer.** 1994. HEN1 Encodes a 20-kilodalton phosphoprotein that binds an extended E-box motif as a homodimer. *Mol. Cell Biol.* **14**: 1245−1255.

1166. **Chakraborty, T. and E. N. Olson.** 1991. Domains outside of the DNA-binding domain impart target gene specificity to myogenin and MRF4. *Mol. Cell Biol.* **11**: 6103−6108.

1167. **Dang, C. V., H. van Dam, M. Buckmire, and W. M. Lee.** 1989. DNA-binding domain of human c-Myc produced in *Escherichia coli. Mol. Cell Biol.* **9**: 2477−2486.

1168. **Davis, R. L., P. F. Cheng, A. B. Lassar, M. Thayer, S. Tapscott, and H. Weintraub.** 1989. MyoD and achaete−scute: 4−5 amino acids distinguishes myogenesis from neurogenesis. *Int. Symp. Princess Takamatsu Cancer Res. Fund.* **20**: 267−278.

1169. **Davis, R. L., P. F. Cheng, A. B. Lassar, and H. Weintraub.** 1990. The MyoD DNA binding domain contains a recognition code for muscle-specific gene activation. *Cell* **60**: 733−746.

1170*. **Davis, R. L. and H. Weintraub.** 1992. Acquisition of myogenic specificity by replacement of three amino acid residues from MyoD into E12. *Science* **256**: 1027−1030.

1171. **Du, H., A. L. Roy, and R. G. Roeder.** 1993. Human transcription factor USF stimulates transcription through the initiator elements of the HIV-1 and the Ad-ML promoters. *EMBO J.* **12**: 501−511.

1172. **Feldmann, T., R. Alex, J. Suckow, R. Dildrop, B. Kisters Woike, and B. Muller Hill.** 1993. Single exchanges of amino acids in the basic region change the specificity of N-Myc. *Nucleic Acids Res.* **21**: 5050−5058.

1173. **Fisher, D. E., L. A. Parent, and P. A. Sharp.** 1992. Myc/Max and other helix−loop−helix/leucine zipper proteins bend DNA toward the minor groove. *Proc. Natl Acad. Sci. USA* **89**: 11779−11783.

1174. **Fisher, D. E., L. A. Parent, and P. A. Sharp.** 1993. High affinity DNA-binding Myc analogs: recognition by an alpha helix. *Cell* **72**: 467−476.

1175. **Fisher, F., D. H. Crouch, P. S. Jayaraman, W. Clark, D. A. Gillespie, and C. R. Goding.** 1993. Transcription activation by Myc and Max: flanking sequences target activation to a subset of CACGTG motifs *in vivo. EMBO J.* **12**: 5075−5082.

1176*. **Fisher, F. and C. R. Goding.** 1992. Single amino acid substitutions alter helix−loop−helix protein specificity for bases flanking the core CANNTG motif. *EMBO J.* **11**: 4103−4109.

1177. **Fisher, F., P. S. Jayaraman, and C. R. Goding.** 1991. C-myc and the yeast transcription factor PHO4 share a common CACGTG-binding motif. *Oncogene* **6**: 1099−1104.

1178. **French, B. A., K. L. Chow, E. N. Olson, and R. J. Schwartz.** 1991. Heterodimers of myogenic helix−loop−helix regulatory factors and E12 bind a complex element governing myogenic induction of the avian cardiac alpha-actin promoter. *Mol. Cell Biol.* **11**: 2439−2450.

1179. **Halazonetis, T. D. and A. N. Kandil.** 1991. Determination of the c-MYC DNA-binding site. *Proc. Natl Acad. Sci. USA* **88**: 6162−6166.

1180. **Hsu, H. L., J. T. Cheng, Q. Chen, and R. Baer.** 1991. Enhancer-binding activity of the tal-1 oncoprotein in association with the E47/E12 helix−loop−helix proteins. *Mol. Cell Biol.* **11**: 3037−3042.

1181. **Hsu, H. L., L. Huang, J. T. Tsan, W. Funk, W. E. Wright, J. S. Hu, R. E. Kingston, and R. Baer.** 1994. Preferred sequences for DNA recognition by the TAL1 helix−loop−helix proteins. *Mol. Cell Biol.* **14**: 1256−1265.

1182. **Johnson, J. E., S. J. Birren, T. Saito, and D. J. Anderson.** 1992. DNA binding and transcriptional regulatory activity of mammalian achaete−scute homologous (MASH) proteins revealed by interaction with a muscle-specific enhancer. *Proc. Natl Acad. Sci. USA* **89**: 3596−3600.

1183. **Kato, G. J., D. S. Wechsler, and C. V. Dang.** 1992. DNA binding by the Myc oncoproteins. *Cancer Treat. Res.* **63**: 313−325.

1184. **Kerkhoff, E., K. Bister, and K. H. Klempnauer.** 1991. Sequence-specific DNA binding by Myc proteins. *Proc. Natl Acad. Sci. USA* **88**: 4323−4327.

1185. **Kurihara, Y., M. Horiuchi, S. Ukita, M. Katahira, and S. Uesugi.** 1993. DNA binding properties of c-Myc-related bHLH/LZ oncoproteins. *Nucleic Acids Symp. Ser.* 169−170.

1186. **Littlewood, T. D., B. Amati, H. Land, and G. I. Evan.** 1992. Max and c-Myc/Max DNA-binding activities in cell extracts. *Oncogene* **7**: 1783−1792.

1187. **Lorenz, U., E. Sock, F. Grummt, and K. Moelling.** 1991. Analysis of DNA sequences present in complexes of v-Myc and cellular DNA. *Oncogene* **6**: 51−57.

1188. **Ma, A., T. Moroy, R. Collum, H. Weintraub, F. W. Alt, and T. K. Blackwell.** 1993. DNA binding by N- and L-Myc proteins. *Oncogene* **8**: 1093−1098.

1189. **Metz, R. and E. Ziff.** 1991. The helix−loop−helix protein rE12 and the C/EBP-related factor rNFIL-6 bind to neighboring sites within the c-fos serum response element. *Oncogene* **6**: 2165−2178.

1190. **Moelling, K., T. Sander, U. Lorenz, P. Beimling, and H. Bading.** 1986. Interaction of the oncogene protein myc with specific DNA fragments. *J. Cancer Res. Clin. Oncol.* **112**: 97−99.

1191. **Negishi, Y., S. M. Iguchi Ariga, and H. Ariga.** 1992. Protein complexes bearing myc-like antigenicity recognize two distinct DNA sequences. *Oncogene* **7**: 543−548.

1192. **Niedenthal, R., R. Stoll, and J. H. Hegemann.** 1991. *In vivo* characterization of the *Saccharomyces cerevisiae* centromere DNA element I, a binding site for the helix−loop− helix protein CPF1. *Mol. Cell Biol.* **11**: 3545−3553.

1193. **Nielsen, A. L., N. Pallisgaard, F. S. Pedersen, and P. Jorgensen.** 1992. Murine helix−loop−helix transcriptional activator proteins binding to the E-box motif of the Akv murine leukemia virus enhancer identified by cDNA cloning. *Mol. Cell Biol.* **12**: 3449−3459.

1194. **Papoulas, O., N. G. Williams, and R. E. Kingston.** 1992. DNA binding activities of c-Myc purified from eukaryotic cells. *J. Biol. Chem.* **267**: 10470−10480.

1195. **Piette, J., J. L. Bessereau, M. Huchet, and J. P. Changeux.** 1990. Two adjacent MyoD1-binding sites regulate expression of the acetylcholine receptor alpha-subunit gene. *Nature* **345**: 353−355.

1196. **Potter, J. J., D. Cheneval, C. V. Dang, L. M. Resar, E. Mezey, and V. W. Yang.** 1991. The upstream stimulatory factor binds to and activates the promoter of the rat class I alcohol dehydrogenase gene. *J. Biol. Chem.* **266**: 15457−15463.

1197. **Prendergast, G. C. and E. B. Ziff.** 1991. Methylation-sensitive sequence-specific DNA binding by the c-Myc basic region. *Science* **251**: 186−189.

1198*. **Prochownik, E. V. and M. E. VanAntwerp.** 1993. Differential patterns of DNA binding by myc and max proteins. *Proc. Natl Acad. Sci. USA* **90**: 960−964.

1199. **Ramsay, G., L. Stanton, M. Schwab, and J. M. Bishop.** 1986. Human proto-oncogene N-myc encodes nuclear proteins that bind DNA. *Mol. Cell Biol.* **6**: 4450−4457.

1200. **Ronen, D., V. Rotter, and D. Reisman.** 1991. Expression from the murine p53 promoter is mediated by factor binding to a downstream helix−loop−helix recognition motif. *Proc. Natl Acad. Sci. USA* **88**: 4128−4132.

1201. **Roth, B. A., S. A. Goff, T. M. Klein, and M. E. Fromm.** 1991. C1- and R-dependent expression of the maize Bz1 gene requires sequences with homology to mammalian myb and myc binding sites. *Plant Cell* **3**: 317−325.

1202. **Sirito, M., S. Walker, Q. Lin, M. T. Kozlowski, W. H. Klein, and M. Sawadogo.** 1992. Members of the USF family of helix−loop−helix proteins bind DNA as homo- as well as heterodimers. *Gene Expr.* **2**: 231−240.

1203. **Solomon, D. L., B. Amati, and H. Land.** 1993. Distinct DNA binding preferences for the c-Myc/Max and Max/Max dimers. *Nucleic Acids Res.* **21**: 5372−5376.

1204. **Sun, X. H., N. G. Copeland, N. A. Jenkins, and D. Baltimore.** 1991. Id proteins Id1 and Id2 selectively inhibit DNA binding by one class of helix−loop−helix proteins. *Mol. Cell Biol.* **11**: 5603−5611.

1205. **Taira, T., Y. Negishi, F. Kihara, S. M. Iguchi Ariga, and H. Ariga.** 1992. c-myc protein complex binds to two sites in human hsp70 promoter region. *Biochim. Biophys. Acta* **1130**: 166−174.

1206. **Thayer, M. J. and H. Weintraub.** 1993. A cellular factor stimulates the DNA-binding activity of MyoD and E47. *Proc. Natl Acad. Sci. USA* **90**: 6483−6487.

1207. **Van Antwerp, M. E., D. G. Chen, C. Chang, and E. V. Prochownik.** 1992. A point mutation in the MyoD basic domain imparts c-Myc-like properties. *Proc. Natl Acad. Sci. USA* **89**: 9010−9014.

1208. **Van Doren, M., H. M. Ellis, and J. W. Posakony.** 1991. The *Drosophila* extramacrochaetae protein antagonizes sequence-specific DNA binding by daughterless/achaete−scute protein complexes. *Development* **113**: 245−255.

1209. **Walsh, K. and A. Gualberto.** 1992. MyoD binds to the guanine tetrad nucleic acid structure. *J. Biol. Chem.* **267**: 13714−13718.

1210. **Wechsler, D. S. and C. V. Dang.** 1992. Opposite orientations of DNA bending by c-Myc and Max. *Proc. Natl Acad. Sci. USA* **89**: 7635−7639.

1211. **Weintraub, H., R. Davis, D. Lockshon, and A. Lassar.** 1990. MyoD binds cooperatively to two sites in a target enhancer sequence: occupancy of two sites is required for activation. *Proc. Natl Acad. Sci. USA* **87**: 5623−5627.

1212. **Wentworth, B. M., M. Donoghue, J. C. Engert, E. B. Berglund, and N. Rosenthal.** 1991. Paired MyoD-binding sites regulate myosin light chain gene expression. *Proc. Natl Acad. Sci. USA* **88**: 1242−1246.

Dimerization partners

1213. **Amati, B., S. Dalton, M. W. Brooks, T. D. Littlewood, G. I. Evan, and H. Land.** 1992. Transcriptional activation by the human c-Myc oncoprotein in yeast requires interaction with Max. *Nature* **359**: 423−426.

1214. **Ayer, D. E., L. Kretzner, and R. N. Eisenman.** 1993. Mad: a heterodimeric partner for Max that antagonizes Myc transcriptional activity. *Cell* **72**: 211−222.

1215*. **Beckmann, H. and T. Kadesch.** 1991. The leucine zipper of TFE3 dictates helix−loop−helix dimerization specificity. *Genes Dev.* **5**: 1057−1066.

1216. **Bengal, E., L. Ransone, R. Scharfmann, V. J. Dwarki, S. J. Tapscott, H. Weintraub, and I. M. Verma.** 1992. Functional antagonism between c-Jun and MyoD proteins: a direct physical association. *Cell* **68**: 507−519.

1217. **Blackwood, E. M., B. Luscher, and R. N. Eisenman.** 1992. Myc and Max associate *in vivo*. *Genes Dev.* **6**: 71−80.

1218. **Blanar, M. A. and W. J. Rutter.** 1992. Interaction cloning: identification of a helix−loop−helix zipper protein that interacts with c-Fos. *Science* **256**: 1014−1018.

1219. **Braun, T. and H. H. Arnold.** 1991. The four human muscle regulatory helix−loop−helix proteins Myf3− Myf6 exhibit similar hetero-dimerization and DNA binding properties. *Nucleic Acids Res.* **19**: 5645−5651.

1220. **Braun, T., K. Gearing, W. E. Wright, and H. H. Arnold.** 1991. Baculovirus-expressed myogenic determination factors require E12 complex formation for binding to the myosin-light-chain enhancer. *Eur. J. Biochem.* **198**: 187−193.

1221*. **Cabrera, C. V. and M. C. Alonso.** 1991. Transcriptional activation by heterodimers of the achaete−scute and daughterless gene products of *Drosophila*. *EMBO J.* **10**: 2965−2973.

1222. **Chakraborty, T., T. J. Brennan, L. Li, D. Edmondson, and E. N. Olson.** 1991. Inefficient homooligomerization contributes to the dependence of myogenin on E2A products for efficient DNA binding. *Mol. Cell Biol.* **11**: 3633−3641.

1223. **Chakraborty, T., J. F. Martin, and E. N. Olson.** 1992. Analysis of the oligomerization of myogenin and E2A products *in vivo* using a two-hybrid assay system. *J. Biol. Chem.* **267**: 17498−17501.

1224. **Corneliussen, B., M. Holm, Y. Waltersson, J. Onions, B. Hallberg, A. Thornell, and T. Grundstrom.** 1994. Calcium/calmodulin inhibition of basic-helix−loop−helix transcription factor domains. *Nature* **368**: 760−764.

1225. **Dang, C. V., J. Barrett, M. Villa Garcia, L. M. Resar, G. J. Kato, and E. R. Fearon.** 1991. Intracellular leucine zipper interactions suggest c-Myc hetero-oligomerization. *Mol. Cell Biol.* **11**: 954−962.

1226. **Fairman, R., R. K. Beran Steed, S. J. Anthony Cahill, J. D. Lear, W. F. Stafford, W. F. DeGrado, P. A. Benfield, and S. L. Brenner.** 1993. Multiple oligomeric states regulate the DNA binding of helix−loop−helix peptides. *Proc. Natl Acad. Sci. USA* **90**: 10429−10433.

1227. **Finkel, T., J. Duc, E. R. Fearon, C. V. Dang, and G. F. Tomaselli.** 1993. Detection and modulation *in vivo* of helix−loop−helix protein−protein interactions. *J. Biol. Chem.* **268**: 5−8.

1228. **Funk, W. D. and W. E. Wright.** 1992. Cyclic amplification and selection of targets for multicomponent complexes: myogenin interacts with factors recognizing binding sites for basic helix−loop−helix, nuclear factor 1, myocyte-specific enhancer-binding factor 2, and COMP1 factor. *Proc. Natl Acad. Sci. USA* **89**: 9484−9488.

1229. **Gillespie, D. A. and R. N. Eisenman.** 1989. Detection of a Myc-associated protein by chemical cross-linking. *Mol. Cell Biol.* **9**: 865−868.

1230*. **Gu, W., K. Bhatia, I. T. Magrath, C. V. Dang, and R. Dalla-Favera.** 1994. Binding and suppression of the Myc transcriptional activation domain by p107. *Science* **264**: 251−254.

1231. **Hainzl, T. and T. Boehm.** 1994. A versatile expression vector for the *in vitro* study of protein—protein interactions: characterization of E47 mutant proteins. *Oncogene* **9**: 885—891.

1232. **Hateboer, G., H. T. Timmers, A. K. Rustgi, M. Billaud, L. J. van't Veer, and R. Bernards.** 1993. TATA-binding protein and the retinoblastoma gene product bind to overlapping epitopes on c-Myc and adenovirus E1A protein. *Proc. Natl Acad. Sci. USA* **90**: 8489—8493.

1233. **Hsu, H. L., I. Wadman, and R. Baer.** 1994. Formation of *in vivo* complexes between the TAL1 and E2A polypeptides of leukemic T cells. *Proc. Natl Acad. Sci. USA* **91**: 3181—3185.

1234*. **Hu, Y. F., B. Luscher, A. Admon, N. Mermod, and R. Tjian.** 1990. Transcription factor AP-4 contains multiple dimerization domains that regulate dimer specificity. *Genes Dev.* **4**: 1741—1752.

1235. **Koskinen, P. J., T. P. Makela, I. Vastrik, and K. Alitalo.** 1993. Myc amplification: regulation of myc function. *Clin. Chim. Acta* **217**: 57—62.

1236*. **Lassar, A. B., R. L. Davis, W. E. Wright, T. Kadesch, C. Murre, A. Voronova, D. Baltimore, and H. Weintraub.** 1991. Functional activity of myogenic HLH proteins requires hetero-oligomerization with E12/E47-like proteins *in vivo*. *Cell* **66**: 305—315.

1237. **Lin, H. and S. F. Konieczny.** 1992. Identification of MRF4, myogenin, and E12 oligomer complexes by chemical cross-linking and two-dimensional gel electrophoresis. *J. Biol. Chem.* **267**: 4773—4780.

1238. **Lin, H., K. E. Yutzey, and S. F. Konieczny.** 1991. Muscle-specific expression of the troponin I gene requires interactions between helix—loop—helix muscle regulatory factors and ubiquitous transcription factors. *Mol. Cell Biol.* **11**: 267—280.

1239*. **Maheswaran, S., H. Lee, and G. E. Sonenshein.** 1994. Intracellular association of the protein product of the c-myc oncogene with the TATA-binding protein. *Mol. Cell Biol.* **14**: 1147—1152.

1240. **Marx, J.** 1990. Partner found for the myc protein. *Science* **249**: 1503—1504.

1241. **Min, S., N. T. Mascarenhas, and E. J. Taparowsky.** 1993. Functional analysis of the carboxy-terminal transforming region of v-Myc: binding to Max is necessary, but not sufficient, for cellular transformation. *Oncogene* **8**: 2691—2701.

1242*. **Murre, C., P. S. McCaw, H. Vaessin, M. Caudy, L. Y. Jan, Y. N. Jan, C. V. Cabrera, J. N. Buskin, S. D. Hauschka, A. B. Lassar** *et al.* 1989. Interactions between heterologous helix—loop—helix proteins generate complexes that bind specifically to a common DNA sequence. *Cell* **58**: 537—544.

1243. **Neuhold, L. A. and B. Wold.** 1993. HLH forced dimers: tethering MyoD to E47 generates a dominant positive myogenic factor insulated from negative regulation by Id. *Cell* **74**: 1033—1042.

1244. **Prendergast, G. C., D. Lawe, and E. B. Ziff.** 1991. Association of Myn, the murine homolog of max, with c-Myc stimulates methylation-sensitive DNA binding and ras cotransformation. *Cell* **65**: 395—407.

1245. **Rashbass, J., M. V. Taylor, and J. B. Gurdon.** 1992. The DNA-binding protein E12 co-operates with XMyoD in the activation of muscle-specific gene expression in *Xenopus* embryos. *EMBO J.* **11**: 2981—2990.

1246. **Roy, A. L., M. Meisterernst, P. Pognonec, and R. G. Roeder.** 1991. Cooperative interaction of an initiator-binding transcription initiation factor and the helix—loop—helix activator USF. *Nature* **354**: 245—248.

1247. **Rustgi, A. K., N. Dyson, and R. Bernards.** 1991. Amino-terminal domains of c-myc and N-myc proteins mediate binding to the retinoblastoma gene product. *Nature* **352**: 541—544.

1248. **Rustgi, A. K., N. Dyson, D. Hill, and R. Bernards.** 1991. The c-myc oncoprotein forms a specific complex with the product of the retinoblastoma gene. *Cold Spring Harb. Symp. Quant. Biol.* **56**: 163—167.

1249*. **Shirakata, M., F. K. Friedman, Q. Wei, and B. M. Paterson.** 1993. Dimerization specificity of myogenic helix—loop—helix DNA-binding factors directed by nonconserved hydrophilic residues. *Genes Dev.* **7**: 2456—2470.

1250. **Shrivastava, A., S. Saleque, G. V. Kalpana, S. Artandi, S. P. Goff, and K. Calame.** 1993. Inhibition of transcriptional regulator Yin-Yang-1 by association with c-Myc. *Science* **262**: 1889—1892.

1251. **Staudinger, J., M. Perry, S. J. Elledge, and E. N. Olson.** 1993. Interactions among vertebrate helix—loop—helix proteins in yeast using the two-hybrid system. *J. Biol. Chem.* **268**: 4608—4611.

1252. **Studzinski, G. P., U. T. Shankavaram, D. C. Moore, and P. V. Reddy.** 1991. Association of c-myc protein with enzymes of DNA replication in high molecular weight fractions from mammalian cells. *J. Cell Physiol.* **147**: 412—419.

1253. **Taylor, D. A., V. B. Kraus, J. J. Schwarz, E. N. Olson, and W. E. Kraus.** 1993. E1A-mediated inhibition of myogenesis correlates with a direct physical interaction of E1A12S and basic helix—loop—helix proteins. *Mol. Cell Biol.* **13**: 4714—4727.

1254. **Tikhonenko, A. T., A. R. Hartman, and M. L. Linial.** 1993. Overproduction of v-Myc in the nucleus and its excess over Max are not required for avian fibroblast transformation. *Mol. Cell Biol.* **13**: 3623—3631.

1255. **Voronova, A. F. and F. Lee.** 1994. The E2A and tal-1 helix−loop−helix proteins associate *in vivo* and are modulated by Id proteins during interleukin 6-induced myeloid differentiation. *Proc. Natl Acad. Sci. USA* **91**: 5952−5956.

1256. **Wenzel, A., C. Cziepluch, U. Hamann, J. Schurmann, and M. Schwab.** 1991. The N-Myc oncoprotein is associated *in vivo* with the phosphoprotein Max(p20/22) in human neuroblastoma cells. *EMBO J.* **10**: 3703−3712.

1257. **Zervos, A. S., J. Gyuris, and R. Brent.** 1993. Mxi1, a protein that specifically interacts with Max to bind Myc−Max recognition sites. *Cell* **72**: 223−232.

Post-transcriptional regulation of the activity of HLH proteins

1258. **Albert, T., B. Urlbauer, F. Kohlhuber, B. Hammersen, and D. Eick.** 1994. Ongoing mutations in the N-terminal domain of c-Myc affect transactivation in Burkitt's lymphoma cell lines. *Oncogene* **9**: 759−763.

1259. **Alvarez, E., I. C. Northwood, F. A. Gonzalez, D. A. Latour, A. Seth, C. Abate, T. Curran, and R. J. Davis.** 1991. Pro-Leu-Ser/Thr-Pro is a consensus primary sequence for substrate protein phosphorylation. Characterization of the phosphorylation of c-myc and c-jun proteins by an epidermal growth factor receptor threonine 669 protein kinase. *J. Biol. Chem.* **266**: 15277−15285.

1260. **Berberich, S. J. and M. D. Cole.** 1992. Casein kinase II inhibits the DNA-binding activity of Max homodimers but not Myc/Max heterodimers. *Genes Dev.* **6**: 166−176.

1261. **Bhatia, K., K. Huppi, G. Spangler, D. Siwarski, R. Iyer, and I. Magrath.** 1993. Point mutations in the c-Myc transactivation domain are common in Burkitt's lymphoma and mouse plasmacytomas. *Nat. Genet.* **5**: 56−61.

1262. **Bousset, K., M. Henriksson, J. M. Luscher Firzlaff, D. W. Litchfield, and B. Luscher.** 1993. Identification of casein kinase II phosphorylation sites in Max: effects on DNA-binding kinetics of Max homo- and Myc/Max heterodimers. *Oncogene* **8**: 3211−3220.

1263. **Bustelo, X. R. and M. Barbacid.** 1992. Tyrosine phosphorylation of the vav proto-oncogene product in activated B cells. *Science* **256**: 1196−1199.

1264. **Bustelo, X. R., J. A. Ledbetter, and M. Barbacid.** 1992. Product of vav proto-oncogene defines a new class of tyrosine protein kinase substrates. *Nature* **356**: 68−71.

1265. **Cheng, J. T., H. L. Hsu, L. Y. Hwang, and R. Baer.** 1993. Products of the TAL1 oncogene: basic helix−loop−helix proteins phosphorylated at serine residues. *Oncogene* **8**: 677−683.

1266. **Dosaka Akita, H., R. K. Rosenberg, J. D. Minna, and M. J. Birrer.** 1991. A complex pattern of translational initiation and phosphorylation in L-myc proteins. *Oncogene* **6**: 371−378.

1267. **Gupta, S., A. Seth, and R. J. Davis.** 1993. Transactivation of gene expression by Myc is inhibited by mutation at the phosphorylation sites Thr-58 and Ser-62. *Proc. Natl Acad. Sci. USA* **90**: 3216−3220.

1268. **Hagiwara, T., K. Nakaya, Y. Nakamura, H. Nakajima, S. Nishimura, and Y. Taya.** 1992. Specific phosphorylation of the acidic central region of the N-myc protein by casein kinase II. *Eur. J. Biochem.* **209**: 945−950.

1269. **Hamann, U., A. Wenzel, R. Frank, and M. Schwab.** 1991. The MYCN protein of human neuroblastoma cells is phosphorylated by casein kinase II in the central region and at serine 367. *Oncogene* **6**: 1745−1751.

1270. **Henriksson, M., A. Bakardjiev, G. Klein, and B. Luscher.** 1993. Phosphorylation sites mapping in the N-terminal domain of c-myc modulate its transforming potential. *Oncogene* **8**: 3199−3209.

1271. **Iijima, S., H. Teraoka, T. Date, and K. Tsukada.** 1992. DNA-activated protein kinase in Raji Burkitt's lymphoma cells. Phosphorylation of c-Myc oncoprotein. *Eur. J. Biochem.* **206**: 595−603.

1272. **Johnston, J. M., M. T. Yu, and W. L. Carroll.** 1991. c-myc hypermutation is ongoing in endemic, but not all Burkitt's lymphoma. *Blood* **78**: 2419−2425.

1273. **Kaffman, A., I. Herskowitz, R. Tjian, and E. K. O'Shea.** 1994. Phosphorylation of the transcription factor PHO4 by a cyclin−CDK complex, PHO80-PHO85. *Science* **263**: 1153−1156.

1274. **Koskinen, P. J., I. Vastrik, T. P. Makela, R. N. Eisenman, and K. Alitalo.** 1994. Max activity is affected by phosphorylation at two NH_2-terminal sites. *Cell Growth Differ.* **5**: 313−320.

1275. **Li, L., R. Heller Harrison, M. Czech, and E. N. Olson.** 1992. Cyclic AMP-dependent protein kinase inhibits the activity of myogenic helix−loop−helix proteins. *Mol. Cell Biol.* **12**: 4478−4485.

1276. **Li, L., J. Zhou, G. James, R. Heller Harrison, M. P. Czech, and E. N. Olson.** 1992. FGF inactivates myogenic helix−loop−helix proteins through phosphorylation of a conserved protein kinase C site in their DNA-binding domains. *Cell* **71**: 1181−1194.

1277. **Luscher, B. and R. N. Eisenman.** 1992. Mitosis-specific phosphorylation of the nuclear oncoproteins Myc and Myb. *J. Cell Biol.* **118**: 775−784.

1278. **Luscher, B., E. A. Kuenzel, E. G. Krebs, and R. N. Eisenman.** 1989. Myc oncoproteins are phosphorylated by casein kinase II. *EMBO J.* **8**: 1111−1119.

1279*. **Lutterbach, B. and S. R. Hann.** 1994. Hierarchical phosphorylation at N-terminal transformation-sensitive sites in c-Myc protein is regulated by mitogens and in mitosis. *Mol. Cell Biol.* **14**: 5510–5522.

1280. **Maheswaran, S., J. E. McCormack, and G. E. Sonenshein.** 1991. Changes in phosphorylation of myc oncogene and RB antioncogene protein products during growth arrest of the murine lymphoma WEHI 231 cell line. *Oncogene* **6**: 1965–1971.

1281. **Margolis, B., P. Hu, S. Katzav, W. Li, J. M. Oliver, A. Ullrich, A. Weiss, and J. Schlessinger.** 1992. Tyrosine phosphorylation of vav proto-oncogene product containing SH2 domain and transcription factor motifs. *Nature* **356**: 71–74.

1282. **Mitsui, K., M. Shirakata, and B. M. Paterson.** 1993. Phosphorylation inhibits the DNA-binding activity of MyoD homodimers but not MyoD-E12 heterodimers. *J. Biol. Chem.* **268**: 24415–24420.

1283. **Pognonec, P., H. Kato, and R. G. Roeder.** 1992. The helix–loop–helix/leucine repeat transcription factor USF can be functionally regulated in a redox-dependent manner. *J. Biol. Chem.* **267**: 24563–24567.

1284. **Pulverer, B. J., C. Fisher, K. Vousden, T. Littlewood, G. Evan, and J. R. Woodgett.** 1994. Site-specific modulation of c-Myc cotransformation by residues phosphorylated *in vivo*. *Oncogene* **9**: 59–70.

1285. **Ramsay, G., M. J. Hayman, and K. Bister.** 1982. Phosphorylation of specific sites in the gag–myc polyproteins encoded by MC29-type viruses correlates with their transforming ability. *EMBO J.* **1**: 1111–1116.

1286. **Saksela, K., T. P. Makela, G. Evan, and K. Alitalo.** 1989. Rapid phosphorylation of the L-myc protein induced by phorbol ester tumor promoters and serum. *EMBO J.* **8**: 149–157.

1287. **Saksela, K., T. P. Makela, K. Hughes, J. R. Woodgett, and K. Alitalo.** 1992. Activation of protein kinase C increases phosphorylation of the L-myc trans-activator domain at a GSK-3 target site. *Oncogene* **7**: 347–353.

1288. **Seth, A., E. Alvarez, S. Gupta, and R. J. Davis.** 1991. A phosphorylation site located in the NH_2-terminal domain of c-Myc increases transactivation of gene expression. *J. Biol. Chem.* **266**: 23521–23524.

1289*. **Seth, A., S. Gupta, and R. J. Davis.** 1993. Cell cycle regulation of the c-Myc transcriptional activation domain. *Mol. Cell Biol.* **13**: 4125–4136.

1290. **Street, A. J., E. Blackwood, B. Luscher, and R. N. Eisenman.** 1990. Mutational analysis of the carboxy-terminal casein kinase II phosphorylation site in human c-myc. *Curr. Top. Microbiol. Immunol.* **166**: 251–258.

1291. **Vandromme, M., G. Carnac, C. Gauthier-Rouviere, D. Fesquet, N. Lamb, and A. Fernandez.** 1994. Nuclear import of the myogenic factor MyoD requires cAMP-dependent protein kinase activity but not the direct phosphorylation of MyoD. *J. Cell Sci.* **107**: 613–620.

1292. **Winter, B., T. Braun, and H. H. Arnold.** 1993. cAMP-dependent protein kinase represses myogenic differentiation and the activity of the muscle-specific helix–loop–helix transcription factors Myf-5 and MyoD. *J. Biol. Chem.* **268**: 9869–9878.

1293. **Xia, Y., L. -Y. Hwang, M. H. Cobb, and R. Baer.** 1994. Products of the TAL2 oncogene in leukemic T cells: bHLH phosphoproteins with DNA-binding activity. *Oncogene* **9**: 1437–1446.

1294*. **Zhou, J. and E. N. Olson.** 1994. Dimerization through the helix–loop–helix motif enhances phosphorylation of the transcription activation domains of myogenin. *Mol. Cell Biol.* **14**: 6232–6243.

New references for third edition

Reviews

1295. **Adams, J. M. and S. Cory.** 1991. Transgenic models for haemopoietic malignancies. *Biochim. Biophys. Acta.* **1072**: 9–31.

1296. **Bernards, R.** 1995. Transcriptional regulation. Flipping the Myc switch. *Curr. Biol.* **5**: 859–861.

1297. **Berns, A., N. van der Lugt, M. Alkema, M. van Lohuizen, J. Domen, D. Acton, J. Allen, P. W. Laird, and J. Jonkers.** 1994. Mouse model systems to study multistep tumorigenesis. *Cold. Spring. Harb. Symp. Quant. Biol.* **59**: 435–447.

1298. **Buckingham, M.** 1994. Muscle differentiation. Which myogenic factors make muscle? *Curr. Biol.* **4**: 61–63.

1299. **Cross, F.** 1995. Transcriptional regulation by a cyclin–cdk. *Trends. Genet.* **11**: 209–211.

1300. **Dias, P., M. Dilling, and P. Houghton.** 1994. The molecular basis of skeletal muscle differentiation. *Semin. Diagn. Pathol.* **11**: 3–14.

1301. **Eisenman, R. N. and J. A. Cooper.** 1995. Signal transduction. Beating a path to Myc. *Nature* **378**: 438–439.

1302. **Evan, G., E. Harrington, A. Fanidi, H. Land, B. Amati, and M. Bennett.** 1994. Integrated control of cell proliferation and cell death by the c-myc oncogene. *Philos. Trans. R. Soc. Lond. B. Biol. Sci.* **345**: 269–275.

1303. **Hankinson, O.** 1993. Research on the aryl hydrocarbon (dioxin) receptor is primed to take off. *Arch. Biochem. Biophys.* **300**: 1−5.

1304. **Hankinson, O.** 1995. The aryl hydrocarbon receptor complex. *Annu. Rev. Pharmacol. Toxicol.* **35**: 307−340.

1305. **Hoffman, B., D. A. Liebermann, M. Selvakumaran, and H. Q. Nguyen.** 1996. Role of c-myc in myeloid differentiation, growth arrest and apoptosis. *Curr. Top. Microbiol. Immunol.* **211**: 17−27.

1306. **Hurlin, P. J., D. E. Ayer, C. Grandori, and R. N. Eisenman.** 1994. The Max transcription factor network: involvement of Mad in differentiation and an approach to identification of target genes. *Cold. Spring. Harb. Symp. Quant. Biol.* **59**: 109−116.

1307. **Kageyama, R., Y. Sasai, C. Akazawa, M. Ishibashi, K. Takebayashi, C. Shimizu, K. Tomita, and S. Nakanishi.** 1995. Regulation of mammalian neural development by helix−loop−helix transcription factors. *Crit. Rev. Neurobiol.* **9**: 177−188.

1308. **Krause, M.** 1995. MyoD and myogenesis in *C. elegans*. *Bioessays* **17**: 219−228.

1309. **Moore, K. J.** 1995. Insight into the microphthalmia gene. *Trends. Genet.* **11**: 442−448.

1310. **Morgenbesser, S. D. and R. A. DePinho.** 1994. Use of transgenic mice to study myc family gene function in normal mammalian development and in cancer. *Semin. Cancer. Biol.* **5**: 21−36.

1311. **Muller, R., D. Mumberg, and F. C. Lucibello.** 1993. Signals and genes in the control of cell-cycle progression. *Biochim. Biophys. Acta.* **1155**: 151−179.

1312. **Murre, C., G. Bain, M. A. van Dijk, I. Engel, B. A. Furnari, M. E. Massari, J. R. Matthews, M. W. Quong, R. R. Rivera, and M. H. Stuiver.** 1994. Structure and function of helix−loop−helix proteins. *Biochim. Biophys. Acta* **1218**: 129−135.

1313. **Muscat, G. E., M. Downes, and D. H. Dowhan.** 1995. Regulation of vertebrate muscle differentiation by thyroid hormone: the role of the myoD gene family. *Bioessays* **17**: 211−218.

1314. **Rudnicki, M. A. and R. Jaenisch.** 1995. The MyoD family of transcription factors and skeletal myogenesis. *Bioessays* **17**: 203−209.

1315. **Skeath, J. B. and S. B. Carroll.** 1994. The achaete−scute complex: generation of cellular pattern and fate within the *Drosophila* nervous system. *FASEB. J.* **8**: 714−721.

1316. **Vastrik, I., T. P. Makela, P. J. Koskinen, J. Klefstrom, and K. Alitalo.** 1994. Myc protein: partners and antagonists. *Crit. Rev. Oncog.* **5**: 59−68.

1317. **Wenzel, A. and M. Schwab.** 1995. The mycN/max protein complex in neuroblastoma. Short review. *Eur. J. Cancer* **31A**: 516−519.

Sequences, expression and functions of HLH proteins

1318. **Abbott, B. D., L. S. Birnbaum, and G. H. Perdew.** 1995. Developmental expression of two members of a new class of transcription factors: I. Expression of aryl hydrocarbon receptor in the C57BL/6N mouse embryo. *Dev. Dyn.* **204**: 133−143.

1319. **Abbott, B. D., M. R. Probst, and G. H. Perdew.** 1994. Immunohistochemical double-staining for Ah receptor and ARNT in human embryonic palatal shelves. *Teratology* **50**: 361−366.

1320. **Adams, J. M., H. Houston, J. Allen, T. Lints, and R. Harvey.** 1992. The hematopoietically expressed vav proto-oncogene shares homology with the dbl GDP−GTP exchange factor, the bcr gene and a yeast gene (CDC24) involved in cytoskeletal organization. *Oncogene.* **7**: 611−618.

1321. **Adams, L., B. M. Carlson, L. Henderson, and D. Goldman.** 1995. Adaptation of nicotinic acetylcholine receptor, myogenin, and MRF4 gene expression to long-term muscle denervation. *J. Cell Biol.* **131**: 1341−1349.

1322. **Adnane, J. and P. D. Robbins.** 1995. The retinoblastoma susceptibility gene product regulates Myc-mediated transcription. *Oncogene.* **10**: 381−387.

1323. **Agrawal, R. S., Y. P. Agrawal, and R. A. Mantyjarvi.** 1994. Flow cytometric quantitation of C-myc and P53 proteins in bovine papillomavirus type 1-transformed primary mouse fibroblasts. *Cytometry.* **17**: 237−245.

1324. **Akazawa, C., M. Ishibashi, C. Shimizu, S. Nakanishi, and R. Kageyama.** 1995. A mammalian helix−loop−helix factor structurally related to the product of *Drosophila* proneural gene atonal is a positive transcriptional regulator expressed in the developing nervous system. *J. Biol. Chem.* **270**: 8730−8738.

1325. **Albanese, I., M. Alberti, V. Bazan, A. Russo, S. Baiamonte, M. Migliavacca, P. Bazan, and M. La Farina.** 1994. Structural analysis of c-myc in human sporadic colorectal carcinomas. *Anticancer. Res.* **14**: 1103−1106.

1326. **Albert, D. A.** 1995. The effect of cyclic-AMP on the regulation of c-myc expression in T lymphoma cells. *J. Clin. Invest.* **95**: 1490−1496.

1327. **Alexandrow, M. G., M. Kawabata, M. Aakre, and H. L. Moses.** 1995. Overexpression of the c-Myc oncoprotein blocks the growth-inhibitory response but is required for the mitogenic effects of transforming growth factor β1. *Proc. Natl. Acad. Sci. U. S. A.* **92**: 3239−3243.

1328. **Allende, M. L. and E. S. Weinberg.** 1994. The expression pattern of two zebrafish achaete−scute homolog (ash) genes is altered in the embryonic brain of the cyclops mutant. *Dev. Biol.* **166**: 509−530.

1329. **Alleva, D. G., D. Askew, C. J. Burger, and K. D. Elgert.** 1994. Macrophage priming and activation during fibrosarcoma growth: expression of c-myb, c-myc, c-fos, and c-fms. *Immunol. Invest.* **23**: 457–472.

1330. **Ambinder, R. F., M. A. Mullen, Y. N. Chang, G. S. Hayward, and S. D. Hayward.** 1991. Functional domains of Epstein–Barr virus nuclear antigen EBNA-1. *J. Virol.* **65**: 1466–1478.

1331. **Ambroziak, J. and S. A. Henry.** 1994. INO2 and INO4 gene products, positive regulators of phospholipid biosynthesis in *Saccharomyces cerevisiae*, form a complex that binds to the INO1 promoter. *J. Biol. Chem.* **269**: 15344–15349.

1332. **Amendola, R.** 1994. Course of c-myc mRNA expression in the regenerating mouse testis determined by competitive reverse transcriptase polymerase chain reaction. *DNA Cell Biol.* **13**: 1099–1107.

1333. **Amundadottir, L. T., M. D. Johnson, G. Merlino, G. H. Smith, and R. B. Dickson.** 1995. Synergistic interaction of transforming growth factor α and c-myc in mouse mammary and salivary gland tumorigenesis. *Cell Growth. Differ.* **6**: 737–748.

1334. **Anderson, D. J.** 1993. MASH genes and the logic of neural crest cell lineage diversification. *C. R. Acad. Sci. III.* **316**: 1082–1096.

1335. **Andres, V. and K. Walsh.** 1996. Myogenin expression, cell cycle withdrawal, and phenotypic differentiation are temporally separable events that precede cell fusion upon myogenesis. *J. Cell Biol.* **132**: 657–666.

1336. **Antonsson, C., V. Arulampalam, M. L. Whitelaw, S. Pettersson, and L. Poellinger.** 1995. Constitutive function of the basic helix–loop–helix/PAS factor Arnt. Regulation of target promoters via the E box motif. *J. Biol. Chem.* **270**: 13968–13972.

1337. **Antonsson, C., M. L. Whitelaw, J. McGuire, J. A. Gustafsson, and L. Poellinger.** 1995. Distinct roles of the molecular chaperone hsp90 in modulating dioxin receptor function via the basic helix–loop–helix and PAS domains. *Mol. Cell Biol.* **15**: 756–765.

1338. **Araki, I., H. Saiga, K. W. Makabe, and N. Satoh.** 1994. Expression of amd1, a gene for a myoD1-related factor in the ascidian *Halocynthia roretzi. Roux's Arch. Devel. Biol.* **203**: 320–327.

1339. **Arbiser, J. L., Z. K. Arbiser, and J. A. Majzoub.** 1993. Effects of hydroxyurea and cyclic adenosine monophosphate/protein kinase A inhibitors on the expression of the human chorionic gonadotropin α subunit and c-myc genes in choriocarcinoma. *J. Endocrinol. Invest.* **16**: 849–856.

1340. **Arcinas, M. and L. M. Boxer.** 1994. Differential protein binding to the c-myc promoter during differentiation of hematopoietic cell lines. *Oncogene.* **9**: 2699–2706.

1341. **Arcinas, M., K. C. Sizer, and L. M. Boxer.** 1994. Activation of c-myc expression by c-Abl is independent of both the DNA binding function of c-Abl and the c-myc EP site. *J. Biol. Chem.* **269**: 21919–21924.

1342. **Arends, M. J., A. H. McGregor, and A. H. Wyllie.** 1994. Apoptosis is inversely related to necrosis and determines net growth in tumors bearing constitutively expressed myc, ras, and HPV oncogenes. *Am. J. Pathol.* **144**: 1045–1057.

1343. **Argenton, F., Y. Arava, A. Aronheim, and M. D. Walker.** 1996. An activation domain of the helix–loop–helix transcription factor E2A shows cell type preference *in vivo* in microinjected Zebra fish embryos. *Mol. Cell. Biol.* **16**: 1714–1721.

1344. **Arnold, T. E., R. A. Worrell, J. L. Barth, J. Morris, and R. Ivarie.** 1994. Dexamethasone-mediated induction of MMTV–myf5 in DD3 myoblasts increases endogenous myogenin expression but does not transactivate myf5. *Exp. Cell Res.* **212**: 321–328.

1345. **Aronheim, A., R. Shiran, A. Rosen, and M. D. Walker.** 1993. The E2A gene product contains two separable and functionally distinct transcription activation domains. *Proc. Natl. Acad. Sci. U. S. A.* **90**: 8063–8067.

1346. **Arsura, M., A. Deshpande, S. R. Hann, and G. E. Sonenshein.** 1995. Variant Max protein, derived by alternative splicing, associates with c-Myc *in vivo* and inhibits transactivation. *Mol. Cell Biol.* **15**: 6702–6709.

1347. **Artandi, S. E., C. Cooper, A. Shrivastava, and K. Calame.** 1994. The basic helix–loop–helix– zipper domain of TFE3 mediates enhancer– promoter interaction. *Mol. Cell Biol.* **14**: 7704–7716.

1348. **Artandi, S. E., K. Merrell, N. Avitahl, K. K. Wong, and K. Calame.** 1995. TFE3 contains two activation domains, one acidic and the other proline-rich, that synergistically activate transcription. *Nucleic Acids Res.* **23**: 3865–3871.

1349. **Asadi, F. K. and R. Sharifi.** 1995. Effects of sex steroids on cell growth and C-myc oncogene expression in LN-CaP and DU-145 prostatic carcinoma cell lines. *Int. Urol. Nephrol.* **27**: 67–80.

1350. **Asai, A., Y. Miyagi, H. Hashimoto, S. H. Lee, K. Mishima, A. Sugiyama, H. Tanaka, T. Mochizuki, T. Yasuda, and Y. Kuchino.** 1994. Modulation of tumor immunogenicity of rat glioma cells by s-Myc expression: eradication of rat gliomas *in vivo. Cell Growth. Differ.* **5**: 1153–1158.

1351. **Asai, A., Y. Miyagi, A. Sugiyama, M. Gamanuma, S. H. Hong, S. Takamoto, K. Nomura, M. Matsutani, K. Takakura, and Y. Kuchino.** 1994. Negative effects of wild-type p53 and s-Myc on cellular growth and tumorigenicity of glioma cells. Implication of the tumor suppressor genes for gene therapy. *J. Neurooncol.* **19**: 259–268.

1352. Asao, H., N. Tanaka, N. Ishii, M. Higuchi, T. Takeshita, M. Nakamura, T. Shirasawa, and K. Sugamura. 1994. Interleukin 2-induced activation of JAK3:possible involvement in signal transduction for c-myc induction and cell proliferation. *FEBS Lett.* **351**: 201−206.

1353. Ashburner, B. P. and J. M. Lopes. 1995. Autoregulated expression of the yeast INO2 and INO4 helix−loop−helix activator genes effects cooperative regulation on their target genes. *Mol. Cell Biol.* **15**: 1709−1715.

1354. Asher, O., S. Fuchs, and M. C. Souroujon. 1994. Acetylcholine receptor and myogenic factor gene expression in *Torpedo* embryonic development. *Neuroreport.* **5**: 1581−1584.

1355. Asker, C. E., K. P. Magnusson, S. P. Piccoli, K. Andersson, G. Klein, M. D. Cole, and K. G. Wiman. 1995. Mouse and rat B-myc share amino acid sequence homology with the c-myc transcriptional activator domain and contain a B-myc specific carboxy terminal region. *Oncogene.* **11**: 1963−1969.

1356. Atchley, W. R. and W. M. Fitch. 1995. Myc and Max:molecular evolution of a family of proto-oncogene products and their dimerization partner. *Proc. Natl. Acad. Sci. U. S. A.* **92**: 10217−10221.

1357. Atchley, W. R., W. M. Fitch, and M. Bronner Fraser. 1994. Molecular evolution of the MyoD family of transcription factors. *Proc. Natl. Acad. Sci. U. S. A.* **91**: 11522−11526.

1358. Aurade, F., C. Pinset, P. Chafey, F. Gros, and D. Montarras. 1994. Myf5, MyoD, myogenin and MRF4 myogenic derivatives of the embryonic mesenchymal cell line C3H10T1/2 exhibit the same adult muscle phenotype. *Differentiation.* **55**: 185−192.

1359. Axelson, H., M. Henriksson, Y. Wang, K. P. Magnusson, and G. Klein. 1995. The amino-terminal phosphorylation sites of C-MYC are frequently mutated in Burkitt's lymphoma lines but not in mouse plasmacytomas and rat immunocytomas. *Eur. J. Cancer* **31A**: 2099−2104.

1360. Axelson, H., Y. Wang, S. Silva, M. G. Mattei, and G. Klein. 1994. Juxtaposition of N-myc and Ig κ through a reciprocal t(6;12) translocation in a mouse plasmacytoma. *Genes. Chromosom. Cancer* **11**: 85−90.

1361. Ayer, D. E., Q. A. Lawrence, and R. N. Eisenman. 1995. Mad−Max transcriptional repression is mediated by ternary complex formation with mammalian homologs of yeast repressor Sin3. *Cell.* **80**: 767−776.

1362. Azzoni, L., I. Anegon, B. Calabretta, and B. Perussia. 1995. Ligand binding to Fc γ R induces c-myc-dependent apoptosis in IL-2-stimulated NK cells. *J. Immunol.* **154**: 491−499.

1363. Bacsi, S. G. and O. Hankinson. 1996. Functional characterization of DNA-binding domains of the subunits of the heterodimeric aryl hydrocarbon receptor complex imputing novel and canonical basic helix−loop−helix protein−DNA interactions. *J. Biol. Chem.* **271**: 8843−8850.

1364. Bai, M. K., J. S. Costopoulos, B. P. Christoforidou, and C. S. Papadimitriou. 1994. Immunohistochemical detection of the c-myc oncogene product in normal, hyperplastic and carcinomatous endometrium. *Oncology.* **51**: 314−319.

1365. Bailey, A. M. and J. W. Posakony. 1995. Suppressor of hairless directly activates transcription of enhancer of split complex genes in response to Notch receptor activity. *Genes. Dev.* **9**: 2609−2622.

1366. Bain, G., E. C. Maandag, D. J. Izon, D. Amsen, A. M. Kruisbeek, B. C. Weintraub, I. Krop, M. S. Schlissel, A. J. Feeney, M. van Roon *et al*. 1994. E2A proteins are required for proper B cell development and initiation of immunoglobulin gene rearrangements. *Cell* **79**: 885−892.

1367. Baker, D. A., J. Maher, I. A. Roberts, and N. J. Dibb. 1994. Evidence that ras and myc mediate the synergy between SCF or M-CSF and other haemopoietic growth factors. *Leukemia* **8**: 1970−1981.

1368. Baker, S. J., M. Pawlita, A. Leutz, and D. Hoelzer. 1994. Essential role of c-myc in ara-C-induced differentiation of human erythroleukemia cells. *Leukemia* **8**: 1309−1317.

1369. Barone, M. V. and S. A. Courtneidge. 1995. Myc but not Fos rescue of PDGF signalling block caused by kinase-inactive Src. *Nature* **378**: 509−512.

1370. Barrera, G., R. Muraca, S. Pizzimenti, A. Serra, C. Rosso, G. Saglio, M. G. Farace, V. M. Fazio, and M. U. Dianzani. 1994. Inhibition of c-myc expression induced by 4-hydroxynonenal, a product of lipid peroxidation, in the HL-60 human leukemic cell line. *Biochem. Biophys. Res. Commun.* **203**: 553−561.

1371. Barrett, J. F., B. C. Lewis, A. T. Hoang, R. J. J. Alvarez, and C. V. Dang. 1995. Cyclin A links c-Myc to adhesion-independent cell proliferation. *J. Biol. Chem.* **270**: 15923−15925.

1372. Barrios, C., J. S. Castresana, U. G. Falkmer, I. Rosendahl, and A. Kreicbergs. 1994. c-myc oncogene amplification and cytometric DNA ploidy pattern as prognostic factors in musculoskeletal neoplasms. *Int. J. Cancer* **58**: 781−786.

1373. Barrios, C., J. S. Castresana, and A. Kreicbergs. 1994. Clinicopathologic correlations and short-term prognosis in musculoskeletal sarcoma with c-myc oncogene amplification. *Am. J. Clin. Oncol.* **17**: 273−276.

1374. Bartholoma, A. and K. A. Nave. 1994. NEX-1: a novel brain-specific helix−loop−helix protein with autoregulation and sustained expression in mature cortical neurons. *Mech. Dev.* **48**: 217−228.

1375. **Basu, A. and J. S. Cline.** 1995. Oncogenic transformation alters cisplatin-induced apoptosis in rat embryo fibroblasts. *Int. J. Cancer* **63**: 597–603.

1376. **Baylies, M. K. and M. Bate.** 1996. *twist*: a myogenic swith in *Drosophila*. *Science* **272**: 1481–1484.

1377. **Bazar, L., V. Harris, I. Sunitha, D. Hartmann, and M. Avigan.** 1995. A transactivator of c-myc is coordinately regulated with the proto-oncogene during cellular growth. *Oncogene.* **10**: 2229–2238.

1378. **Bazar, L., D. Meighen, V. Harris, R. Duncan, D. Levens, and M. Avigan.** 1995. Targeted melting and binding of a DNA regulatory element by a transactivator of c-myc. *J. Biol. Chem.* **270**: 8241–8248.

1379. **Ben Baruch, N., W. C. Reinhold, N. Alexandrova, I. Ichinose, M. Blake, J. B. Trepel, and M. Zajac Kaye.** 1994. c-myc down-regulation in suramin-treated HL60 cells precedes growth inhibition but does not trigger differentiation. *Mol. Pharmacol.* **46**: 73–78.

1380. **Benharroch, D., T. Yermiahu, D. B. Geffen, I. Prinsloo, J. Gopas, S. Segal, and M. Aboud.** 1995. Expression of c-myc and c-ras oncogenes in the neoplastic and non-neoplastic cells of Hodgkin's disease. *Eur. J. Haematol.* **55**: 178–183.

1381. **Bennett, M. K., J. M. Lopez, H. B. Sanchez, and T. F. Osborne.** 1995. Sterol regulation of fatty acid synthase promoter. Coordinate feedback regulation of two major lipid pathways. *J. Biol. Chem.* **270**: 25578–25583.

1382. **Bennett, M. R., D. F. Gibson, S. M. Schwartz, and J. F. Tait.** 1995. Binding and phagocytosis of apoptotic vascular smooth muscle cells is mediated in part by exposure of phosphatidylserine. *Circ. Res.* **77**: 1136–1142.

1383. **Bennett, M. R., T. D. Littlewood, D. C. Hancock, G. I. Evan, and A. C. Newby.** 1994. Down-regulation of the c-myc proto-oncogene in inhibition of vascular smooth-muscle cell proliferation: a signal for growth arrest? *Biochem. J.* **302**: 701–708.

1384. **Bentley, N. J., T. Eisen, and C. R. Goding.** 1994. Melanocyte-specific expression of the human tyrosinase promoter: activation by the microphthalmia gene product and role of the initiator. *Mol. Cell Biol.* **14**: 7996–8006.

1385. **Berberich, S., A. Trivedi, D. C. Daniel, E. M. Johnson, and M. Leffak.** 1995. *In vitro* replication of plasmids containing human c-myc DNA. *J. Mol. Biol.* **245**: 92–109.

1386. **Berberich, S. J. and E. H. Postel.** 1995. PuF/NM23-H2/NDPK-B transactivates a human c-myc promoter-CAT gene via a functional nuclease hypersensitive element. *Oncogene.* **10**: 2343–2347.

1387. **Berebbi, M., C. Cajean Feroldi, F. Apiou, J. Couturier, M. Garcette, R. Emanoil Ravier, J. Cabannes, M. Perricaudet, and D. Blangy.** 1995. Integration of viral sequences into the c-myc gene in two mammary adenocarcinomas induced by polyomavirus in athymic nude mice. *J. Virol.* **69**: 5935–5945.

1388. **Berghard, A., K. Gradin, I. Pongratz, M. Whitelaw, and L. Poellinger.** 1993. Cross-coupling of signal transduction pathways: the dioxin receptor mediates induction of cytochrome P-450IA1 expression via a protein kinase C-dependent mechanism. *Mol. Cell Biol.* **13**: 677–689.

1389. **Bernard, M., L. Smit, E. Macintyre, D. Matthieu Mahul, and K. Pulford.** 1995. Nuclear localization of the SCL/TAL1 basic helix–loop–helix protein is not dependent on the presence of the basic domain. *Blood.* **85**: 3356–3357.

1390. **Bhatia, K., G. Spangler, G. Gaidano, N. Hamdy, R. Dalla Favera, and I. Magrath.** 1994. Mutations in the coding region of c-myc occur frequently in acquired immunodeficiency syndrome-associated lymphomas. *Blood.* **84**: 883–888.

1391. **Bhatia, K., G. Spangler, N. Hamdy, A. Neri, G. Brubaker, A. Levin, and I. Magrath.** 1995. Mutations in the coding region of c-myc occur independently of mutations in the regulatory regions and are predominantly associated with myc/Ig translocation. *Curr. Top. Microbiol. Immunol.* **194**: 389–398.

1392. **Bieche, I., M. H. Champeme, and R. Lidereau.** 1994. A tumor suppressor gene on chromosome 1p32-pter controls the amplification of MYC family genes in breast cancer. *Cancer Res.* **54**: 4274–4276.

1393. **Black, B. L., J. F. Martin, and E. N. Olson.** 1995. The mouse MRF4 promoter is trans-activated directly and indirectly by muscle-specific transcription factors. *J. Biol. Chem.* **270**: 2889–2892.

1394. **Blackwood, E. M., T. G. Lugo, L. Kretzner, M. W. King, A. J. Street, O. N. Witte, and R. N. Eisenman.** 1994. Functional analysis of the AUG- and CUG-initiated forms of the c-Myc protein. *Mol. Biol. Cell* **5**: 597–609.

1395. **Blanar, M. A., P. H. Crossley, K. G. Peters, E. Steingrimsson, N. G. Copeland, N. A. Jenkins, G. R. Martin, and W. J. Rutter.** 1995. Meso1, a basic-helix–loop–helix protein involved in mammalian presomitic mesoderm development. *Proc. Natl. Acad. Sci. U. S. A.* **92**: 5870–5874.

1396. **Blaugrund, E., T. D. Pham, V. M. Tennyson, L. Lo, L. Sommer, D. J. Anderson, and M. D. Gershon.** 1996. Distinct subpopulations of enteric neuronal progenitors defined by time of development, sympathoadrenal lineage markers and Mash-1-dependence. *Development.* **122**: 309–320.

1397. **Blyth, K., A. Terry, M. O'Hara, E. W. Baxter, M. Campbell, M. Stewart, L. A. Donehower, D. E. Onions, J. C. Neil, and E. R. Cameron.** 1995. Synergy between a human c-myc transgene and p53 null genotype in murine thymic lymphomas: contrasting effects of homozygous and heterozygous p53 loss. *Oncogene*. **10**: 1717–1723.

1398. **Bock, K. W.** 1994. Aryl hydrocarbon or dioxin receptor: biologic and toxic responses. *Rev. Physiol. Biochem. Pharmacol.* **125**: 1–42.

1399. **Bockamp, E. O., F. McLaughlin, A. M. Murrell, B. Gottgens, L. Robb, C. G. Begley, and A. R. Green.** 1995. Lineage-restricted regulation of the murine SCL/TAL-1 promoter. *Blood*. **86**: 1502–1514.

1400. **Bodrug, S. E., B. J. Warner, M. L. Bath, G. J. Lindeman, A. W. Harris, and J. M. Adams.** 1994. Cyclin D1 transgene impedes lymphocyte maturation and collaborates in lymphomagenesis with the myc gene. *EMBO J.* **13**: 2124–2130.

1401. **Bogenmann, E., M. Torres, and H. Matsushima.** 1995. Constitutive N-myc gene expression inhibits trkA mediated neuronal differentiation. *Oncogene*. **10**: 1915–1925.

1402. **Boguski, M. S., A. Bairoch, T. K. Attwood, and G. S. Michaels.** 1992. Proto-vav and gene expression. *Nature* **358**: 113.

1403. **Bolufer, P., R. Molina, A. Ruiz, M. Hernandez, C. Vazquez, and A. Lluch.** 1994. Estradiol receptors in combination with neu or myc oncogene amplifications might define new subtypes of breast cancer. *Clin. Chim. Acta* **229**: 107–122.

1404. **Bonven, B. J., A. L. Nielsen, P. L. Norby, F. S. Pedersen, and P. Jorgensen.** 1995. E-box variants direct formation of distinct complexes with the basic helix–loop–helix protein ALF1. *J. Mol. Biol.* **249**: 564–575.

1405. **Bordow, S. B., M. Haber, J. Madafiglio, B. Cheung, G. M. Marshall, and M. D. Norris.** 1994. Expression of the multidrug resistance-associated protein (MRP) gene correlates with amplification and overexpression of the N-myc oncogene in childhood neuroblastoma. *Cancer Res.* **54**: 5036–5040.

1406. **Borkowski, O. M., N. H. Brown, and M. Bate.** 1995. Anterior-posterior subdivision and the diversification of the mesoderm in *Drosophila. Development*. **121**: 4183–4193.

1407. **Brand, M., A. P. Jarman, L. Y. Jan, and Y. N. Jan.** 1993. asense is a *Drosophila* neural precursor gene and is capable of initiating sense organ formation. *Development*. **119**: 1–17.

1408. **Braun, T. and H. -H. Arnold.** 1996. *myf*-5 and *myoD* genes are activated in distinct mesenchymal stem cells and determine different skeletal muscle cell lineages. *EMBO. J.* **15**: 310–318.

1409. **Braun, T. and H. H. Arnold.** 1994. ES-cells carrying two inactivated myf-5 alleles form skeletal muscle cells: activation of an alternative myf-5-independent differentiation pathway. *Dev. Biol.* **164**: 24–36.

1410. **Braun, T. and H. H. Arnold.** 1995. Inactivation of Myf-6 and Myf-5 genes in mice leads to alterations in skeletal muscle development. *EMBO J.* **14**: 1176–1186.

1411. **Braun, T., E. Bober, M. A. Rudnicki, R. Jaenisch, and H. H. Arnold.** 1994. MyoD expression marks the onset of skeletal myogenesis in Myf-5 mutant mice. *Development*. **120**: 3083–3092.

1412. **Brennscheidt, U., D. Eick, R. Kunzmann, U. Martens, M. Kiehntopf, R. Mertelsmann, and F. Herrmann.** 1994. Burkitt-like mutations in the c-myc gene locus in prolymphocytic leukemia. *Leukemia* **8**: 897–902.

1413. **Breuer, B., I. DeVivo, J. C. Luo, S. Smith, M. R. Pincus, A. H. Tatum, J. Daucher, C. R. Minick, D. G. Miller, E. J. Nowak** *et al*. 1994. erbB-2 and myc oncoproteins in sera and tumors of breast cancer patients. *Cancer Epidemiol. Biomarkers. Prev.* **3**: 63–66.

1414. **Brough, D. E., T. J. Hofmann, K. B. Ellwood, R. A. Townley, and M. D. Cole.** 1995. An essential domain of the c-myc protein interacts with a nuclear factor that is also required for E1A-mediated transformation. *Mol. Cell Biol.* **15**: 1536–1544.

1415. **Brown, N. L., C. A. Sattler, S. W. Paddock, and S. B. Carroll.** 1995. Hairy and emc negatively regulate morphogenetic furrow progression in the *Drosophila* eye. *Cell*. **80**: 879–887.

1416. **Brys, A. and N. Maizels.** 1994. LR1 regulates c-myc transcription in B-cell lymphomas. *Proc. Natl. Acad. Sci. U. S. A.* **91**: 4915–4919.

1417. **Bungert, J., I. Kober, F. During, and K. H. Seifart.** 1992. Transcription factor eUSF is an essential component of isolated transcription complexes on the duck histone H5 gene and it mediates the interaction of TFIID with a TATA-deficient promoter *J. Mol. Biol.* **223**: 885–898. [Published erratum appears in 1992. *J. Mol. Biol.* **227**:978.]

1418. **Burgess, R., P. Cserjesi, K. L. Ligon, and E. N. Olson.** 1995. Paraxis: a basic helix–loop– helix protein expressed in paraxial mesoderm and developing somites. *Dev. Biol.* **168**: 296–306.

1419. **Burgess, T. L., E. F. Fisher, S. L. Ross, J. V. Bready, Y. X. Qian, L. A. Bayewitch, A. M. Cohen, C. J. Herrera, S. S. Hu, T. B. Kramer** *et al*. 1995. The antiproliferative activity of c-myb and c-myc antisense oligonucleotides in smooth muscle cells is caused by a nonantisense mechanism. *Proc. Natl. Acad. Sci. U. S. A.* **92**: 4051–4055.

1420. **Bustelo, X. R., S. D. Rubin, K. L. Suen, D. Carrasco, and M. Barbacid.** 1993. Developmental expression of the vav protooncogene. *Cell Growth. Differ.* **4**: 297–308.

1421. **Butterworth, B. E., C. S. Sprankle, S. M. Goldsworthy, D. M. Wilson, and T. L. Goldsworthy.** 1994. Expression of myc, fos, and Ha-ras in the livers of furan-treated F344 rats and B6C3F1 mice. *Mol. Carcinog.* **9**: 24–32.

1422. **Cameron, E. R., M. Campbell, K. Blyth, S. A. Argyle, L. Keanie, J. C. Neil, and D. E. Onions.** 1996. Apparent bypass of negative selection in CD8$^+$ tumours in CD2-myc transgenic mice. *Br. J. Cancer* **73**: 13–17.

1423. **Campos Ortega, J. A.** 1995. Genetic mechanisms of early neurogenesis in *Drosophila melanogaster. Mol. Neurobiol.* **10**: 75–89.

1424. **Carmena, A., M. Bate, and F. Jimenez.** 1995. Lethal of scute, a proneural gene, participates in the specification of muscle progenitors during *Drosophila* embryogenesis. *Genes. Dev.* **9**: 2373–2383.

1425. **Carney, M. E., R. C. O'Reilly, B. Sholevar, O. I. Buiakova, L. D. Lowry, W. M. Keane, F. L. Margolis, and J. L. Rothstein.** 1995. Expression of the human Achaete-scute 1 gene in olfactory neuroblastoma (esthesioneuroblastoma). *J. Neurooncol.* **26**: 35–43.

1426. **Carrier, F., C. Y. Chang, J. L. Duh, D. W. Nebert, and A. Puga.** 1994. Interaction of the regulatory domains of the murine Cyp1a1 gene with two DNA-binding proteins in addition to the Ah receptor and the Ah receptor nuclear translocator (ARNT). *Biochem. Pharmacol.* **48**: 1767–1778.

1427. **Carver, L. A., V. Jackiw, and C. A. Bradfield.** 1994. The 90-kDa heat shock protein is essential for Ah receptor signaling in a yeast expression system. *J. Biol. Chem.* **269**: 30109–30112.

1428. **Castresana, J. S., C. Barrios, L. Gomez, and A. Kreicbergs.** 1994. No association between c-myc amplification and TP53 mutation in sarcoma tumorigenesis. *Cancer Genet. Cytogenet.* **76**: 47–49.

1429. **Chakrabarti, D., S. Mukhopadhyay, and A. K. Duttagupta.** 1995. A novel genetic interaction between daughterless and a variegating rearrangement strain of *Drosophila melanogaster. Genome.* **38**: 105–111.

1430. **Chan, W. K., R. Chu, S. Jain, J. K. Reddy, and C. A. Bradfield.** 1994. Baculovirus expression of the Ah receptor and Ah receptor nuclear translocater. Evidence for additional dioxin responsive element-binding species and factors required for signaling. *J. Biol. Chem.* **269**: 26464–26471.

1431. **Chang, H., J. A. Blondal, S. Benchimol, M. D. Minden, and H. A. Messner.** 1995. p53 mutations, c-myc and bcl-2 rearrangements in human non-Hodgkin's lymphoma cell lines. *Leuk. Lymphoma.* **19**: 165–171.

1432. **Chaouchi, N., C. Wallon, J. Taieb, M. T. Auffredou, G. Tertian, F. M. Lemoine, J. F. Delfraissy, and A. Vazquez.** 1994. Interferon-α-mediated prevention of *in vitro* apoptosis of chronic lymphocytic leukemia B cells: role of bcl-2 and c-myc. *Clin. Immunol. Immunopathol.* **73**: 197–204.

1433. **Chattopadhyay, P., M. Banerjee, C. Sarkar, M. Mathur, A. K. Mohapatra, and S. Sinha.** 1995. Infrequent alteration of the c-myc gene in human glial tumours associated with increased numbers of c-myc positive cells. *Oncogene.* **11**: 2711–2714.

1434. **Chaudhary, D. and D. M. Miller.** 1995. The c-myc promoter binding protein (MBP-1) and TBP bind simultaneously in the minor groove of the c-myc P2 promoter. *Biochemistry* **34**: 3438–3445.

1435. **Chavany, C., Y. Connell, and L. Neckers.** 1995. Contribution of sequence and phosphorothioate content to inhibition of cell growth and adhesion caused by c-myc antisense oligomers. *Mol. Pharmacol.* **48**: 738–746.

1436. **Chen, C. H., J. Zhang, and C. C. Ling.** 1994. Transfected c-myc and c-Ha-ras modulate radiation-induced apoptosis in rat embryo cells. *Radiat. Res.* **139**: 307–315.

1437. **Chen, H., B. Li, and J. L. Workman.** 1994. A histone-binding protein, nucleoplasmin, stimulates transcription factor binding to nucleosomes and factor-induced nucleosome disassembly. *EMBO J.* **13**: 380–390.

1438. **Chen, J., T. Liu, and A. H. Ross.** 1994. Down-regulation of c-myc oncogene during NGF-induced differentiation of neuroblastoma cell lines. *Chin. Med. Sci. J.* **9**: 152–156.

1439. **Chen, J., T. Willingham, L. R. Margraf, N. Schreiber Agus, R. A. DePinho, and P. D. Nisen.** 1995. Effects of the MYC oncogene antagonist, MAD, on proliferation, cell cycling and the malignant phenotype of human brain tumour cells. *Nat. Med.* **1**: 638–643.

1440. **Chen, L., M. Krause, M. Sepanski, and A. Fire.** 1994. The *Caenorhabditis elegans* MYOD homologue HLH-1 is essential for proper muscle function and complete morphogenesis. *Development.* **120**: 1631–1641.

1441. **Cheng, J. M., J. L. Hiemstra, S. S. Schneider, B. A. Kaufman, A. Naumova, N. K. Cheung, S. L. Cohn, L. Diller, C. Sapienza, and G. M. Brodeur.** 1994. Preferential amplification of the paternal allele in neuroblastomas with N-myc amplification. *Prog. Clin. Biol. Res.* **385**: 43–49.

1442. **Cheng, N. C., N. Van Roy, A. Chan, M. Beitsma, A. Westerveld, F. Speleman, and R. Versteeg.** 1995. Deletion mapping in neuroblastoma cell lines suggests two distinct tumor suppressor genes in the 1p35–36 region, only one of which is associated with N-myc amplification. *Oncogene.* **10**: 291–297.

1443. Cherney, B. W., K. Bhatia, and G. Tosato. 1994. A role for deregulated c-Myc expression in apoptosis of Epstein–Barr virus-immortalized B cells. *Proc. Natl. Acad. Sci. U. S. A.* **91**: 12967–12971.

1444. Chetty, R., L. Cerroni, K. Pulford, A. Giatromanolaki, S. Biddolph, L. Kaklamanis, and K. Gatter. 1995. TAL1 gene deletions and TAL1 protein expression in sporadic melanoma. *Melanoma. Res.* **5**: 251–254.

1445. Chetty, R., K. Pulford, M. Jones, D. Mathieu Mahul, P. Close, S. Hussein, G. Pallesen, E. Ralfkiaer, H. Stein, K. Gatter *et al.* 1995. SCL/Tal-1 expression in T-acute lymphoblastic leukemia: an immunohistochemical and genotypic study. *Hum. Pathol.* **26**: 994–998.

1446. Chieffi, P., S. Minucci, G. Cobellis, S. Fasano, and R. Pierantoni. 1995. Changes in proto-oncogene activity in the testis of the frog, *Rana esculenta*, during the annual reproductive cycle. *Gen. Comp. Endocrinol.* **99**: 127–136.

1447. Chien, C. H., F. F. Wang, and T. C. Hamilton. 1994. Transcriptional activation of c-myc proto-oncogene by estrogen in human ovarian cancer cells. *Mol. Cell Endocrinol.* **99**: 11–19.

1448. Chin, L., N. Schreiber Agus, I. Pellicer, K. Chen, H. W. Lee, M. Dudast, C. Cordon Cardo, and R. A. DePinho. 1995. Contrasting roles for Myc and Mad proteins in cellular growth and differentiation. *Proc. Natl. Acad. Sci. U. S. A.* **92**: 8488–8492.

1449. Chou, T. Y., G. W. Hart, and C. V. Dang. 1995. c-Myc is glycosylated at threonine 58, a known phosphorylation site and a mutational hot spot in lymphomas. *J. Biol. Chem.* **270**: 18961–18965.

1450. Christiansen, H., O. Delattre, S. Fuchs, M. Theobald, N. M. Christiansen, F. Berthold, and F. Lampert. 1994. Loss of the putative tumor suppressor-gene locus 1p36 as investigated by a PCR-assay and N-myc amplification in 48 neuroblastomas: results of the German Neuroblastoma Study Group. *Prog. Clin. Biol. Res.* **385**: 19–25.

1451. Chu, E., T. Takechi, K. L. Jones, D. M. Voeller, S. M. Copur, G. F. Maley, F. Maley, S. Segal, and C. J. Allegra. 1995. Thymidylate synthase binds to c-myc RNA in human colon cancer cells and *in vitro*. *Mol. Cell Biol.* **15**: 179–185.

1452. Clark, H. M., T. Yano, T. Otsuki, E. S. Jaffe, D. Shibata, and M. Raffeld. 1994. Mutations in the coding region of c-MYC in AIDS-associated and other aggressive lymphomas. *Cancer Res.* **54**: 3383–3386.

1453. Clevenger, C. V., W. Ngo, D. L. Sokol, S. M. Luger, and A. M. Gewirtz. 1995. Vav is necessary for prolactin-stimulated proliferation and is translocated into the nucleus of a T-cell line. *J. Biol. Chem.* **270**: 13246–13253.

1454. Cogswell, J. P., M. M. Godlevski, M. Bonham, J. Bisi, and L. Babiss. 1995. Upstream stimulatory factor regulates expression of the cell cycle-dependent cyclin B1 gene promoter. *Mol. Cell Biol.* **15**: 2782–2790.

1455. Cohn, S. L., A. T. Look, V. V. Joshi, T. Holbrook, H. Salwen, D. Chagnovich, L. Chesler, S. T. Rowe, M. B. Valentine, H. Komuro *et al.* 1995. Lack of correlation of N-myc gene amplification with prognosis in localized neuroblastoma: a Pediatric Oncology Group study. *Cancer Res.* **55**: 721–726.

1456. Collins, V. P. 1995. Gene amplification in human gliomas. *Glia.* **15**: 289–296.

1457. Combaret, V., N. Gross, C. Lasset, D. Frappaz, G. Peruisseau, T. Philip, D. Beck, and M. C. Favrot. 1996. Clinical relevance of CD44 cell-surface expression and N-myc gene amplification in a multicentric analysis of 121 pediatric neuroblastomas. *J. Clin. Oncol.* **14**: 25–34.

1458. Consonni, G., F. Geuna, G. Gavazzi, and C. Tonelli. 1993. Molecular homology among members of the R gene family in maize. *Plant. J.* **3**: 335–346.

1459. Consonni, G., A. Viotti, S. L. Dellaporta, and C. Tonelli. 1992. cDNA nucleotide sequence of Sn, a regulatory gene in maize. *Nucleic Acids Res.* **20**: 373.

1460. Contegiacomo, A., C. Pizzi, L. De Marchis, M. Alimandi, P. Delrio, E. Di Palma, G. Petrella, L. Ottini, D. French, L. Frati *et al.* 1995. High cell kinetics is associated with amplification of the int-2, bcl-1, myc and erbB-2 proto-oncogenes and loss of heterozygosity at the DF3 locus in primary breast cancers. *Int. J. Cancer* **61**: 1–6.

1461. Coppola, J., S. Bryant, T. Koda, D. Conway, and M. Barbacid. 1991. Mechanism of activation of the vav protooncogene. *Cell Growth. Differ.* **2**: 95–105.

1462. Corbo, L., F. Le Roux, and A. Sergeant. 1994. The EBV early gene product EB2 transforms rodent cells through a signalling pathway involving c-Myc. *Oncogene.* **9**: 3299–3304.

1463. Corvi, R., L. Savelyeva, L. Amler, R. Handgretinger, and M. Schwab. 1995. Cytogenetic evolution of MYCN and MDM2 amplification in the neuroblastoma LS tumour and its cell line. *Eur. J. Cancer* **31A**: 520–523.

1464. Corvi, R., L. Savelyeva, and M. Schwab. 1995. Duplication of N-MYC at its resident site 2p24 may be a mechanism of activation alternative to amplification in human neuroblastoma cells. *Cancer Res.* **55**: 3471–3474.

1465. Coumailleau, P., L. Poellinger, J. A. Gustafsson, and M. L. Whitelaw. 1995. Definition of a minimal domain of the dioxin receptor that is associated with Hsp90 and maintains wild type ligand binding affinity and specificity. *J. Biol. Chem.* **270**: 25291–25300.

1466. **Cowley, C. G., W. L. Carroll, and J. M. Johnston.** 1996. The absence of ongoing immunoglobulin gene hypermutation suggests a distinct mechanism for c-myc mutation in endemic Burkitt's lymphoma. *J. Pediatr. Hematol. Oncol.* **18**: 29–35.

1467. **Crescenzi, M., D. H. Crouch, and F. Tato.** 1994. Transformation by myc prevents fusion but not biochemical differentiation of C2C12 myoblasts: mechanisms of phenotypic correction in mixed culture with normal cells. *J. Cell Biol.* **125**: 1137–1145.

1468. **Cross, J. C., M. L. Flannery, M. A. Blanar, E. Steingrimsson, N. A. Jenkins, N. G. Copeland, W. J. Rutter, and Z. Werb.** 1995. Hxt encodes a basic helix–loop–helix transcription factor that regulates trophoblast cell development. *Development.* **121**: 2513–2523.

1469. **Cserjesi, P., D. Brown, K. L. Ligon, G. E. Lyons, N. G. Copeland, D. J. Gilbert, N. A. Jenkins, and E. N. Olson.** 1995. Scleraxis: a basic helix–loop–helix protein that prefigures skeletal formation during mouse embryogenesis. *Development.* **121**: 1099–1110.

1470. **Cserjesi, P., D. Brown, G. E. Lyons, and E. N. Olson.** 1995. Expression of the novel basic helix–loop–helix gene eHAND in neural crest derivatives and extraembryonic membranes during mouse development. *Dev. Biol.* **170**: 664–678.

1471. **Cutrona, G., M. Ulivi, F. Fais, S. Roncella, and M. Ferrarini.** 1995. Transfection of the c-myc oncogene into normal Epstein–Barr virus-harboring B cells results in new phenotypic and functional features resembling those of Burkitt lymphoma cells and normal centroblasts. *J. Exp. Med.* **181**: 699–711.

1472. **Dajani, O. F., M. Refsnes, T. K. Guren, R. S. Horn, G. H. Thoresen, and T. Christoffersen.** 1994. Elevated glucose concentrations inhibit DNA synthesis and expression of c-myc in cultured hepatocytes. *Biochem. Biophys. Res. Commun.* **202**: 1476–1482.

1473. **Daksis, J. I., R. Y. Lu, L. M. Facchini, W. W. Marhin, and L. J. Penn.** 1994. Myc induces cyclin D1 expression in the absence of *de novo* protein synthesis and links mitogen-stimulated signal transduction to the cell cycle. *Oncogene.* **9**: 3635–3645.

1474. **Damiani, R. D. J. and S. R. Wessler.** 1993. An upstream open reading frame represses expression of Lc, a member of the R/B family of maize transcriptional activators. *Proc. Natl. Acad. Sci. U. S. A.* **90**: 8244–8248.

1475. **Datta, P. K., A. K. Ghosh, and S. T. Jacob.** 1995. The RNA polymerase I promoter-activating factor CPBF is functionally and immunologically related to the basic helix–loop–helix–zipper DNA-binding protein USF. *J. Biol. Chem.* **270**: 8637–8641.

1476. **Davidoff, A. N. and B. V. Mendelow.** 1994. Protein synthesis inhibition is not a requisite for puromycin- and cycloheximide-induced c-myc mRNA superinduction. *Anticancer. Res.* **14**: 1199–1201.

1477. **Dawson, S. R., D. L. Turner, H. Weintraub, and S. M. Parkhurst.** 1995. Specificity for the hairy/enhancer of split basic helix–loop–helix (bHLH) proteins maps outside the bHLH domain and suggests two separable modes of transcriptional repression. *Mol. Cell Biol.* **15**: 6923–6931.

1478. **de Celis, J. F., A. Baonza, and A. Garcia Bellido.** 1995. Behavior of extramacrochaetae mutant cells in the morphogenesis of the *Drosophila* wing. *Mech. Dev.* **53**: 209–221.

1479. **de Celis, J. F., A. Garcia Bellido, and S. J. Bray.** 1996. Activation and function of Notch at the dorsal–ventral boundary of the wing imaginal disc. *Development.* **122**: 359–369.

1480. **De Winde, J. H. and L. A. Grivell.** 1995. Regulation of mitochondrial biogenesis in *Saccharomyces cerevisiae*. Intricate interplay between general and specific transcription factors in the promoter of the QCR8 gene. *Eur. J. Biochem.* **233**: 200–208.

1481. **Deed, R. W., M. Jasiok, and J. D. Norton.** 1994. Nucleotide sequence of the cDNA encoding human helix–loop–helix Id-1 protein: identification of functionally conserved residues common to Id proteins. *Biochim. Biophys. Acta* **1219**: 160–162.

1482. **Deguchi, T. and H. C. Pitot.** 1995. Expression of c-myc in altered hepatic foci induced in rats by various single doses of diethylnitrosamine and promotion by 0.05% phenobarbital. *Mol. Carcinog.* **14**: 152–159.

1483. **Delgado, M. D., A. Lerga, M. Canelles, M. T. Gomez Casares, and J. Leon.** 1995. Differential regulation of Max and role of c-Myc during erythroid and myelomonocytic differentiation of K562 cells. *Oncogene.* **10**: 1659–1665.

1484. **Deltour, L., P. Leduque, N. Blume, O. Madsen, P. Dubois, J. Jami, and D. Bucchini.** 1993. Differential expression of the two nonallelic proinsulin genes in the developing mouse embryo. *Proc. Natl. Acad. Sci. U. S. A.* **90**: 527–531.

1485. **Denis, N., S. Blanc, M. P. Leibovitch, N. Nicolaiew, F. Dautry, M. Raymondjean, J. Kruh, and A. Kitzis.** 1987. c-myc oncogene expression inhibits the initiation of myogenic differentiation. *Exp. Cell. Res.* **172**: 212–217.

1486. **Desbarats, L., S. Gaubatz, and M. Eilers.** 1996. Discrimination between different E-box-binding proteins at an endogenous target gene of c-*myc*. *Genes. Dev.* **10**: 447–460.

1487. **Desprez, P. Y., E. Hara, M. J. Bissell, and J. Campisi.** 1995. Suppression of mammary epithelial cell differentiation by the helix–loop–helix protein Id-1. *Mol. Cell Biol.* **15**: 3398–3404.

1488. **Dewanjee, M. K., A. K. Ghafouripour, M. Kapadvanjwala, S. Dewanjee, A. N. Serafini, D. M. Lopez, and G. N. Sfakianakis.** 1994. Noninvasive imaging of c-myc oncogene messenger RNA with indium-111-antisense probes in a mammary tumor-bearing mouse model. *J. Nucl. Med.* **35**: 1054–1063.

1489. **Dewanjee, M. K., A. K. Ghafouripour, M. Kapadvanjwala, and A. T. Samy.** 1994. Kinetics of hybridization of mRNA of c-myc oncogene with ^{111}In-labeled antisense oligodeoxynucleotide probes by high-pressure liquid chromatography. *Biotechniques.* **16**: 844–6, 848, 850.

1490. **Di Fagagna, F. D., G. Marzio, M. I. Gutierrez, L. Y. Kang, A. Falaschi, and M. Giacca.** 1995. Molecular and functional interactions of transcription factor USF with the long terminal repeat of human immunodeficiency virus type 1. *J. Virol.* **69**: 2765–2775.

1491. **Diaz Guerra, M. J., M. O. Bergot, A. Martinez, M. H. Cuif, A. Kahn, and M. Raymondjean.** 1993. Functional characterization of the L-type pyruvate kinase gene glucose response complex. *Mol. Cell Biol.* **13**: 7725–7733.

1492. **Djondjurov, L. P., M. M. Andreeva, D. Z. Markova, and R. M. Donev.** 1994. Spatial and structural segregation of the transcribed and nontranscribed alleles of c-myc in Namalva-S cells. *Oncol. Res.* **6**: 347–356.

1493. **Dolwick, K. M., H. I. Swanson, and C. A. Bradfield.** 1993. *In vitro* analysis of Ah receptor domains involved in ligand-activated DNA recognition. *Proc. Natl. Acad. Sci. U. S. A.* **90**: 8566–8570.

1494. **Dooley, S., I. Wundrack, N. Blin, and C. Welter.** 1995. Coexpression pattern of c-myc associated genes in a small cell lung cancer cell line with high steady state c-myc transcription. *Biochem. Biophys. Res. Commun.* **213**: 789–795.

1495. **Dorsman, J. C., A. Gozdzicka Jozefiak, W. C. van Heeswijk, and L. A. Grivell.** 1991. Multi-functional DNA proteins in yeast: the factors GFI and GFII are identical to the ARS-binding factor ABFI and the centromere-binding factor CPF1 respectively. *Yeast.* **7**: 401–412.

1496. **Dosaka Akita, H., K. Akie, H. Hiroumi, I. Kinoshita, Y. Kawakami, and A. Murakami.** 1995. Inhibition of proliferation by L-myc antisense DNA for the translational initiation site in human small cell lung cancer. *Cancer Res.* **55**: 1559–1564.

1497. **Dowell, S. J., J. S. Tsang, and J. Mellor.** 1992. The centromere and promoter factor 1 of yeast contains a dimerisation domain located carboxy-terminal to the bHLH domain. *Nucleic Acids Res.* **20**: 4229–4236.

1498. **Downes, M., L. Mynett Johnson, and G. E. Muscat.** 1994. The retinoic acid and retinoid X receptors are differentially expressed during myoblast differentiation. *Endocrinology* **134**: 2658–2661.

1499. **Duivenvoorden, W. C., R. Schafer, A. M. Pfeifer, D. Piquet, and P. Maier.** 1995. Nuclear matrix condensation and c-myc and c-fos expression are specifically altered in culture rat hepatocytes after exposure to cyproterone acetate and phenobarbital. *Biochem. Biophys. Res. Commun.* **215**: 598–605.

1500. **Duncan, M. K., T. Shimamura, and K. Chada.** 1994. Expression of the helix–loop–helix protein, Id, during branching morphogenesis in the kidney. *Kidney. Int.* **46**: 324–332.

1501. **Eagle, L. R., X. Yin, A. R. Brothman, B. J. Williams, N. B. Atkin, and E. V. Prochownik.** 1995. Mutation of the *Mxi1* gene in prostate cancer. *Nat. Genet.* **9**: 249–255.

1502. **Eckhardt, S. G., A. Dai, K. K. Davidson, B. J. Forseth, G. M. Wahl, and D. D. Von Hoff.** 1994. Induction of differentiation in HL60 cells by the reduction of extrachromosomally amplified c-myc. *Proc. Natl. Acad. Sci. U. S. A.* **91**: 6674–6678.

1503. **Edelman, E. R., M. Simons, M. G. Sirois, and R. D. Rosenberg.** 1995. c-myc in vasculoproliferative disease. *Circ. Res.* **76**: 176–182.

1504. **Edmondson, D. G. and E. N. Olson.** 1989. A gene with homology to the myc similarity region of MyoD1 is expressed during myogenesis and is sufficient to activate the muscle differentiation program. *Genes. Dev.* **3**: 628–640. [Published erratum appears in 1990. *Genes Dev.* **4**:1450.]

1505. **Einarson, M. B. and M. V. Chao.** 1995. Regulation of Id1 and its association with basic helix–loop–helix proteins during nerve growth factor-induced differentiation of PC12 cells. *Mol. Cell Biol.* **15**: 4175–4183.

1506. **Elferink, C. J. and J. P. J. Whitlock.** 1994. Dioxin-dependent, DNA sequence-specific binding of a multiprotein complex containing the Ah receptor. *Receptor.* **4**: 157–173.

1507. **Eliopoulos, A. G., D. J. Kerr, H. R. Maurer, P. Hilgard, and D. A. Spandidos.** 1995. Induction of the c-myc but not the cH-ras promoter by platinum compounds. *Biochem. Pharmacol.* **50**: 33–38.

1508. **Ellis, H. M.** 1994. Embryonic expression and function of the *Drosophila* helix–loop–helix gene, extramacrochaetae. *Mech. Dev.* **47**: 65–72.

1509. **Ellis, H. M., D. R. Spann, and J. W. Posakony.** 1990. extramacrochaetae, a negative regulator of sensory organ development in *Drosophila*, defines a new class of helix–loop–helix proteins. *Cell* **61**: 27–38.

1510. **Ellmeier, W. and A. Weith.** 1995. Expression of the helix–loop–helix gene Id3 during murine embryonic development. *Dev. Dyn.* **203**: 163–173.

1511. **Elson, A., C. Deng, J. Campos Torres, L. A. Donehower, and P. Leder.** 1995. The MMTV/c-myc transgene and p53 null alleles collaborate to induce T-cell lymphomas, but not mammary carcinomas in transgenic mice. *Oncogene.* **11**: 181–190.

1512. **Elwood, N. J. and C. G. Begley.** 1995. Reconstitution of mice with bone marrow cells expressing the SCL gene is insufficient to cause leukemia. *Cell Growth. Differ.* **6**: 19–25.

1513. **Elwood, N. J., W. D. Cook, D. Metcalf, and C. G. Begley.** 1993. SCL, the gene implicated in human T-cell leukaemia, is oncogenic in a murine T-lymphocyte cell line. *Oncogene.* **8**: 3093–3101.

1514. **Elwood, N. J., A. R. Green, A. Melder, C. G. Begley, and N. Nicola.** 1994. The SCL protein displays cell-specific heterogeneity in size. *Leukemia* **8**: 106–114.

1515. **Ema, M., M. Suzuki, M. Morita, K. Hirose, K. Sogawa, Y. Matsuda, O. Gotoh, Y. Saijoh, H. Fujii, H. Hamada, and Y. Fujii Kuriyama.** 1996. cDNA cloning of a murine homologue of *Drosophila* single-minded, its mRNA expression in mouse development, and chromosome localization. *Biochem. Biophys. Res. Commun.* **218**: 588–594.

1516. **Emery, J. F. and E. Bier.** 1995. Specificity of CNS and PNS regulatory subelements comprising pan-neural enhancers of the deadpan and scratch genes is achieved by repression. *Development.* **121**: 3549–3560.

1517. **Enan, E. and F. Matsumura.** 1995. Evidence for a second pathway in the action mechanism of 2,3,7,8-tetrachlorodibenzo-*p*-dioxin (TCDD). Significance of Ah-receptor mediated activation of protein kinase under cell-free conditions. *Biochem. Pharmacol.* **49**: 249–261.

1518. **Ericsson, J., S. M. Jackson, B. C. Lee, and P. A. Edwards.** 1996. Sterol regulatory element binding protein binds to a cis element in the promoter of the farnesyl diphosphate synthase gene. *Proc. Natl. Acad. Sci. U. S. A.* **93**: 945–950.

1519. **Ernst, C. W., D. A. Vaske, R. G. Larson, M. E. White, and M. F. Rothschild.** 1994. Rapid communication: MspI restriction fragment length polymorphism at the swine MYF6 locus. *J. Anim. Sci.* **72**: 799.

1520. **Evans, S. M., W. Yan, M. P. Murillo, J. Ponce, and N. Papalopulu.** 1995. tinman, a *Drosophila* homeobox gene required for heart and visceral mesoderm specification, may be represented by a family of genes in vertebrates: XNkx-2.3, a second vertebrate homologue of tinman. *Development.* **121**: 3889–3899.

1521. **Fegan, C. D., D. White, and M. Sweeney.** 1995. C-myc amplification, double minutes and homogenous staining regions in a case of AML. *Br. J. Haematol.* **90**: 486–488.

1522. **Feinman, R., W. Q. Qiu, R. N. Pearse, B. S. Nikolajczyk, R. Sen, M. Sheffery, and J. V. Ravetch.** 1994. PU.1 and an HLH family member contribute to the myeloid-specific transcription of the Fc γ RIIIA promoter. *EMBO J.* **13**: 3852–3860.

1523. **Fernandez, A., M. C. Marin, T. McDonnell, and H. N. Ananthaswamy.** 1994. Differential sensitivity of normal and Ha-ras-transformed C3H mouse embryo fibroblasts to tumor necrosis factor: induction of bcl-2, c-myc, and manganese superoxide dismutase in resistant cells. *Oncogene.* **9**: 2009–2017.

1524. **Finnegan, M. C., D. W. Hammond, B. W. Hancock, and M. H. Goyns.** 1995. Activation of MYCN in a case of non-Hodgkin's lymphoma. *Leuk. Lymphoma.* **18**: 511–514.

1525. **Fischer, K. D., A. Zmuldzinas, S. Gardner, M. Barbacid, A. Bernstein, and C. Guidos.** 1995. Defective T-cell receptor signalling and positive selection of Vav-deficient CD4$^+$ CD8$^+$ thymocytes. *Nature* **374**: 474–477.

1526. **Fisher, A. L., S. Ohsako, and M. Caudy.** 1996. The WRPW motif of the Hairy-related proteins acts as a 4-amino-acid transcription repression and protein-protein interaction domain. *Mol. Cell. Biol.* **16**: 2670–2677.

1527. **Flickinger, K. S., R. Judware, R. Lechner, W. G. Carter, and L. A. Culp.** 1994. Integrin expression in human neuroblastoma cells with or without N-myc amplification and in ectopic/orthotopic nude mouse tumors. *Exp. Cell Res.* **213**: 156–163.

1528. **Floss, T., H. -H. Arnold, and T. Braun.** 1996. Myf-5^{m1}/Myf-6^{m1} compound heterozygous mouse mutants down-regulate Myf-5 expression and exert rib defects: evidence for long-range *cis* effects on Myc-5 transcription. *Dev. Biol.* **174**: 140–147.

1529. **Fodor, E., S. L. Weinrich, A. Meister, N. Mermod, and W. J. Rutter.** 1991. A pancreatic exocrine cell factor and AP4 bind overlapping sites in the amylase 2A enhancer. *Biochemistry* **30**: 8102–8108.

1530. **Fornari, F. A. J., W. D. Jarvis, S. Grant, M. S. Orr, J. K. Randolph, F. K. White, V. R. Mumaw, E. T. Lovings, R. H. Freeman, and D. A. Gewirtz.** 1994. Induction of differentiation and growth arrest associated with nascent (nonoligosomal) DNA fragmentation and reduced c-myc expression in MCF-7 human breast tumor cells after continuous exposure to a sublethal concentration of doxorubicin. *Cell Growth. Differ.* **5**: 723–733.

1531. **Fraser, H. M., S. F. Lunn, G. M. Cowen, and P. J. Illingworth.** 1995. Induced luteal regression in the primate: evidence for apoptosis and changes in c-myc protein. *J. Endocrinol.* **147**: 131–137.

1532. **Frazier, K. S., M. E. Hines, A. I. Hurvitz, P. G. Robinson, and A. J. Herron.** 1993. Analysis of DNA aneuploidy and c-myc oncoprotein content of canine plasma cell tumors using flow cytometry. *Vet. Pathol.* **30**: 505–511.

1533. **Frost, G. H., K. Rhee, T. Ma, and E. A. Thompson.** 1994. Expression of c-Myc in glucocorticoid-treated fibroblastic cells. *J. Steroid. Biochem. Mol. Biol.* **50**: 109–119.

1534. **Fuchtbauer, E. M.** 1995. Expression of M-twist during postimplantation development of the mouse. *Dev. Dyn.* **204**: 316–322.

1535. **Fujii Kuriyama, Y., M. Ema, J. Mimura, N. Matsushita, and K. Sogawa.** 1995. Polymorphic forms of the Ah receptor and induction of the CYP1A1 gene. *Pharmacogenetics.* 5 Spec **No**:S149-S153.

1536. **Fujii Kuriyama, Y., M. Ema, J. Mimura, and K. Sogawa.** 1994. Ah receptor: a novel ligand-activated transcription factor. *Exp. Clin. Immunogenet.* **11**: 65–74.

1537. **Fujimoto, J., M. Hori, S. Ichigo, M. Nishigaki, and T. Tamaya.** 1994. Tissue differences in the expression of mRNAs of Ha-ras, c-myc, fos and jun in human uterine endometrium, myometrium and leiomyoma under the influence of estrogen/progesterone. *Tumour. Biol.* **15**: 311–317.

1538. **Fukamizu, A., M. Sagara, F. Sugiyama, H. Horiguchi, H. Kamma, T. Hatae, T. Ogata, K. Yagami, and K. Murakami.** 1994. Neuroectodermal tumors expressing c-, L-, and N-myc in transgenic mice that carry the E1A/E1B gene of human adenovirus type 12. *J. Biol. Chem.* **269**: 31252–31258.

1539. **Fukunaga, B. N. and O. Hankinson.** 1996. Identification of a novel domain in the aryl hydrocarbon receptor required for DNA binding. *J. Biol. Chem.* **271**: 3743–3749.

1540. **Fukunaga, B. N., M. R. Probst, S. Reisz Porszasz, and O. Hankinson.** 1995. Identification of functional domains of the aryl hydrocarbon receptor. *J. Biol. Chem.* **270**: 29270–29278.

1541. **Fulton, R., R. Gallagher, D. Crouch, and J. C. Neil.** 1996. Apparent uncoupling of oncogenicity from fibroblast transformation and apoptosis in a mutant myc gene transduced by feline leukemia virus. *J. Virol.* **70**: 1154–1162.

1542. **Furihata, C., A. Yamakoshi, A. Hatta, M. Tatematsu, H. Iwata, K. Hayashi, K. Umezawa, and T. Matsushima.** 1994. Induction of c-fos and c-myc oncogene expression in the pyloric mucosa of rat stomach by N-methyl-N'-nitro-N-nitrosoguanidine and taurocholate. *Cancer Lett.* **83**: 215–220.

1543. **Gaffey, M. J., H. F. J. Frierson, and M. E. Williams. 1993. Chromosome 11q13, c-erbB-2, and c-myc amplification in invasive breast carcinoma: clinicopathologic correlations.** *Mod. Pathol.* **6**: 654–659.

1544. **Gallagher, R. C., J. C. Neil, and R. Fulton.** 1995. Cloning and sequence of the feline max, and max 9 transcripts. *DNA Seq.* **5**: 269–271.

1545. **Galland, F., S. Katzav, and D. Birnbaum.** 1992. The products of the mcf-2 and vav proto-oncogenes and of the yeast gene cdc-24 share sequence similarities. *Oncogene.* **7**: 585–587.

1545a. **Gallant, P., Shiio, Y., Cheng, P. F., Parkhurst, S. M. and Eisenman, R. N.** 1996. Myc and Max homologs in *Drosophila. Science* **274**: 1523–1527.

1546. **Gandarillas, A. and F. M. Watt.** 1995. Changes in expression of members of the fos and jun families and myc network during terminal differentiation of human keratinocytes. *Oncogene.* **11**: 1403–1407.

1547. **Gaubatz, S., A. Imhof, R. Dosch, O. Werner, P. Mitchell, R. Buettner, and M. Eilers.** 1995. Transcriptional activation by Myc is under negative control by the transcription factor AP-2. *EMBO J.* **14**: 1508–1519.

1548. **Gazzeri, S., E. Brambilla, C. Caron de Fromentel, V. Gouyer, D. Moro, P. Perron, F. Berger, and C. Brambilla.** 1994. p53 genetic abnormalities and myc activation in human lung carcinoma. *Int. J. Cancer* **58**: 24–32.

1549. **George Weinstein, M., J. Gerhart, R. Reed, J. Flynn, B. Callihan, M. Mattiacci, C. Miehle, G. Foti, J. W. Lash, and H. Weintraub.** 1996. Skeletal myogenesis: the preferred pathway of chick embryo epiblast cells *in vitro. Dev. Biol.* **173**: 279–291.

1550. **Gerber, A. N. and S. J. Tapscott.** 1996. Tumor cell complementation groups based on myogenic potential: evidence for inactivation of loci required for basic helix–loop–helix protein activity. *Mol. Cell. Biol.* **16**: 3901–3908.

1551. **Gibson, A. W., T. Cheng, and R. N. Johnston.** 1995. Apoptosis induced by c-myc overexpression is dependent on growth conditions. *Exp. Cell Res.* **218**: 351–358.

1552. **Givol, I., D. Givol, S. Rulong, J. Resau, I. Tsarfaty, and S. H. Hughes.** 1995. Overexpression of human p21waf1/cip1 arrests the growth of chicken embryo fibroblasts transformed by individual oncogenes. *Oncogene.* **11**: 2609–2618.

1553. **Goldfarb, A. N. and J. M. Greenberg.** 1994. T-cell acute lymphoblastic leukemia and the associated basic helix–loop–helix gene SCL/tal. *Leuk. Lymphoma.* **12**: 157–166.

1554. **Goldfarb, A. N. and K. Lewandowska.** 1994. Nuclear redirection of a cytoplasmic helix–loop–helix protein via heterodimerization with a nuclear localizing partner. *Exp. Cell. Res.* **214**: 481–485.

1555. **Goldfarb, A. N. and K. Lewandowska.** 1995. Inhibition of cellular differentiation by the SCL/tal oncoprotein: transcriptional repression by an Id-like mechanism. *Blood.* **85**: 465–471.

1556. **Goldhamer, D. J., B. P. Brunk, A. Faerman, A. King, M. Shani, and C. P. J. Emerson.** 1995. Embryonic activation of the myoD gene is regulated by a highly conserved distal control element. *Development.* **121**: 637–649.

1557. **Goswami, S. K. and M. A. Siddiqui.** 1995. Transactivation of cardiac MLC-2 promoter by MyoD in 10T1/2 fibroblast cells is independent of E-box requirement but depends upon new proteins that recognize MEF-2 site. *Cell Mol. Biol. Res.* **41**: 199–205.

1558. **Gradin, K., R. Toftgard, and A. Berghard.** 1995. Differential effects of a topoisomerase I inhibitor on dioxin inducibility and high-level expression of the cytochrome P450IA1 gene. *Mol. Pharmacol.* **48**: 610–615.

1559. **Gradin, K., M. L. Whitelaw, R. Toftgard, L. Poellinger, and A. Berghard.** 1994. A tyrosine kinase-dependent pathway regulates ligand-dependent activation of the dioxin receptor in human keratinocytes. *J. Biol. Chem.* **269**: 23800–23807.

1560. **Grass, S., H. H. Arnold, and T. Braun.** 1996. Alterations in somite patterning of Myf-5-deficient mice: a possible role for FGF-4 and FGF-6. *Development.* **122**: 141–150.

1561. **Grauer, A., R. Baier, R. Ziegler, and F. Raue.** 1995. Crucial role of c-myc in $1,25(OH)_2D_3$ control of C-cell-carcinoma proliferation. *Biochem. Biophys. Res. Commun.* **213**: 922–927.

1562. **Gray, I. C., S. M. Phillips, S. J. Lee, J. P. Neoptolemos, J. Weissenbach, and N. K. Spurr.** 1995. Loss of the chromosomal region 10q23–25 in prostate cancer. *Cancer Res.* **55**: 4800–4803.

1563. **Greene, D. R., S. R. Taylor, M. Aihara, K. Yoshida, S. Egawa, S. H. Park, T. L. Timme, G. Yang, P. T. Scardino, and T. C. Thompson.** 1995. DNA ploidy and clonal selection in ras + myc-induced mouse prostate cancer. *Int. J. Cancer* **60**: 395–399.

1564. **Grens, A., E. Mason, J. L. Marsh, and H. R. Bode.** 1995. Evolutionary conservation of a cell fate specification gene: the *Hydra* achaete–scute homolog has proneural activity in *Drosophila*. *Development.* **121**: 4027–4035.

1565. **Griffioen, M., L. T. Peltenburg, D. A. van Oorschot, and P. I. Schrier.** 1995. C-myc represses transiently transfected HLA class I promoter sequences not locus-specifically. *Immunobiology* **193**: 238–247.

1566. **Gromova, I. I., B. Thomsen, and S. V. Razin.** 1995. Different topoisomerase II antitumor drugs direct similar specific long-range fragmentation of an amplified c-MYC gene locus in living cells and in high-salt-extracted nuclei. *Proc. Natl. Acad. Sci. U. S. A.* **92**: 102–106.

1567. **Guillemot, F.** 1995. Analysis of the role of basic-helix–loop–helix transcription factors in the development of neural lineages in the mouse. *Biol. Cell* **84**: 3–6.

1568. **Guillemot, F., A. Nagy, A. Auerbach, J. Rossant, and A. L. Joyner.** 1994. Essential role of Mash-2 in extraembryonic development. *Nature* **371**: 333–336.

1569. **Gulbins, E., K. Schlottmann, B. Brenner, F. Lang, and K. M. Coggeshall.** 1995. Molecular analysis of Ras activation by tyrosine phosphorylated Vav. *Biochem. Biophys. Res. Commun.* **217**: 876–885.

1570. **Gundersen, K., I. Rabben, B. J. Klocke, and J. P. Merlie.** 1995. Overexpression of myogenin in muscles of transgenic **mice**: interaction with Id-1, negative crossregulation of myogenic factors, and induction of extrasynaptic acetylcholine receptor expression. *Mol. Cell Biol.* **15**: 7127–7134.

1571. **Guo, K., J. Wang, V. Andres, R. C. Smith, and K. Walsh.** 1995. MyoD-induced expression of p21 inhibits cyclin-dependent kinase activity upon myocyte terminal differentiation. *Mol. Cell. Biol.* **15**: 3823–3829.

1572. **Hale, T. K. and A. W. Braithwaite.** 1995. Identification of an upstream region of the mouse p53 promoter critical for transcriptional expression. *Nucleic Acids Res.* **23**: 663–669.

1573. **Halevy, O., B. G. Novitch, D. B. Spicer, S. X. Skapek, J. Rhee, G. J. Hannon, D. Beach, and A. B. Lassar.** 1995. Correlation of terminal cell cycle arrest of skeletal muscle with induction of p21 by MyoD. *Science* **267**: 1018–1021.

1574. **Halle, J. P., C. Schmidt, and G. Adam.** 1995. Changes of the methylation pattern of the c-myc gene during *in vitro* aging of IMR90 human embryonic fibroblasts. *Mutat. Res.* **316**: 157–171.

1575. **Halle, J. P., G. Stelzer, A. Goppelt, and M. Meisterernst.** 1995. Activation of transcription by recombinant upstream stimulatory factor 1 is mediated by a novel positive cofactor. *J. Biol. Chem.* **270**: 21307–21311.

1576. **Hann, S. R.** 1994. Regulation and function of non-AUG-initiated proto-oncogenes. *Biochimie.* **76**: 880–886.

1577. **Hann, S. R.** 1995. Methionine deprivation regulates the translation of functionally-distinct c-Myc proteins. *Adv. Exp. Med. Biol.* **375**: 107–116.

1578. **Hann, S. R., M. Dixit, R. C. Sears, and L. Sealy.** 1994. The alternatively initiated c-Myc proteins differentially regulate transcription through a noncanonical DNA-binding site. *Genes. Dev.* **8**: 2441–2452.

1579. **Harlow, S. P. and C. C. Stewart.** 1993. Quantitation of c-myc gene amplification by a competitive PCR assay system. *PCR. Methods Appl.* **3**: 163–168.

1580. **Harrington, E. A., M. R. Bennett, A. Fanidi, and G. I. Evan.** 1994. c-Myc-induced apoptosis in fibroblasts is inhibited by specific cytokines. *EMBO J.* **13**: 3286–3295.

1581. **Harris, L. J., K. Currie, and V. L. Chandler.** 1994. Large tandem duplication associated with a Mu2 insertion in *Zea mays* B-Peru gene. *Plant. Mol. Biol.* **25**: 817–828.

1582. **Hartley, D. A., A. Preiss, and S. Artavanis Tsakonas.** 1988. A deduced gene product from the *Drosophila* neurogenic locus, enhancer of split, shows homology to mammalian G-protein β subunit. *Cell.* **55**: 785−795.

1583. **Harvey, W. H., O. S. Harb, S. T. Kosak, J. C. Sheaffer, L. R. Lowe, and N. A. Heerema.** 1994. Interferon-α-2b downregulation of oncogenes H-ras, c-raf-2, c-kit, c-myc, c-myb and c-fos in ESKOL, a hairy cell leukemic line, results in temporal perturbation of signal transduction cascade. *Leuk. Res.* **18**: 577−585.

1584. **Hatton, K. S., K. Mahon, L. Chin, F-C. Chiu, H-W. Lee, D. Peng, S. D. Morgenbesser, J. Horner, and R. A. DePinho.** 1996. Expression and activity of L-Myc in normal mouse development. *Mol. Cell. Biol.* **16**: 1794−1804.

1585. **Hayashi, N. and Y. Oshima.** 1991. Specific cis-acting sequence for PHO8 expression interacts with PHO4 protein, a positive regulatory factor, in *Saccharomyces cerevisiae*. *Mol. Cell Biol.* **11**: 785−794.

1586. **Hayashi, S., J. Okabe Kado, Y. Honma, and K. Kawajiri.** 1995. Expression of Ah receptor (TCDD receptor) during human monocytic differentiation. *Carcinogenesis* **16**: 1403−1409.

1587. **Hebrok, M., K. Wertz, and E. M. Fuchtbauer.** 1994. M-twist is an inhibitor of muscle differentiation. *Dev. Biol.* **165**: 537−544.

1588. **Heitzler, P., M. Bourouis, L. Ruel, C. Carteret, and P. Simpson.** 1996. Genes of the Enhancer of split and achaete−scute complexes are required for a regulatory loop between Notch and Delta during lateral signalling in *Drosophila*. *Development.* **122**: 161−171.

1589. **Helms, J. A., S. Kuratani, and G. D. Maxwell.** 1994. Cloning and analysis of a new developmentally regulated member of the basic helix−loop−helix family. *Mech. Dev.* **48**: 93−108.

1590. **Hemmi, H., K. Yamada, U. H. Yoon, M. Kato, F. Taniguchi, Y. Tsuchida, and H. Shimatake.** 1995. Coexpression of the myc gene family members in human neuroblastoma cell lines. *Biochem. Mol. Biol. Int.* **36**: 1135−1141.

1591. **Henrion, A. A., A. Martinez, M. G. Mattei, A. Kahn, and M. Raymondjean.** 1995. Structure, sequence, and chromosomal location of the gene for USF2 transcription factors in mouse. *Genomics.* **25**: 36−43.

1592. **Henske, E. P., M. P. Short, S. Jozwiak, C. M. Bovey, S. Ramlakhan, J. L. Haines, and D. J. Kwiatkowski.** 1995. Identification of VAV2 on 9q34 and its exclusion as the tuberous sclerosis gene TSC1. *Ann. Hum. Genet.* **59**: 25−37.

1593. **Henthorn, P. S., C. C. Stewart, T. Kadesch, and J. M. Puck.** 1991. The gene encoding human TFE3, a transcription factor that binds the immunoglobulin heavy-chain enhancer, maps to Xp11.22. *Genomics.* **11**: 374−378.

1594. **Hermeking, H. and D. Eick.** 1994. Mediation of c-Myc-induced apoptosis by p53. *Science* **265**: 2091−2093.

1595. **Hermeking, H., J. O. Funk, M. Reichert, J. W. Ellwart, and D. Eick.** 1995. Abrogation of p53-induced cell cycle arrest by c-Myc: evidence for an inhibitor of p21WAF1/CIP1/SDI1. *Oncogene.* **11**: 1409−1415.

1596. **Hermeking, H., D. A. Wolf, F. Kohlhuber, A. Dickmanns, M. Billaud, E. Fanning, and D. Eick.** 1994. Role of c-myc in simian virus 40 large tumor antigen-induced DNA synthesis in quiescent 3T3-L1 mouse fibroblasts. *Proc. Natl. Acad. Sci. U. S. A.* **91**: 10412−10416.

1597. **Heruth, D. P., L. A. Wetmore, A. Leyva, and P. G. Rothberg.** 1995. Influence of protein tyrosine phosphorylation on the expression of the c-myc oncogene in cancer of the large bowel. *J. Cell Biochem.* **58**: 83−94.

1598. **Hesketh, J., G. Campbell, M. Piechaczyk, and J. M. Blanchard.** 1994. Targeting of c-myc and β-globin coding sequences to cytoskeletal-bound polysomes by c-myc 3' untranslated region. *Biochem. J.* **298**: 143−148.

1599. **Heufelder, A. E. and R. S. Bahn.** 1995. Modulation of cellular functions in retroorbital fibroblasts using antisense oligonucleotides targeting the c-myc protooncogene. *Invest. Ophthalmol. Vis. Sci.* **36**: 1420−1432.

1600. **Hewitt, S. M., S. Hamada, T. J. McDonnell, F. J. Rauscher, and G. F. Saunders.** 1995. Regulation of the proto-oncogenes bcl-2 and c-myc by the Wilms' tumor suppressor gene WT1. *Cancer Res.* **55**: 5386−5389.

1601. **Hiemstra, J. L., S. S. Schneider, and G. M. Brodeur.** 1994. High-resolution mapping of the N-myc amplicon core domain in neuroblastomas. *Prog. Clin. Biol. Res.* **385**: 51−57.

1602. **Higuchi, T., H. Kanzaki, M. Fujimoto, H. Hatayama, H. Watanabe, M. Fukumoto, Y. Kaneko, H. Higashitsuji, M. Kishishita, T. Mori** *et al.* 1995. Expression of vav proto-oncogene by nonhematopoietic trophoblast cells at the human uteroplacental interface. *Biol. Reprod.* **53**: 840−846.

1603. **Hirose, K., M. Morita, M. Ema, J. Mimura, H. Hamada, H. Fujii, Y. Saijo, O. Gotoh, K. Sogawa, and Y. Fujii-Kuriyama.** 1996. cDNA cloning and tissue-specific expression of a novel basic helix−loop−helix/PAS factor (Arnt2) with close sequence similarity to the aryl hydrocarbon receptor nuclear translocator (Arnt). *Mol. Cell. Biol.* **16**: 1706−1713.

1604. **Hirst, K., F. Fisher, P. C. McAndrew, and C. R. Goding.** 1994. The transcription factor, the Cdk, its cyclin and their regulator: directing the transcriptional response to a nutritional signal. *EMBO J.* **13**: 5410−5420.

1605. **Hoang, A. T., B. Lutterbach, B. C. Lewis, T. Yano, T. Y. Chou, J. F. Barrett, M. Raffeld, S. R. Hann, and C. V. Dang.** 1995. A link between increased transforming activity of lymphoma-derived MYC mutant alleles, their defective regulation by p107, and altered phosphorylation of the c-Myc transactivation domain. *Mol. Cell Biol.* **15**: 4031–4042.

1606. **Hoang, T., E. Paradis, G. Brady, F. Billia, K. Nakahara, N. N. Iscove, and I. R. Kirsch.** 1996. Opposing effects of the basic helix–loop–helix transcription factor SCL on erythroid and monocytic differentiation. *Blood.* **87**: 102–111.

1607. **Hoffman, P. W. and J. M. Chernak.** 1995. DNA binding and regulatory effects of transcription factors SP1 and USF at the rat amyloid precursor protein gene promoter. *Nucleic Acids Res.* **23**: 2229–2235.

1608. **Hollenberg, S. M., R. Sternglanz, P. F. Cheng, and H. Weintraub.** 1995. Identification of a new family of tissue-specific basic helix–loop–helix proteins with a two-hybrid system. *Mol. Cell Biol.* **15**: 3813–3822.

1609. **Hoover, R. G., V. Kaushal, C. Lary, P. Travis, and T. Sneed.** 1995. c-myc transcription is initiated from P_0 in 70% of patients with multiple myeloma. *Curr. Top. Microbiol. Immunol.* **194**: 257–264.

1610. **Hopewell, R. and E. B. Ziff.** 1995. The nerve growth factor-responsive PC12 cell line does not express the Myc dimerization partner Max. *Mol. Cell Biol.* **15**: 3470–3478.

1611. **Hopwood, N. D., A. Pluck, and J. B. Gurdon.** 1989. A *Xenopus* mRNA related to *Drosophila* twist is expressed in response to induction in the mesoderm and the neural crest. *Cell.* **59**: 893–903.

1612. **Hord, N. G. and G. H. Perdew.** 1994. Physicochemical and immunocytochemical analysis of the aryl hydrocarbon receptor nuclear translocator: characterization of two monoclonal antibodies to the aryl hydrocarbon receptor nuclear translocator. *Mol. Pharmacol.* **46**: 618–626.

1613. **Hori, M., R. Kamijo, K. Takeda, and M. Nagumo.** 1994. Downregulation of c-myc expression by tumor necrosis factor-α in combination with transforming growth factor-β or interferon-γ with concomitant inhibition of proliferation in human cell lines. *J. Interferon. Res.* **14**: 49–55.

1614. **Hortnagel, K., J. Mautner, L. J. Strobl, D. A. Wolf, B. Christoph, C. Geltinger, and A. Polack.** 1995. The role of immunoglobulin κ elements in c-myc activation. *Oncogene.* **10**: 1393–1401.

1615. **Hortnagel, K., A. Polack, J. Mautner, R. Feederle, and G. W. Bornkamm.** 1995. Regulatory elements in the immunoglobulin κ locus induce c-myc activation in Burkitt's lymphoma cells. *Curr. Top. Microbiol. Immunol.* **194**: 415–422.

1616. **Hoshizaki, D. K., J. E. Hill, and S. A. Henry.** 1990. The *Saccharomyces cerevisiae* INO4 gene encodes a small, highly basic protein required for derepression of phospholipid biosynthetic enzymes. *J. Biol. Chem.* **265**: 4736–4745.

1617. **Hovland, R., G. Campbell, I. Pryme, and J. Hesketh.** 1995. The mRNAs for cyclin A, c-myc and ribosomal proteins L4 and S6 are associated with cytoskeletal-bound polysomes in HepG2 cells. *Biochem. J.* **310**: 193–196.

1618. **Hsu, B., M. C. Marin, A. K. el Naggar, L. C. Stephens, S. Brisbay, and T. J. McDonnell.** 1995. Evidence that c-myc mediated apoptosis does not require wild-type p53 during lymphomagenesis. *Oncogene.* **11**: 175–179.

1619. **Hu, P., B. Margolis, and J. Schlessinger.** 1993. Vav: a potential link between tyrosine kinases and ras-like GTPases in hematopoietic cell signaling. *Bioessays* **15**: 179–183.

1620. **Huang, W., S. Q. Kuang, Q. H. Huang, S. Dong, T. Zhang, L. J. Gu, L. M. Ching, S. J. Chen, L. C. Chang, and Z. Chen.** 1995. RT/PCR detection of SIL-TAL-1 fusion mRNA in Chinese T-cell acute lymphoblastic leukemia (T-ALL). *Cancer Genet. Cytogenet.* **81**: 76–82.

1621. **Huang, Y., R. Snyder, M. Kligshteyn, and E. Wickstrom.** 1995. Prevention of tumor formation in a mouse model of Burkitt's lymphoma by 6 weeks of treatment with anti-c-myc DNA phosphorothioate. *Mol. Med.* **1**: 647–658.

1622. **Huby, R. D., G. W. Carlile, and S. C. Ley.** 1995. Interactions between the protein-tyrosine kinase ZAP-70, the proto-oncoprotein Vav, and tubulin in Jurkat T cells. *J. Biol. Chem.* **270**: 30241–30244.

1623. **Hurlin, P. J., K. P. Foley, D. E. Ayer, R. N. Eisenman, D. Hanahan, and J. M. Arbeit.** 1995. Regulation of Myc and Mad during epidermal differentiation and HPV-associated tumorigenesis. *Oncogene.* **11**: 2487–2501.

1624. **Hurlin, P. J., C. Queva, P. J. Koskinen, E. Steingrimsson, D. E. Ayer, N. G. Copeland, N. A. Jenkins, and R. N. Eisenman.** 1995. Mad3 and Mad4:novel Max-interacting transcriptional repressors that suppress c-myc dependent transformation and are expressed during neural and epidermal differentiation. *EMBO. J.* **14**: 5646–5659.

1626. **Huynen, L., J. Bass, R. C. Gardner, and A. R. Bellamy.** 1992. Nucleotide sequence of the sheep MyoD1 gene. *Nucleic. Acids. Res.* **20**: 374.

1627. **Ikegaki, N., M. Katsumata, Y. Tsujimoto, A. Nakagawara, and G. M. Brodeur.** 1995. Relationship between bcl-2 and myc gene expression in human neuroblastoma. *Cancer Lett.* **91**: 161–168.

1628. Imreh, S., Y. Wang, C. K. Panda, M. Babonits, H. Axelson, S. Silva, A. Szeles, F. Wiener, and G. Klein. 1994. Hypersomy of chromosome 15 with retrovirally rearranged c-myc, loss of germline c-myc and IgK/c-myc juxtaposition in a macrophage-monocytic tumour line. *Eur. J. Cancer* **30A**: 994–1002.

1629. Inagaki, T., S. Matsuwari, R. Takahashi, K. Shimada, K. Fujie, and S. Maeda. 1994. Establishment of human oral-cancer cell lines (KOSC-2 and -3) carrying p53 and c-myc abnormalities by geneticin treatment. *Int. J. Cancer* **56**: 301–308.

1630. Inghirami, G., L. Macri, E. Cesarman, A. Chadburn, J. Zhong, and D. M. Knowles. 1994. Molecular characterization of CD30$^+$ anaplastic large-cell lymphoma: high frequency of c-myc proto-oncogene activation. *Blood.* **83**: 3581–3590.

1631. Ingvarsson, S., C. Asker, H. Axelson, G. Klein, and J. Sumegi. 1988. Structure and expression of B-myc, a new member of the myc gene family. *Mol. Cell. Biol.* **8**: 3168–3174.

1632. Inoue, N., S. Harada, T. Honma, T. Kitamura, and K. Yanagi. 1991. The domain of Epstein–Barr virus nuclear antigen 1 essential for binding to oriP region has a sequence fitted for the hypothetical basic-helix–loop–helix structure. *Virology.* **182**: 84–93.

1633. Isaac, D. D. and D. J. Andrew. 1996. Tubulogenesis in *Drosophila*: a requirement for the *trachealess* gene product. *Genes. Dev.* **10**: 103–117.

1634. Ishibashi, M., S. L. Ang, K. Shiota, S. Nakanishi, R. Kageyama, and F. Guillemot. 1995. Targeted disruption of mammalian hairy and Enhancer of split homolog-1 (HES-1) leads to up-regulation of neural helix–loop–helix factors, premature neurogenesis, and severe neural tube defects. *Genes. Dev.* **9**: 3136–3148.

1635. Ishida, S., K. Shudo, S. Takada, and K. Koike. 1994. Transcription from the P2 promoter of human protooncogene myc is suppressed by retinoic acid through an interaction between the E2F element and its binding proteins. *Cell Growth. Differ.* **5**: 287–294.

1636. Ishida, S., K. Shudo, S. Takada, and K. Koike. 1995. A direct role of transcription factor E2F in c-myc gene expression during granulocytic and macrophage-like differentiation of HL60 cells. *Cell Growth. Differ.* **6**: 229–237.

1637. Islas, A. L. and P. C. Hanawalt. 1995. DNA repair in the MYC and FMS proto-oncogenes in ultraviolet light-irradiated human HL60 promyelocytic cells during differentiation. *Cancer Res.* **55**: 336–341.

1638. Jackson, S. M., A. Gutierrez Hartmann, and J. P. Hoeffler. 1995. Upstream stimulatory factor, a basic-helix–loop–helix–zipper protein, regulates the activity of the α-glycoprotein hormone subunit gene in pituitary cells. *Mol. Endocrinol.* **9**: 278–291.

1639. Jacobs El, J., M. Y. Zhou, and B. Russell. 1995. MRF4, Myf-5, and myogenin mRNAs in the adaptive responses of mature rat muscle. *Am. J. Physiol.* **268**:C1045-C1052.

1640. Jacobsen, K. A., V. S. Prasad, C. L. Sidman, and D. G. Osmond. 1994. Apoptosis and macrophage-mediated deletion of precursor B cells in the bone marrow of E μ-myc transgenic mice. *Blood.* **84**: 2784–2794.

1641. Jain, S., K. M. Dolwick, J. V. Schmidt, and C. A. Bradfield. 1994. Potent transactivation domains of the Ah receptor and the Ah receptor nuclear translocator map to their carboxyl termini. *J. Biol. Chem.* **269**: 31518–31524.

1642. Janicke, R. U., F. H. Lee, and A. G. Porter. 1994. Nuclear c-Myc plays an important role in the cytotoxicity of tumor necrosis factor α in tumor cells. *Mol. Cell Biol.* **14**: 5661–5670.

1643. Janz, S., G. M. Jones, J. R. Muller, and M. Potter. 1995. Genomic instability in B-cells and diversity of recombinations that activate c-myc. *Curr. Top. Microbiol. Immunol.* **194**: 373–380.

1644. Jarman, A. P., M. Brand, L. Y. Jan, and Y. N. Jan. 1993. The regulation and function of the helix–loop–helix gene, asense, in *Drosophila* neural precursors. *Development.* **119**: 19–29.

1645. Jarman, A. P., Y. Grau, L. Y. Jan, and Y. N. Jan. 1993. atonal is a proneural gene that directs chordotonal organ formation in the *Drosophila* peripheral nervous system. *Cell.* **73**: 1307–1321.

1646. Jarman, A. P., E. H. Grell, L. Ackerman, L. Y. Jan, and Y. N. Jan. 1994. Atonal is the proneural gene for *Drosophila* photoreceptors. *Nature.* **369**: 398–400.

1647. Jarriault, S., C. Brou, F. Logeat, E. H. Schroeter, R. Kopan, and A. Israel. 1995. Signalling downstream of activated mammalian Notch. *Nature* **377**: 355–358.

1648. Jeffers, M. D., J. A. Richmond, and E. M. Macaulay. 1995. Overexpression of the c-myc proto-oncogene occurs frequently in uterine sarcomas. *Mod. Pathol.* **8**: 701–704.

1649. Ji, L., M. Arcinas, and L. M. Boxer. 1994. NF-κ B sites function as positive regulators of expression of the translocated c-myc allele in Burkitt's lymphoma. *Mol. Cell Biol.* **14**: 7967–7974.

1650. Ji, L., M. Arcinas, and L. M. Boxer. 1995. The transcription factor, Nm23H2, binds to and activates the translocated c-myc allele in Burkitt's lymphoma. *J. Biol. Chem.* **270**: 13392–13398.

1651. Johnson, B., B. A. Brooks, C. Heinzmann, A. Diep, T. Mohandas, R. S. Sparkes, H. Reyes, E. Hoffman, E. Lange, R. A. Gatti *et al.* 1993. The Ah receptor nuclear translocator gene (ARNT) is located on q21 of human chromosome 1 and on mouse chromosome 3 near Cf-3. *Genomics.* **17**: 592–598.

1652. **Jones, D. E. J., D. M. Cui, and D. M. Miller.** 1995. Expression of β-galactosidase under the control of the human c-myc promoter in transgenic mice is inhibited by mithramycin. *Oncogene.* **10**: 2323–2330.

1653. **Jones, G. J., N. S. Heiss, R. B. Veale, and A. L. Thornley.** 1993. Amplification and expression of the TGF-α, EGF receptor and c-myc genes in four human oesophageal squamous cell carcinoma lines. *Biosci. Rep.* **13**: 303–312.

1654. **Judware, R. and L. A. Culp.** 1995. Over-expression of transfected N-myc oncogene in human SKNSH neuroblastoma cells down-regulates expression of β_1 integrin subunit. *Oncogene.* **11**: 2599–2607.

1655. **Judware, R., R. Lechner, and L. A. Culp.** 1995. Inverse expressions of the N-myc oncogene and β_1 integrin in human neuroblastoma: relationships to disease progression in a nude mouse model system. *Clin. Exp. Metastasis.* **13**: 123–133.

1656. **Kakar, S. S. and D. Roy.** 1994. Curcumin inhibits TPA induced expression of c-fos, c-jun and c-myc proto-oncogenes messenger RNAs in mouse skin. *Cancer Lett.* **87**: 85–89.

1657. **Kanavaros, P., D. Ioannidou, M. Tzardi, G. Datseris, J. Katsantonis, G. Delidis, and A. Tosca.** 1994. Mycosis fungoides: expression of C-myc p62 p53, bcl-2 and PCNA proteins and absence of association with Epstein–Barr virus. *Pathol. Res. Pract.* **190**: 767–774.

1658. **Kato, J., Y. Kohgo, H. Kondo, K. Sasaki, and Y. Niitsu.** 1994. Antisense oligodeoxynucleotides for IL-2, c-myc and transferrin receptor synchronize mitogen-activated lymphocytes in the G1 phase. *Scand. J. Immunol.* **39**: 499–504.

1659. **Katsaros, D., C. Theillet, P. Zola, G. Louason, B. Sanfilippo, E. Isaia, R. Arisio, G. Giardina, and P. Sismondi.** 1995. Concurrent abnormal expression of erbB-2, myc and ras genes is associated with poor outcome of ovarian cancer patients. *Anticancer. Res.* **15**: 1501–1510.

1660. **Katzav, S.** 1992. vav:a molecule for all haemopoiesis? *Br. J. Haematol.* **81**: 141–144.

1661. **Katzav, S.** 1993. Single point mutations in the SH2 domain impair the transforming potential of vav and fail to activate proto-vav. *Oncogene.* **8**: 1757–1763.

1662. **Katzav, S., G. Packham, M. Sutherland, P. Aroca, E. Santos, and J. L. Cleveland.** 1995. Vav and Ras induce fibroblast transformation by overlapping signaling pathways which require c-Myc function. *Oncogene.* **11**: 1079–1088.

1663. **Kaushal, S., J. W. Schneider, B. Nadal Ginard, and V. Mahdavi.** 1994. Activation of the myogenic lineage by MEF2A, a factor that induces and cooperates with MyoD. *Science* **266**: 1236–1240.

1664. **Kawabe, Y., M. Honda, Y. Wada, Y. Yazaki, T. Suzuki, Y. Ohba, H. Nabata, A. Endo, A. Matsumoto, H. Itakura** *et al.* 1994. Sterol mediated regulation of SREBP-1a,1b,1c and SREBP-2 in cultured human cells. *Biochem. Biophys. Res. Commun.* **202**: 1460–1467.

1665. **Kazanietz, M. G., X. R. Bustelo, M. Barbacid, W. Kolch, H. Mischak, G. Wong, G. R. Pettit, J. D. Bruns, and P. M. Blumberg.** 1994. Zinc finger domains and phorbol ester pharmacophore. Analysis of binding to mutated form of protein kinase C ζ and the vav and c-raf proto-oncogene products. *J. Biol. Chem.* **269**: 11590–11594.

1666. **Kent, N. A., J. S. Tsang, D. J. Crowther, and J. Mellor.** 1994. Chromatin structure modulation in *Saccharomyces cerevisiae* by centromere and promoter factor 1. *Mol. Cell Biol.* **14**: 5229–5241.

1667. **Kerkhoff, E. and E. B. Ziff.** 1995. Deregulated messenger RNA expression during T cell apoptosis. *Nucleic Acids Res.* **23**: 4857–4863.

1668. **Khosla, S., M. J. Oursler, M. J. Schroeder, and N. L. Eberhardt.** 1994. Transforming growth factor-β_1 induces growth inhibition of a human medullary thyroid carcinoma cell line despite an increase in steady state c-myc messenger ribonucleic acid levels. *Endocrinology* **135**: 1887–1893.

1669. **Khosravi Far, R., M. Chrzanowska Wodnicka, P. A. Solski, A. Eva, K. Burridge, and C. J. Der.** 1994. Dbl and Vav mediate transformation via mitogen-activated protein kinase pathways that are distinct from those activated by oncogenic Ras. *Mol. Cell Biol.* **14**: 6848–6857.

1670. **Kim, H. G. and D. M. Miller.** 1995. Inhibition of *in vitro* transcription by a triplex-forming oligonucleotide targeted to human c-myc P2 promoter. *Biochemistry* **34**: 8165–8171.

1671. **Kim, J. B. and B. M. Spiegelman.** 1996. ADD1/SREBP1 promotes adipocyte differentiation and gene expression linked to fatty acid metabolism. *Genes Dev.* **10**: 1096–1107.

1672. **Kimura, S., T. Maekawa, K. Hirakawa, A. Murakami, and T. Abe.** 1995. Alterations of c-myc expression by antisense oligodeoxynucleotides enhance the induction of apoptosis in HL-60 cells. *Cancer Res.* **55**: 1379–1384.

1673. **Kinniburgh, A. J., A. B. Firulli, and R. Kolluri.** 1994. DNA triplexes and regulation of the c-myc gene. *Gene* **149**: 93–100.

1674. **Klefstrom, J., I. Vastrik, E. Saksela, J. Valle, M. Eilers, and K. Alitalo.** 1994. c-Myc induces cellular susceptibility to the cytotoxic action of TNF-α. *EMBO J.* **13**: 5442–5450.

1675. **Klein, G.** 1994. Role of EBV and Ig/myc translocation in Burkitt lymphoma. *Antibiot. Chemother.* **46**: 110–116.

1676. **Kleman, M. I., L. Poellinger, and J. A. Gustafsson.** 1994. Regulation of human dioxin receptor function by indolocarbazoles, receptor ligands of dietary origin. *J. Biol. Chem.* **269**: 5137—5144.

1677. **Ko, H. P., S. T. Okino, Q. Ma, and J. P. J. Whitlock.** 1996. Dioxin-induced CYP1A1 transcription *in vivo*: the aromatic hydrocarbon receptor mediates transactivation, enhancer-promoter communication, and changes in chromatin structure. *Mol. Cell Biol.* **16**: 430—436.

1678. **Kobayashi, A., K. Sogawa, and Y. Fujii-Kuriyama.** 1996. Cooperative interaction between AhR.Arnt and Sp1 for the drug-inducible expression of *CYP1A1* gene. *J. Biol. Chem.* **271**: 12310—12316.

1679. **Kohlhuber, F., H. Hermeking, A. Graessmann, and D. Eick.** 1995. Induction of apoptosis by the c-Myc helix—loop—helix/leucine zipper domain in mouse 3T3-L1 fibroblasts. *J. Biol. Chem.* **270**: 28797—28805.

1680. **Kokubo, T., R. Takada, S. Yamashita, D. W. Gong, R. G. Roeder, M. Horikoshi, and Y. Nakatani.** 1993. Identification of TFIID components required for transcriptional activation by upstream stimulatory factor. *J. Biol. Chem.* **268**: 17554—17558.

1681. **Koskinen, P. J., D. E. Ayer, and R. N. Eisenman.** 1995. Repression of Myc-Ras cotransformation by Mad is mediated by multiple protein-protein interactions. *Cell. Growth. Differ.* **6**: 623—629.

1682. **Kovacs, D. M., W. Wasco, J. Witherby, K. M. Felsenstein, F. Brunel, R. G. Roeder, and R. E. Tanzi.** 1995. The upstream stimulatory factor functionally interacts with the Alzheimer amyloid β-protein precursor gene. *Hum. Mol. Genet.* **4**: 1527—1533.

1683. **Kozma, L., I. Kiss, S. Szakall, and I. Ember.** 1994. Investigation of c-myc oncogene amplification in colorectal cancer. *Cancer Lett.* **81**: 165—169.

1684. **Krajewski, S., J. Chatten, M. Hanada, and J. C. Reed.** 1995. Immunohistochemical analysis of the Bcl-2 oncoprotein in human neuroblastomas. Comparisons with tumor cell differentiation and N-Myc protein. *Lab. Invest.* **72**: 42—54.

1685. **Krause, M., A. Fire, S. W. Harrison, J. Priess, and H. Weintraub.** 1990. CeMyoD accumulation defines the body wall muscle cell fate during *C. elegans* embryogenesis. *Cell* **63**: 907—919.

1686. **Krause, M., S. W. Harrison, S. Q. Xu, L. Chen, and A. Fire.** 1994. Elements regulating cell- and stage-specific expression of the *C. elegans* MyoD family homolog hlh-1. *Dev. Biol.* **166**: 133—148.

1687. **Krishnan, V., W. Porter, M. Santostefano, X. Wang, and S. Safe.** 1995. Molecular mechanism of inhibition of estrogen-induced cathepsin D gene expression by 2,3,7,8-tetrachlorodibenzo-*p*-dioxin (TCDD) in MCF-7 cells. *Mol. Cell Biol.* **15**: 6710—6719.

1688. **Krupitza, G., R. Fritsche, E. Dittrich, H. Harant, H. Huber, T. Grunt, and C. Dittrich.** 1995. Macrophage colony-stimulating factor is expressed by an ovarian carcinoma subline and stimulates the c-myc proto-oncogene. *Br. J. Cancer* **72**: 35—40.

1689. **Krupitza, G., W. Hulla, H. Harant, E. Dittrich, E. Kallay, H. Huber, T. Grunt, and C. Dittrich.** 1995. Retinoic acid induced death of ovarian carcinoma cells correlates with c-myc stimulation. *Int. J. Cancer* **61**: 649—657.

1690. **Kumagai, T., Y. Tanio, T. Osaki, S. Hosoe, I. Tachibana, K. Ueno, T. Kijima, T. Horai, and T. Kishimoto.** 1996. Eradication of Myc-overexpressing small cell lung cancer cells transfected with herpes simplex virus thymidine kinase gene containing Myc-Max response elements. *Cancer Res.* **56**: 354—358.

1691. **Kumakura, S., H. Ishikura, K. Tsumura, H. Hayashi, J. Endo, and T. Tsunematsu.** 1994. c-myc protein expression during cell cycle phases in differentiating HL-60 cells. *Leuk. Lymphoma.* **14**: 171—180.

1692. **Kurabayashi, M., R. Jeyaseelan, and L. Kedes.** 1995. Sequences of the $5'$-flanking region of the human helix—loop—helix protein-encoding Id2A gene, and promoter activity regulated by serum and c-Jun/AP-1. *Gene* **156**: 311—312.

1693. **Kwong, Y. L., D. Chan, and R. Liang.** 1995. SIL/TAL1 recombination in adult T-acute lymphoblastic leukemia and T-lymphoblastic lymphoma. *Cancer Genet. Cytogenet.* **85**: 159—160.

1694. **La Cava, A., E. Carbone, A. Moscarella, M. Barcova, S. Salzano, S. Zappacosta, and S. Fontana.** 1994. A novel strategy of c-myc oncogene in NK activity regulation not related to the W6/32 MHC class-I epitope. *Int. J. Cancer* **58**: 123—128.

1695. **La Rocca, S. A., D. H. Crouch, and D. A. Gillespie.** 1994. c-Myc inhibits myogenic differentiation and myoD expression by a mechanism which can be dissociated from cell transformation. *Oncogene.* **9**: 3499—3508.

1696. **Land, H., A. C. Chen, J. P. Morgenstern, L. F. Parada, and R. A. Weinberg.** 1986. Behavior of myc and ras oncogenes in transformation of rat embryo fibroblasts. *Mol. Cell. Biol.* **6**: 1917—1925.

1697. **Land, H., L. F. Parada, and R. A. Weinberg.** 1983. Cellular oncogenes and multistep carcinogenesis. *Science.* **222**: 771—778.

1698. **Larminat, F., E. J. Beecham, C. J. J. Link, A. May, and V. A. Bohr.** 1995. DNA repair in the endogenous and episomal amplified c-myc oncogene loci in human tumor cells. *Oncogene.* **10**: 1639—1645.

1699. **Lasorella, A., A. Iavarone, and M. A. Israel.** 1996. Id2 specifically alters regulation of the cell cycle by tumor suppressor proteins. *Mol. Cell. Biol.* **16**: 2570—2578.

1700. **Lavenu, A., S. Pistoi, S. Pournin, C. Babinet, and D. Morello.** 1995. Both coding exons of the c-myc gene contribute to its posttranscriptional regulation in the quiescent liver and regenerating liver and after protein synthesis inhibition. *Mol. Cell Biol.* **15**: 4410–4419.

1701. **Le Jossic, C., G. P. Ilyin, P. Loyer, D. Glaise, S. Cariou, and C. Guguen Guillouzo.** 1994. Expression of helix–loop–helix factor Id-1 is dependent on the hepatocyte proliferation and differentiation status in rat liver and in primary culture. *Cancer Res.* **54**: 6065–6068.

1702. **Lecourtois, M. and F. Schweisguth.** 1995. The neurogenic suppressor of hairless DNA-binding protein mediates the transcriptional activation of the enhancer of split complex genes triggered by Notch signaling. *Genes. Dev.* **9**: 2598–2608.

1703. **Lee, H., M. Arsura, M. Wu, M. Duyao, A. J. Buckler, and G. E. Sonenshein.** 1995. Role of Rel-related factors in control of c-myc gene transcription in receptor-mediated apoptosis of the murine B cell WEHI 231 line. *J. Exp. Med.* **181**: 1169–1177.

1704. **Lee, H., M. Wu, F. A. La Rosa, M. P. Duyao, A. J. Buckler, and G. E. Sonenshein.** 1995. Role of the Rel-family of transcription factors in the regulation of c-myc gene transcription and apoptosis of WEHI 231 murine B-cells. *Curr. Top. Microbiol. Immunol.* **194**: 247–255.

1705. **Lee, J. E., S. M. Hollenberg, L. Snider, D. L. Turner, N. Lipnick, and H. Weintraub.** 1995. Conversion of *Xenopus* ectoderm into neurons by NeuroD, a basic helix–loop–helix protein. *Science* **268**: 836–844.

1706. **Lee, L. A., L. M. Resar, and C. V. Dang.** 1995. Cell density and paradoxical transcriptional properties of c-Myc and Max in cultured mouse fibroblasts. *J. Clin. Invest.* **95**: 900–904.

1707. **Lefrancois Martinez, A. M., A. Martinez, B. Antoine, M. Raymondjean, and A. Kahn.** 1995. Upstream stimulatory factor proteins are major components of the glucose response complex of the L-type pyruvate kinase gene promoter. *J. Biol. Chem.* **270**: 2640–2643.

1708. **Lemaitre, J. M., S. Bocquet, R. Buckle, and M. Mechali.** 1995. Selective and rapid nuclear translocation of a c-Myc-containing complex after fertilization of *Xenopus laevis* eggs. *Mol. Cell Biol.* **15**: 5054–5062.

1709. **Lemaitre, J. M., S. Bocquet, N. Thierry, R. Buckle, and M. Mechali.** 1994. Production of a functional full-length *Xenopus laevis* c-Myc protein in insect cells. *Gene* **150**: 325–330.

1710. **Lenahan, M. K. and H. L. Ozer.** 1996. Induction of c-myc mediated apoptosis in SV40-transformed rat fibroblasts. *Oncogene* **12**: 1847–1854.

1711. **Lens, D., E. Matutes, N. Farahat, R. Morilla, and D. Catovsky.** 1994. Differential expression of c-myc protein in B and T lymphocytes. *Leukemia* **8**: 2102–2110.

1712. **Lerga, A., B. Belandia, M. D. Delgado, M. A. Cuadrado, C. Richard, J. M. Ortiz, J. Martin Perez, and J. Leon.** 1995. Down-regulation of c-Myc and Max genes is associated to inhibition of protein phosphatase 2A in K562 human leukemia cells. *Biochem. Biophys. Res. Commun.* **215**: 889–895.

1713. **Leroy Viard, K., M. A. Vinit, N. Lecointe, H. Jouault, U. Hibner, P. H. Romeo, and D. Mathieu Mahul.** 1995. Loss of TAL-1 protein activity induces premature apoptosis of Jurkat leukemic T cells upon medium depletion. *EMBO J.* **14**: 2341–2349.

1714. **Leroy Viard, K., M. A. Vinit, N. Lecointe, D. Mathieu Mahul, and P. H. Romeo.** 1994. Distinct DNase-I hypersensitive sites are associated with TAL-1 transcription in erythroid and T-cell lines. *Blood.* **84**: 3819–3827.

1715. **Levasseur, M., P. G. Middleton, B. Angus, S. J. Proctor, J. Norden, and M. R. Howard.** 1995. c-MYC gene abnormalities in high grade and centroblastic–centrocytic non-Hodgkins lymphoma. *Leuk. Lymphoma.* **18**: 131–136.

1716. **Lewin, I., J. Jacob Hirsch, Z. C. Zang, V. Kupershtein, Z. Szallasi, J. Rivera, and E. Razin.** 1996. Aggregation of the Fc epsilon RI in mast cells induces the synthesis of Fos-interacting protein and increases its DNA binding-activity: the dependence on protein kinase C-β. *J. Biol. Chem.* **271**: 1514–1519.

1717. **Lewin, I., H. Nechushtan, Q. Ke, and E. Razin.** 1993. Regulation of AP-1 expression and activity in antigen-stimulated mast cells: the role played by protein kinase C and the possible involvement of Fos interacting protein. *Blood.* **82**: 3745–3751.

1718. **Leygue, E., R. Gol Winkler, A. Gompel, C. Louis Sylvestre, L. Soquet, S. Staub, F. Kuttenn, and P. Mauvais Jarvis.** 1995. Estradiol stimulates c-myc proto-oncogene expression in normal human breast epithelial cells in culture. *J. Steroid. Biochem. Mol. Biol.* **52**: 299–305.

1719. **Li, H., L. Dong, and J. P. J. Whitlock.** 1994. Transcriptional activation function of the mouse Ah receptor nuclear translocator. *J. Biol. Chem.* **269**: 28098–28105.

1720. **Li, L., P. Cserjesi, and E. N. Olson.** 1995. Dermo-1: a novel twist-related bHLH protein expressed in the developing dermis. *Dev. Biol.* **172**: 280–292.

1721. **Li, S., T. Maruo, C. A. Ladines Llave, H. Kondo, and M. Mochizuki.** 1994. Stage-limited expression of myc oncoprotein in the human ovary during follicular growth, regression and atresia. *Endocr. J.* **41**: 83–92.

1722. **Lim, K. and B. D. Hwang.** 1995. Follicle-stimulating hormone transiently induces expression of protooncogene c-myc in primary Sertoli cell cultures of early pubertal and prepubertal rat. *Mol. Cell Endocrinol.* **111**: 51−56.

1723. **Lim, K., J. H. Yoo, K. Y. Kim, G. R. Kweon, S. T. Kwak, and B. D. Hwang.** 1994. Testosterone regulation of proto-oncogene c-myc expression in primary Sertoli cell cultures from prepubertal rats. *J. Androl.* **15**: 543−550.

1724. **Lin, H., R. Goodman, and A. Shirley Henderson.** 1994. Specific region of the c-myc promoter is responsive to electric and magnetic fields. *J. Cell Biochem.* **54**: 281−288.

1725. **Lin, Q., X. Luo, and M. Sawadogo.** 1994. Archaic structure of the gene encoding transcription factor USF. *J. Biol. Chem.* **269**: 23894−23903.

1726. **Lindeman, G. J., A. W. Harris, M. L. Bath, R. N. Eisenman, and J. M. Adams.** 1995. Overexpressed max is not oncogenic and attenuates myc-induced lymphoproliferation and lymphomagenesis in transgenic mice. *Oncogene.* **10**: 1013−1017.

1727. **Lipponen, P., M. Eskelinen, and K. Syrjanen.** 1995. Expression of tumour-suppressor gene Rb, apoptosis-suppressing protein Bcl-2 and c-Myc have no independent prognostic value in renal adenocarcinoma. *Br. J. Cancer* **71**: 863−867.

1728. **Lipponen, P. K.** 1995. Expression of c-myc protein is related to cell proliferation and expression of growth factor receptors in transitional cell bladder cancer. *J. Pathol.* **175**: 203−210.

1729. **Lister, J., W. C. Forrester, and M. H. Baron.** 1995. Inhibition of an erythroid differentiation switch by the helix−loop−helix protein Id1. *J. Biol. Chem.* **270**: 17939−17946.

1730. **Lo, L., F. Guillemot, A. L. Joyner, and D. J. Anderson.** 1994. MASH-1: a marker and a mutation for mammalian neural crest development. *Perspect. Dev. Neurobiol.* **2**: 191−201.

1731. **Lonn, U., S. Lonn, B. Nilsson, and B. Stenkvist.** 1995. Prognostic value of erb-B2 and myc amplification in breast cancer imprints. *Cancer* **75**: 2681−2687.

1732. **Lopez, J. M., M. K. Bennett, H. B. Sanchez, J. M. Rosenfeld, and T. E. Osborne.** 1996. Sterol regulation of acetyl coenzyme A carboxylase: a mechanism for coordinate control of cellular lipid. *Proc. Natl. Acad. Sci. U. S. A.* **93**: 1049−1053.

1733. **Lotem, J. and L. Sachs.** 1995. A mutant p53 antagonizes the deregulated c-myc-mediated enhancement of apoptosis and decrease in leukemogenicity. *Proc. Natl. Acad. Sci. U. S. A.* **92**: 9672−9676.

1734. **Lovec, H., A. Grzeschiczek, M. B. Kowalski, and T. Moroy.** 1994. Cyclin D1/bcl-1 cooperates with myc genes in the generation of B-cell lymphoma in transgenic mice. *EMBO J.* **13**: 3487−3495.

1735. **Lovec, H., A. Sewing, F. C. Lucibello, R. Muller, and T. Moroy.** 1994. Oncogenic activity of cyclin D1 revealed through cooperation with Ha-ras: link between cell cycle control and malignant transformation. *Oncogene.* **9**: 323−326.

1736. **Ludolph, D. C., A. W. Neff, A. L. Mescher, G. M. Malacinski, M. A. Parker, and R. C. Smith.** 1994. Overexpression of XMyoD or XMyf5 in *Xenopus* embryos induces the formation of enlarged myotomes through recruitment of cells of nonsomitic lineage. *Dev. Biol.* **166**: 18−33.

1737. **Luo, X. and M. Sawadogo.** 1996. Functional domains of the transcription factor **USF2**:atypical nuclear localization signals and context-dependent transcriptional activation domains. *Mol. Cell. Biol.* **16**: 1367−1375.

1738. **Luo, X. and M. Sawadogo.** 1996. Antiproliferative properties of the USF family of helix−loop−helix transcription factors. *Proc. Natl. Acad. Sci. U. S. A.* **93**: 1308−1313.

1739. **Luo, Y. and M. O. Krause.** 1994. Changes in promoter utilization in human and mouse c-myc genes upon transformation induction in temperature-sensitive cell lines. *J. Cell Physiol.* **160**: 303−315.

1740. **Ma, Q., L. Dong, and J. P. J. Whitlock.** 1995. Transcriptional activation by the mouse Ah receptor. Interplay between multiple stimulatory and inhibitory functions. *J. Biol. Chem.* **270**: 12697−12703.

1741. **Macchi, P., L. Notarangelo, S. Giliani, D. Strina, M. Repetto, M. G. Sacco, P. Vezzoni, and A. Villa.** 1995. The genomic organization of the human transcription factor 3 (TFE3) gene. *Genomics.* **28**: 491−494.

1742. **MacLean Hunter, S., T. P. Makela, A. Grzeschiczek, K. Alitalo, and T. Moroy.** 1994. Expression of a rlf/L-myc minigene inhibits differentiation of embryonic stem cells and embroid body formation. *Oncogene.* **9**: 3509−3517.

1743. **Madisen, L. and M. Groudine.** 1994. Identification of a locus control region in the immunoglobulin heavy-chain locus that deregulates c-myc expression in plasmacytoma and Burkitt's lymphoma cells. *Genes. Dev.* **8**: 2212−2226.

1744. **Mai, S.** 1994. Overexpression of c-myc precedes amplification of the gene encoding dihydrofolate reductase. *Gene* **148**: 253−260.

1745. **Mai, S., J. Hanley Hyde, A. Coleman, D. Siwarski, and K. Huppi.** 1995. Amplified extrachromosomal elements containing c-Myc and Pvt 1 in a mouse plasmacytoma. *Genome.* **38**: 780−785.

1746. **Mai, S., J. Hanley Hyde, and M. Fluri.** 1996. c-Myc overexpression associated DHFR gene amplification in hamster, rat, mouse and human cell lines. *Oncogene.* **12:** 277–288.

1747. **Mai, S. and I. L. Martensson.** 1995. The c-myc protein represses the λ 5 and TdT initiators. *Nucleic Acids Res.* **23:** 1–9.

1748. **Majello, B., P. De Luca, G. Suske, and L. Lania.** 1995. Differential transcriptional regulation of c-myc promoter through the same DNA binding sites targeted by Sp1-like proteins. *Oncogene.* **10:** 1841–1848.

1749. **Makela, T. P., E. Hellsten, J. Vesa, H. Hirvonen, A. Palotie, L. Peltonen, and K. Alitalo.** 1995. The rearranged L-myc fusion gene (RLF) encodes a Zn-15 related zinc finger protein. *Oncogene.* **11:** 2699–2704.

1750. **Makino, R., K. Akiyama, J. Yasuda, S. Mashiyama, S. Honda, T. Sekiya, and K. Hayashi.** 1994. Cloning and characterization of a c-myc intron binding protein (MIBP1). *Nucleic Acids Res.* **22:** 5679–5685.

1751. **Malde, P. and M. K. Collins.** 1994. Disregulation of Myc expression in murine bone marrow cells results in an inability to proliferate in sub-optimal growth factor and an increased sensitivity to DNA damage. *Int. Immunol.* **6:** 1169–1176.

1752. **Mallo, M., M. Gendron Maguire, M. L. Harbison, and T. Gridley.** 1995. Protein characterization and targeted disruption of Grg, a mouse gene related to the groucho transcript of the *Drosophila* Enhancer of split complex. *Dev. Dyn.* **204:** 338–347.

1753. **Malynn, B. A., J. Demengeot, V. Stewart, J. Charron, and F. W. Alt.** 1995. Generation of normal lymphocytes derived from N-myc-deficient embryonic stem cells. *Int. Immunol.* **7:** 1637–1647.

1754. **Manohar, C. F., H. R. Salwen, G. M. Brodeur, and S. L. Cohn.** 1995. Co-amplification and concomitant high levels of expression of a DEAD box gene with MYCN in human neuroblastoma. *Genes. Chromosomes. Cancer* **14:** 196–203.

1755. **Marhin, W. W., Y. J. Hei, S. Chen, Z. Jiang, B. L. Gallie, R. A. Phillips, and L. Z. Penn.** 1996. Loss of Rb and Myc activation co-operate to suppress cyclin D1 and contribute to transformation. *Oncogene.* **12:** 43–52.

1756. **Marin, M. C., B. Hsu, L. C. Stephens, S. Brisbay, and T. J. McDonnell.** 1995. The functional basis of c-myc and bcl-2 complementation during multistep lymphomagenesis *in vivo. Exp. Cell Res.* **217:** 240–247.

1757. **Marsh, A. G. and C. W. Walker.** 1995. Effect of estradiol and progesterone on c-myc expression in the sea star testis and the seasonal regulation of spermatogenesis. *Mol. Reprod. Dev.* **40:** 62–68.

1758. **Martel, C., D. Lallemand, and C. Cremisi.** 1995. Specific c-myc and max regulation in epithelial cells. *Oncogene.* **10:** 2195–2205.

1759. **Martelli, F., C. Cenciarelli, G. Santarelli, B. Polikar, A. Felsani, and M. Caruso.** 1994. MyoD induces retinoblastoma gene expression during myogenic differentiation. *Oncogene.* **9:** 3579–3590.

1760. **Martin, C., A. Prescott, S. Mackay, J. Bartlett, and E. Vrijlandt.** 1991. Control of anthocyanin biosynthesis in flowers of *Antirrhinum majus. Plant. J.* **1:** 37–49.

1761. **Massari, M. E., P. A. Jennings, and C. Murre.** 1996. The AD1 transactivation domain of E2A contains a highly conserved helix which is required for its activity in both *Saccharomyces cerevisiae* and mammalian cells. *Mol. Cell Biol.* **16:** 121–129.

1762. **Matsunaga, T., H. Shirasawa, M. Tanabe, N. Ohnuma, K. Kawamura, T. Etoh, H. Takahashi, and B. Simizu.** 1994. Expression of neuronal src mRNA as a favorable marker and inverse correlation to N-myc gene amplification in human neuroblastomas. *Int. J. Cancer* **58:** 793–798.

1763. **Matsunaga, T., H. Takahashi, N. Ohnuma, M. Tanabe, H. Yoshida, H. Enomoto, H. Horie, H. Shirasawa, and B. Simizu.** 1993. Paratesticular neuroblastoma with N-myc activation. *J. Pediatr. Surg.* **28:** 1612–1614.

1764. **Mautner, J., S. Joos, T. Werner, D. Eick, G. W. Bornkamm, and A. Polack.** 1995. Identification of two enhancer elements downstream of the human c-myc gene. *Nucleic Acids Res.* **23:** 72–80.

1765. **McKenna, W. G., E. J. Bernhard, D. A. Markiewicz, M. S. Rudoltz, A. Maity, and R. J. Muschel.** 1996. Regulation of radiation-induced apoptosis in oncogene-transfected fibroblasts: influence of H-ras on the G2 delay. *Oncogene.* **12:** 237–245.

1766. **McKenney, D. W., H. Onodera, L. Gorman, T. Mimura, and D. M. Rothstein.** 1995. Distinct isoforms of the CD45 protein-tyrosine phosphatase differentially regulate interleukin 2 secretion and activation signal pathways involving Vav in T cells. *J. Biol. Chem.* **270:** 24949–24954.

1767. **McKenzie, E. A., N. A. Kent, S. J. Dowell, F. Moreno, L. E. Bird, and J. Mellor.** 1993. The centromere and promoter factor, 1, CPF1, of *Saccharomyces cerevisiae* modulates gene activity through a family of factors including SPT21, RPD1 (SIN3), RPD3 and CCR4. *Mol. Gen. Genet.* **240:** 374–386.

1768. **Megeney, L. A., B. Kablar, K. Garrett, J. E. Anderson, and M. A. Rudnicki.** 1996. MyoD is required for myogenic stem cell function in adult skeletal muscle. *Genes. Dev.* **10:** 1173–1183.

1769. **Meier, J. L. and S. E. Straus.** 1995. Interactions between varicella-zoster virus IE62 and cellular transcription factor USF in the coordinate activation of genes 28 and 29. *Neurology.* **45:** S30–S32.

1770. **Meinhardt, G. and R. Hass.** 1995. Differential expression of c-myc, max and mxi1 in human myeloid leukemia cells during retrodifferentiation and cell death. *Leuk. Res.* **19**: 699−705.

1771. **Meluh, P. B. and D. Koshland.** 1995. Evidence that the MIF2 gene of *Saccharomyces cerevisiae* encodes a centromere protein with homology to the mammalian centromere protein CENP-C. *Mol. Biol. Cell* **6**: 793−807.

1772. **Mermod, N., T. J. Williams, and R. Tjian.** 1988. Enhancer binding factors AP-4 and AP-1 act in concert to activate SV40 late transcription *in vitro. Nature* **332**: 557−561.

1773. **Metz, T., A. W. Harris, and J. M. Adams.** 1995. Absence of p53 allows direct immortalization of hematopoietic cells by the myc and raf oncogenes. *Cell* **82**: 29−36.

1774. **Meyer, K. B., M. Skogberg, C. Margenfeld, J. Ireland, and S. Pettersson.** 1995. Repression of the immunoglobulin heavy chain 3′ enhancer by helix−loop−helix protein Id3 via a functionally important E47/E12 binding site: implications for developmental control of enhancer function. *Eur. J. Immunol.* **25**: 1770−1777.

1775. **Michelotti, E. F., T. Tomonaga, H. Krutzsch, and D. Levens.** 1995. Cellular nucleic acid binding protein regulates the CT element of the human c-myc protooncogene. *J. Biol. Chem.* **270**: 9494−9499.

1776. **Michelson, A. M.** 1996. A new turn (or two) for Twist. *Science* **272**: 1449−1450.

1777. **Miller, B. A., J. Floros, J. Y. Cheung, D. M. Wojchowski, L. Bell, C. G. Begley, N. J. Elwood, J. Kreider, and C. Christian.** 1994. Steel factor affects SCL expression during normal erythroid differentiation. *Blood.* **84**: 2971−2976.

1778. **Miltenberger, R. J., K. A. Sukow, and P. J. Farnham.** 1995. An E-box-mediated increase in cad transcription at the G_1/S-phase boundary is suppressed by inhibitory c-Myc mutants. *Mol. Cell Biol.* **15**: 2527−2535.

1779. **Mironov, N. M., A. M. Aguelon, G. I. Potapova, O. V. Gorbunov, A. A. Klimenkov, and H. Yamasaki.** 1994. L-myc allele polymorphism and prognosis for metastases in Russian gastric cancer patients. *Eur. J. Cancer* **30A**: 1732.

1780. **Miyamoto, A., X. Cui, L. Naumovski, and M. L. Cleary.** 1996. Helix−loop−helix proteins Lyl1 and E2a form heterodimeric complexes with distinctive DNA-binding properties in hematolymphoid cells. *Mol. Cell. Biol.* **16**: 2394−2401.

1781. **Miyazaki, T., Z. J. Liu, A. Kawahara, Y. Minami, K. Yamada, Y. Tsujimoto, E. L. Barsoumian, R. M. Permutter, and T. Taniguchi.** 1995. Three distinct IL-2 signaling pathways mediated by bcl-2, c-myc, and lck cooperate in hematopoietic cell proliferation. *Cell* **81**: 223−231.

1782. **Mizuguchi, J., C. H. Hu, Z. Cao, K. R. Loeb, D. W. Chung, and E. W. Davie.** 1995. Characterization of the 5′-flanking region of the gene for the γ chain of human fibrinogen. *J. Biol. Chem.* **270**: 28350−28356.

1783. **Mizushima, Y., T. Kashii, and M. Kobayashi.** 1995. Reduction of cisplatin cytotoxicity on human lung cancer cell lines with N-myc amplification by pretreatment with N-myc antisense oligodeoxynucleotides. *Anticancer. Res.* **15**: 37−43.

1784. **Mizutani, Y., M. Fukumoto, B. Bonavida, and O. Yoshida.** 1994. Enhancement of sensitivity of urinary bladder tumor cells to cisplatin by c-myc antisense oligonucleotide. *Cancer* **74**: 2546−2554.

1785. **Mol, P. C., R. H. Wang, D. W. Batey, L. A. Lee, C. V. Dang, and S. L. Berger.** 1995. Do products of the myc proto-oncogene play a role in transcriptional regulation of the prothymosin α gene? *Mol. Cell Biol.* **15**: 6999−7009.

1786. **Molkentin, J. D., B. L. Black, J. F. Martin, and E. N. Olson.** 1995. Cooperative activation of muscle gene expression by MEF2 and myogenic bHLH proteins. *Cell* **83**: 1125−1136.

1787. **Monk, B. J., J. A. Chapman, G. A. Johnson, B. K. Brightman, S. P. Wilczynski, M. J. Schell, and H. Fan.** 1994. Correlation of C-myc and HER-2/neu amplification and expression with histopathologic variables in uterine corpus cancer. *Am. J. Obstet. Gynecol.* **171**: 1193−1198.

1788. **Morgenbesser, S. D., N. Schreiber Agus, M. Bidder, K. A. Mahon, P. A. Overbeek, J. Horner, and R. A. DePinho.** 1995. Contrasting roles for c-Myc and L-Myc in the regulation of cellular growth and differentiation *in vivo. EMBO J.* **14**: 743−756.

1789. **Muller Wieland, D., P. Lochow, N. Banskota, and W. Krone.** 1995. Increase of protooncogene c-myc mRNA levels by low density lipoprotein in vascular smooth muscle cells. *Biochem. Mol. Biol. Int.* **35**: 1169−1173.

1790. **Muller, J. R., S. Janz, J. J. Goedert, M. Potter, and C. S. Rabkin.** 1995. Persistence of immunoglobulin heavy chain/c-myc recombination-positive lymphocyte clones in the blood of human immunodeficiency virus-infected homosexual men. *Proc. Natl. Acad. Sci. U. S. A.* **92**: 6577−6581.

1791. **Muller, J. R., S. Janz, and M. Potter.** 1995. Differences between Burkitt's lymphomas and mouse plasmacytomas in the immunoglobulin heavy chain/c-myc recombinations that occur in their chromosomal translocations. *Cancer Res.* **55**: 5012−5018.

1792. **Muller, J. R., S. Janz, and M. Potter.** 1995. Illegitimate recombinations between c-myc and immunoglobulin loci are remodeled by deletions in mouse plasmacytomas but not in Burkitt's lymphomas. *Curr. Top. Microbiol. Immunol.* **194**: 425−429.

1793. **Muller, J. R., G. M. Jones, M. Potter, and S. Janz.** 1996. Detection of immunoglobulin/c-myc recombinations in mice that are resistant to plasmacytoma induction. *Cancer Res.* **56**: 419–423.

1794. **Muller, J. R., M. Potter, and S. Janz.** 1994. Differences in the molecular structure of c-myc-activating recombinations in murine plasmacytomas and precursor cells. *Proc. Natl. Acad. Sci. U. S. A.* **91**: 12066–12070.

1795. **Mullick, A., N. Groulx, D. Trasler, and P. Gros.** 1995. Nhlh1, a basic helix–loop–helix transcription factor, is very tightly linked to the mouse looptail (Lp) mutation. *Mamm. Genome.* **6**: 700–704.

1796. **Munsterberg, A. E., J. Kitajewski, D. A. Bumcrot, A. P. McMahon, and A. B. Lassar.** 1995. Combinatorial signaling by Sonic hedgehog and Wnt family members induces myogenic bHLH gene expression in the somite. *Genes. Dev.* **9**: 2911–2922.

1797. **Murrell, A. M., E. O. Bockamp, B. Gottgens, Y. S. Chan, M. A. Cross, C. M. Heyworth, and A. R. Green.** 1995. Discordant regulation of SCL/TAL-1 mRNA and protein during erythroid differentiation. *Oncogene.* **11**: 131–139.

1798. **Musaro, A., M. G. Cusella De Angelis, A. Germani, C. Ciccarelli, M. Molinaro, and B. M. Zani.** 1995. Enhanced expression of myogenic regulatory genes in aging skeletal muscle. *Exp. Cell Res.* **221**: 241–248.

1799. **Muscat, G. E., S. Rea, and M. Downes.** 1995. Identification of a regulatory function for an orphan receptor in muscle: COUP-TF II affects the expression of the myoD gene family during myogenesis. *Nucleic Acids Res.* **23**: 1311–1318.

1800. **Naidu, P. S., D. C. Ludolph, R. Q. To, T. J. Hinterberger, and S. F. Konieczny.** 1995. Myogenin and MEF2 function synergistically to activate the MRF4 promoter during myogenesis. *Mol. Cell Biol.* **15**: 2707–2718.

1801. **Nakai, J. S. and N. J. Bunce.** 1995. Characterization of the Ah receptor from human placental tissue. *J. Biochem. Toxicol.* **10**: 151–159.

1802. **Namciu, S., G. E. Lyons, B. K. Micales, H. C. Heyman, C. Colmenares, and E. Stavnezer.** 1995. Enhanced expression of mouse c-ski accompanies terminal skeletal muscle differentiation *in vivo* and *in vitro*. *Dev. Dyn.* **204**: 291–300.

1803. **Navankasattusas, S., M. Sawadogo, M. van Bilsen, C. V. Dang, and K. R. Chien.** 1994. The basic helix–loop–helix protein upstream stimulating factor regulates the cardiac ventricular myosin light-chain 2 gene via independent cis regulatory elements. *Mol. Cell Biol.* **14**: 7331–7339.

1804. **Naya, F. J., C. M. Stellrecht, and M. J. Tsai.** 1995. Tissue-specific regulation of the insulin gene by a novel basic helix–loop–helix transcription factor. *Genes. Dev.* **9**: 1009–1019.

1805. **Naz, R. K., G. Kumar, and B. S. Minhas.** 1994. Expression and role of c-myc protooncogene in murine preimplantation embryonic development. *J. Assist. Reprod. Genet.* **11**: 208–216.

1806. **Nebert, D. W., A. Puga, and V. Vasiliou.** 1993. Role of the Ah receptor and the dioxin-inducible [Ah] gene battery in toxicity, cancer, and signal transduction. *Ann. N. Y. Acad. Sci.* **685**: 624–640.

1807. **Neiman, P. E., J. Summers, S. J. Thomas, S. Xuereb, and G. Loring.** 1994. Genetic instability and apoptotic cell death during neoplastic progression of v-myc-initiated B-cell lymphomas in the bursa of Fabricius. *Cold. Spring. Harb. Symp. Quant. Biol.* **59**: 509–515.

1808. **Neri, A., N. S. Fracchiolla, E. Roscetti, S. Garatti, D. Trecca, A. Boletini, L. Perletti, L. Baldini, A. T. Maiolo, and E. Berti.** 1995. Molecular analysis of cutaneous B- and T-cell lymphomas. *Blood.* **86**: 3160–3172.

1809. **Nervi, C., L. Benedetti, A. Minasi, M. Molinaro, and S. Adamo.** 1995. Arginine– vasopressin induces differentiation of skeletal myogenic cells and up-regulation of myogenin and Myf-5. *Cell Growth. Differ.* **6**: 81–89.

1810. **Neuman, K., H. O. Nornes, and T. Neuman.** 1995. Helix–loop–helix transcription factors regulate Id2 gene promoter activity. *FEBS Lett.* **374**: 279–283.

1811. **Nguyen, H. Q., M. Selvakumaran, D. A. Liebermann, and B. Hoffman.** 1995. Blocking c-Myc and Max expression inhibits proliferation and induces differentiation of normal and leukemic myeloid cells. *Oncogene.* **11**: 2439–2444.

1812. **Nieborowska Skorska, M., M. Z. Ratajczak, B. Calabretta, and T. Skorski.** 1994. The role of c-Myc protooncogene in chronic myelogenous leukemia. *Folia. Histochem. Cytobiol.* **32**: 231–234.

1813. **Nikoloff, D. M. and S. A. Henry.** 1994. Functional characterization of the INO2 gene of *Saccharomyces cerevisiae*. A positive regulator of phospholipid biosynthesis. *J. Biol. Chem.* **269**: 7402–7411.

1814. **Nikoloff, D. M., P. McGraw, and S. A. Henry.** 1992. The INO2 gene of *Saccharomyces cerevisiae* encodes a helix–loop–helix protein that is required for activation of phospholipid synthesis. *Nucleic. Acids. Res.* **20**: 3253.

1815. **Niwa, O., K. Kamiya, C. Furihata, Y. Nitta, Z. Wang, Y. J. Fan, Y. Ninomiya, N. Kotomura, M. Numoto, and R. Kominami.** 1995. Association of minisatellite instability with c-myc amplification and K-ras mutation in methylcholanthrene-induced mouse sarcomas. *Cancer Res.* **55**: 5670–5676.

1816. **Norris, M. D., M. Haber, J. Gilbert, M. Kavallaris, G. M. Marshall, and B. W. Stewart.** 1994. N-myc gene amplification in neuroblastoma determined by the polymerase chain reaction. *Prog. Clin. Biol. Res.* **385**: 27–33.

1817. **Nourse, J., J. D. Mellentin, N. Galili, J. Wilkinson, E. Stanbridge, S. D. Smith, and M. L. Cleary.** 1990. Chromosomal translocation t(1;19) results in synthesis of a homeobox fusion mRNA that codes for a potential chimeric transcription factor. *Cell* **60**: 535–545.

1818. **Numoto, M., K. Yokoro, K. Yanagihara, K. Kamiya, and O. Niwa.** 1995. Over-expressed ZF5 gene product, a c-myc-binding protein related to GL1-Kruppel protein, has a growth-suppressive activity in mouse cell lines. *Jpn. J. Cancer Res.* **86**: 277–283.

1819. **O'Connell, K. F. and R. E. Baker.** 1992. Possible cross-regulation of phosphate and sulfate metabolism in *Saccharomyces cerevisiae*. *Genetics* **132**: 63–73.

1820. **O'Connell, T. D. and R. U. Simpson.** 1995. 1,25-Dihydroxyvitamin D_3 regulation of myocardial growth and c-myc levels in the rat heart. *Biochem. Biophys. Res. Commun.* **213**: 59–65.

1821. **Ohsako, S., J. Hyer, G. Panganiban, I. Oliver, and M. Caudy.** 1994. Hairy function as a DNA-binding helix–loop–helix repressor of *Drosophila* sensory organ formation. *Genes. Dev.* **8**: 2743–2755.

1822. **Olson, E. N., H-H. Arnold, P. W. J. Rigby, and B. J. Wold.** 1996. Know your neighbors: Three phenotypes in null mutants of the myogenic bHLH gene *MRF4*. *Cell* **85**: 1–4.

1823. **Olson, E. N., M. Perry, and R. A. Schulz.** 1995. Regulation of muscle differentiation by the MEF2 family of MADS box transcription factors. *Dev. Biol.* **172**: 2–14.

1824. **Onoda, N., K. Maeda, Y. S. Chung, Y. Yano, I. Matsui Yuasa, S. Otani, and M. Sowa.** 1996. Overexpression of c-myc messenger RNA in primary and metastatic lesions of carcinoma of the stomach. *J. Am. Coll. Surg.* **182**: 55–59.

1825. **Orr, M. S., F. A. Fornari, J. K. Randolph, and D. A. Gewitz.** 1995. Transcriptional down-regulation of c-myc expression in the MCF-7 breast tumor cell line by the topoisomerase II inhibitor, VM-26. *Biochim. Biophys. Acta* **1262**: 139–145.

1826. **Oswald, F., H. Lovec, T. Moroy, and M. Lipp.** 1994. E2F-dependent regulation of human **MYC**:transactivation by cyclins D1 and A overrides tumour suppressor protein functions. *Oncogene.* **9**: 2029–2036.

1827. **Outram, S. V. and M. J. Owen.** 1994. The helix–loop–helix containing transcription factor USF activates the promoter of the CD2 gene. *J. Biol. Chem.* **269**: 26525–26530.

1828. **Paatero, G. I., T. Trydal, K. A. Karlstedt, D. Aarskog, and J. R. Lillehaug.** 1994. Time-course study of 1,25-$(OH)_2$-vitamin D_3 induction of homologous receptor and c-myc in nontransformed and transformed C3H/10T1/2 cell clones. *Int. J. Biochem.* **26**: 367–374.

1829. **Packham, G., C. Bello Fernandez, and J. L. Cleveland.** 1994. Position and orientation independent transactivation by c-Myc. *Cell Mol. Biol. Res.* **40**: 699–706.

1830. **Packham, G. and J. L. Cleveland.** 1995. The role of ornithine decarboxylase in c-Myc-induced apoptosis. *Curr. Top. Microbiol. Immunol.* **194**: 283–290.

1831. **Packham, G. and J. L. Cleveland.** 1995. c-Myc and apoptosis. *Biochim. Biophys. Acta* **1242**: 11–28.

1832. **Pagliuca, A., P. C. Bartoli, S. Saccone, G. Della Valle, and L. Lania.** 1995. Molecular cloning of ID4, a novel dominant negative helix–loop–helix human gene on chromosome 6p21.3-p22. *Genomics.* **27**: 200–203.

1833. **Pai, J. T., M. S. Brown, and J. L. Goldstein.** 1996. Purification and cDNA cloning of a second apoptosis-related cysteine protease that cleaves and activates sterol regulatory element binding proteins. *Proc. Natl. Acad. Sci. U. S. A.* **93**: 5437–5442.

1834. **Pallavicini, M. G., T. George, P. S. DeTeresa, R. Amendola, and J. W. Gray.** 1994. Intracellular dynamics of c-myc mRNA traffic in single cells *in situ*. *J. Cell Physiol.* **158**: 223–230.

1835. **Pandey, S. and E. Wang.** 1995. Cells en route to apoptosis are characterized by the upregulation of c-fos, c-myc, c-jun, cdc2, and RB phosphorylation, resembling events of early cell-cycle traverse. *J. Cell Biochem.* **58**: 135–150.

1836. **Panno, J. P. and B. A. McKeown.** 1995. Cloning and expression of a myc family member from the pituitary gland of the Rainbow trout, *Oncorhynchus mykiss*. *Biochim. Biophys. Acta* **1264**: 7–11.

1837. **Papas, T. S. and J. A. Lautenberger.** 1985. Sequence curiosity in v-myc oncogene. *Nature.* **318**: 237.

1838. **Paroush, Z., R. L. J. Finley, T. Kidd, S. M. Wainwright, P. W. Ingham, R. Brent, and D. Ish Horowicz.** 1994. Groucho is required for *Drosophila* neurogenesis, segmentation, and sex determination and interacts directly with hairy-related bHLH proteins. *Cell* **79**: 805–815.

1839. **Parr, E. J., A. W. Gibson, and K. A. Sharkey.** 1994. c-Myc antigens in the mammalian enteric nervous system. *Neuroscience.* **58**: 807–816.

1840. **Pasqualini, J. R., T. A. Chen, C. Maloche, G. Chetrite, E. Valentin, and V. Allfrey.** 1995. Transcriptional activation of the c-myc oncogene in the T-47D mammary cancer cells by conditioned media from embryonic mouse fibroblasts (BALB/c-3T3). Effect of the antiestrogen ICI 164,384. *Anticancer. Res.* **15**: 671–674.

1841. **Pastorek, J., S. Pastorekova, I. Callebaut, J. P. Mornon, V. Zelnik, R. Opavsky, M. Zat'ovicova, S. Liao, D. Portetelle, E. J. Stanbridge et al.** 1994. Cloning and characterization of MN, a human tumor-associated protein with a domain homologous to carbonic anhydrase and a putative helix–loop–helix DNA binding segment. *Oncogene.* **9**: 2877–2888.

1842. **Patapoutian, A., J. K. Yoon, J. H. Miner, S. Wang, K. Stark, and B. Wold.** 1995. Disruption of the mouse MRF4 gene identifies multiple waves of myogenesis in the myotome. *Development*. **121**: 3347–3358.

1843. **Paterson, J. M., C. F. Morrison, S. C. Mendelson, J. McAllister, and J. P. Quinn.** 1995. An upstream stimulatory factor (USF) binding motif is critical for rat preprotachykinin-A promoter activity in PC12 cells. *Biochem. J.* **310**: 401–406.

1844. **Patterson, G. I., L. J. Harris, V. Walbot, and V. L. Chandler.** 1991. Genetic analysis of B-Peru, a regulatory gene in maize. *Genetics* **127**: 205–220.

1845. **Patterson, G. I., K. M. Kubo, T. Shroyer, and V. L. Chandler.** 1995. Sequences required for paramutation of the maize b gene map to a region containing the promoter and upstream sequences. *Genetics* **140**: 1389–1406.

1846. **Patterson, G. I., C. J. Thorpe, and V. L. Chandler.** 1993. Paramutation, an allelic interaction, is associated with a stable and heritable reduction of transcription of the maize b regulatory gene. *Genetics* **135**: 881–894.

1847. **Pechoux, C., Y. Chardonnet, M. C. Chignol, and P. Noel.** 1994. Heterogeneous immunoreactivity of frozen human benign and malignant breast lesions to C-MYC and C-Ha-ras cellular oncogenes. *Histol. Histopathol.* **9**: 35–44.

1848. **Peers, B., J. Leonard, S. Sharma, G. Teitelman, and M. R. Montminy.** 1994. Insulin expression in pancreatic islet cells relies on cooperative interactions between the helix loop helix factor E47 and the homeobox factor STF-1. *Mol. Endocrinol.* **8**: 1798–1806.

1849. **Peleg, Y. and R. L. Metzenberg.** 1994. Analysis of the DNA-binding and dimerization activities of *Neurospora crassa* transcription factor NUC-1. *Mol. Cell Biol.* **14**: 7816–7826.

1850. **Peltenburg, L. T. and P. I. Schrier.** 1994. Transcriptional suppression of HLA-B expression by c-Myc is mediated through the core promoter elements. *Immunogenetics*. **40**: 54–61.

1851. **Pena, A., S. Wu, N. J. Hickok, D. R. Soprano, and K. J. Soprano.** 1995. Regulation of human ornithine decarboxylase expression following prolonged quiescence: role for the c-Myc/Max protein complex. *J. Cell Physiol.* **162**: 234–245.

1852. **Perdew, G. H., B. Abbott, and L. H. Stanker.** 1995. Production and characterization of monoclonal antibodies directed against the Ah receptor. *Hybridoma*. **14**: 279–283.

1853. **Peverali, F. A., D. Orioli, L. Tonon, P. Ciana, G. Bunone, M. Negri, and G. Della Valle.** 1996. Retinoic acid-induced growth arrest and differentiation of neuroblastoma cells are counteracted by N-myc and enhanced by max overexpressions. *Oncogene*. **12**: 457–462.

1854. **Peverali, F. A., T. Ramqvist, R. Saffrich, R. Pepperkok, M. V. Barone, and L. Philipson.** 1994. Regulation of G1 progression by E2A and Id helix–loop–helix proteins. *EMBO J.* **13**: 4291–4301.

1855. **Peyton, M., C. M. Stellrecht, F. J. Naya, H. P. Huang, P. J. Samora, and M. J. Tsai.** 1996. BETA3, a novel helix–loop–helix protein, can act as a negative regulator of BETA2 and MyoD-responsive genes. *Mol. Cell Biol.* **16**: 626–633.

1856. **Pica, F., O. Franzese, C. D'Onofrio, L. Paganini, C. Favalli, E. Bonmassar, and E. Garaci.** 1995. Effect of PGE2 on c-Myc and Bcl-2 production and programmed cell death in human lymphocytes. *Adv. Prostaglandin. Thromboxane. Leukot. Res.* **23**: 457–459.

1857. **Pietilainen, T., P. Lipponen, S. Aaltomaa, M. Eskelinen, V. M. Kosma, and K. Syrjanen.** 1995. Expression of c-myc proteins in breast cancer as related to established prognostic factors and survival. *Anticancer. Res.* **15**: 959–964.

1858. **Plet, A., D. Eick, and J. M. Blanchard.** 1995. Elongation and premature termination of transcripts initiated from c-fos and c-myc promoters show dissimilar patterns. *Oncogene*. **10**: 319–328.

1859. **Pollenz, R. S., C. A. Sattler, and A. Poland.** 1994. The aryl hydrocarbon receptor and aryl hydrocarbon receptor nuclear translocator protein show distinct subcellular localizations in Hepa 1c1c7 cells by immunofluorescence microscopy. *Mol. Pharmacol.* **45**: 428–438.

1860. **Polly, P. and R. C. Nicholson.** 1994. High levels of c-myc gene expression precede point mutational activation of Ki-ras in mouse lung cancer. *Cancer Lett.* **76**: 87–92.

1861. **Porteus, M. H., A. Bulfone, J. K. Liu, L. Puelles, L. C. Lo, and J. L. Rubenstein.** 1994. DLX-2, MASH-1, and MAP-2 expression and bromodeoxyuridine incorporation define molecularly distinct cell populations in the embryonic mouse forebrain. *J. Neurosci.* **14**: 6370–6383.

1862. **Preisler, H. D., A. Raza, R. Larson, J. Goldberg, G. Tricot, G. Browman, and J. Bennett.** 1994. The relationship of the *in vivo* cell cycle characteristics and treatment outcome in acute myelogenous leukemia to the expression of the FMS and MYC proto-oncogenes. *Leuk. Lymphoma*. **14**: 273–278.

1863. **Preiss, A., D. A. Hartley, and S. Artavanis Tsakonas.** 1988. The molecular genetics of Enhancer of split, a gene required for embryonic neural development in *Drosophila*. *EMBO. J.* **7**: 3917–3927.

1864. **Presnell, S. C., M. T. Thompson, and S. C. Strom.** 1995. Investigation of the cooperative effects of transforming growth factor α and c-myc overexpression in rat liver epithelial cells. *Mol. Carcinog.* **13**: 233–244.

1865. **Probst, M. R., S. Reisz Porszasz, R. V. Agbunag, M. S. Ong, and O. Hankinson.** 1993. Role of the aryl hydrocarbon receptor nuclear translocator protein in aryl hydrocarbon (dioxin) receptor action. *Mol. Pharmacol.* **44**: 511−518.

1866. **Prokipcak, R. D., D. J. Herrick, and J. Ross.** 1994. Purification and properties of a protein that binds to the C-terminal coding region of human c-myc mRNA. *J. Biol. Chem.* **269**: 9261−9269.

1867. **Puck, J. M., C. C. Stewart, and P. S. Henthorn.** 1991. A high-frequency RFLP at the human TFE3 locus on the X chromosome. *Nucleic Acids Res.* **19**: 684.

1868. **Pulford, K., N. Lecointe, K. Leroy Viard, M. Jones, D. Mathieu Mahul, and D. Y. Mason.** 1995. Expression of TAL-1 proteins in human tissues. *Blood.* **85**: 675−684.

1869. **Raffeld, M., T. Yano, A. T. Hoang, B. Lewis, H. M. Clark, T. Otsuki, and C. V. Dang.** 1995. Clustered mutations in the transcriptional activation domain of Myc in 8q24 translocated lymphomas and their functional consequences. *Curr. Top. Microbiol. Immunol.* **194**: 265−272.

1870. **Rao, G., L. Alland, P. Guida, N. Schreiber-Agus, K. Chen, L. Chin, J. M. Rochelle, M. F. Seldin, A. I. Skoultchi, and R. A. DePinho.** 1996. Mouse Sin3A interacts with and can functionally substitute for the amino-terminal repression domain of the Myc antagonist Mxi1. *Oncogene.* **12**: 1165−1172.

1871. **Raschella, G., A. Romeo, A. Negroni, S. Pucci, C. Dominici, M. A. Castello, P. Bevilacqua, A. Felsani, and B. Calabretta.** 1994. Lack of correlation between N-myc and MAX expression in neuroblastoma tumors and in cell lines: implication for N-myc-MAX complex formation. *Cancer Res.* **54**: 2251−2255.

1872. **Rawls, A., J. H. Morris, M. Rudnicki, T. Braun, H. H. Arnold, W. H. Klein, and E. N. Olson.** 1995. Myogenin's functions do not overlap with those of MyoD or Myf-5 during mouse embryogenesis. *Dev. Biol.* **172**: 37−50.

1873. **Ray, R. B.** 1995. Induction of cell death in murine fibroblasts by a c-myc promoter binding protein. *Cell Growth. Differ.* **6**: 1089−1096.

1874. **Reach, M., L. X. Xu, and C. S. Young.** 1991. Transcription from the adenovirus major late promoter uses redundant activating elements. *EMBO J.* **10**: 3439−3446.

1875. **Reddoch, J. F. and D. M. Miller.** 1995. Inhibition of nuclear protein binding to two sites in the murine c-myc promoter by intermolecular triplex formation. *Biochemistry* **34**: 7659−7667.

1876. **Reisz Porszasz, S., M. R. Probst, B. N. Fukunaga, and O. Hankinson.** 1994. Identification of functional domains of the aryl hydrocarbon receptor nuclear translocator protein (ARNT). *Mol. Cell Biol.* **14**: 6075−6086.

1877. **Reisz Porszasz, S., H. Reyes, H. F. DeLuca, J. M. Prahl, and O. Hankinson.** 1993. Investigation on the potential role of the Ah receptor nuclear translocator protein in vitamin D receptor action. *J. Recept. Res.* **13**: 1147−1159.

1878. **Rescan, P. Y., L. Gauvry, G. Paboeuf, and B. Fauconneau.** 1994. Identification of a muscle factor related to MyoD in a fish species. *Biochim. Biophys. Acta* **1218**: 202−204.

1879. **Reynolds, J. E., T. Yang, L. Qian, J. D. Jenkinson, P. Zhou, A. Eastman, and R. W. Craig.** 1994. Mcl-1, a member of the Bcl-2 family, delays apoptosis induced by c-Myc overexpression in Chinese hamster ovary cells. *Cancer Res.* **54**: 6348−6352.

1880. **Rhee, K., W. Bresnahan, A. Hirai, M. Hirai, and E. A. Thompson.** 1995. c-Myc and cyclin D3 (CcnD3) genes are independent targets for glucocorticoid inhibition of lymphoid cell proliferation. *Cancer Res.* **55**: 4188−4195.

1881. **Rhee, K., T. Ma, and E. A. Thompson.** 1994. The macromolecular state of the transcription factor E2F and glucocorticoid regulation of c-myc transcription. *J. Biol. Chem.* **269**: 17035−17042.

1882. **Rhoer Moja, S., H. Bazin, S. Sauvaigo, C. Chypre, and M. Vindimian.** 1994. Solid support quantitation of c-myc PCR products using a cleavable reporter. *Nucleic Acids Res.* **22**: 547−548.

1883. **Rideout, W. M., P. Eversole Cire, C. H. Spruck, C. M. Hustad, G. A. Coetzee, F. A. Gonzales, and P. A. Jones.** 1994. Progressive increases in the methylation status and heterochromatinization of the myoD CpG island during oncogenic transformation. *Mol. Cell Biol.* **14**: 6143−6152.

1884. **Riechmann, V. and F. Sablitzky.** 1995. Mutually exclusive expression of two dominant-negative helix−loop−helix (dnHLH) genes, ld4 and ld3, in the developing brain of the mouse suggests distinct regulatory roles of these dnHLH proteins during cellular proliferation and differentiation of the nervous system. *Cell. Growth. Differ.* **6**: 837−843.

1885. **Righi, M., O. Letari, P. Sacerdote, F. Marangoni, A. Miozzo, and S. Nicosia.** 1995. myc-immortalized microglial cells express a functional platelet-activating factor receptor. *J. Neurochem.* **64**: 121−129.

1886. **Rochefort, H.** 1995. Oestrogen- and anti-oestrogen-regulated genes in human breast cancer. *Ciba. Found. Symp.* **191**: 254−265.

1887. **Rohwedel, J., V. Maltsev, E. Bober, H. H. Arnold, J. Hescheler, and A. M. Wobus.** 1994. Muscle cell differentiation of embryonic stem cells reflects myogenesis *in vivo*:developmentally regulated expression of myogenic determination genes and functional expression of ionic currents. *Dev. Biol.* **164**: 87−101.

1888. **Roman, C., L. Cohn, and K. Calame.** 1991. A dominant negative form of transcription activator mTFE3 created by differential splicing. *Science* **254**: 94—97.

1889. **Romand, R., U. Hirning Folz, and G. Ehret.** 1994. N-myc expression in the embryonic cochlea of the mouse. *Hear. Res.* **72**: 53—58.

1890. **Roncalli, M., G. Bulfamante, G. Viale, D. R. Springall, R. Alfano, A. Comi, M. Maggioni, J. M. Polak, and G. Coggi.** 1994. C-myc and tumour suppressor gene product expression in developing and term human trophoblast. *Placenta.* **15**: 399—409.

1891. **Roncalli, M., G. Viale, L. Grimelius, H. Johansson, E. Wilander, R. M. Alfano, D. Springall, P. M. Battezzati, J. M. Polak, and G. Coggi.** 1994. Prognostic value of N-myc immunoreactivity in medullary thyroid carcinoma. *Cancer* **74**: 134—141.

1892. **Ronchi, A., K. Petroni, and C. Tonelli.** 1995. The reduced expression of endogenous duplications (REED) in the maize R gene family is mediated by DNA methylation. *EMBO J.* **14**: 5318—5328.

1893. **Rosenthal, S. M. and Z. Q. Cheng.** 1995. Opposing early and late effects of insulin-like growth factor I on differentiation and the cell cycle regulatory retinoblastoma protein in skeletal myoblasts. *Proc. Natl. Acad. Sci. U. S. A.* **92**: 10307—10311.

1894. **Rosolen, A., J. Toretsky, and L. Neckers.** 1994. Antisense inhibition of CHP100 C-myc expression results in reduced *in vitro* growth kinetics and loss of *in vivo* tumorigenesis. *Prog. Clin. Biol. Res.* **385**: 95—101.

1895. **Rothberg, P. G. and Y. M. Otto.** 1995. A polymorphic variant of human c-Myc: Asn11 → Ser. *Mamm. Genome.* **6**: 209—211.

1896. **Rothermel, B. A., A. W. Shyjan, J. L. Etheredge, and R. A. Butow.** 1995. Transactivation by Rtg1p, a basic helix—loop—helix protein that functions in communication between mitochondria and the nucleus in yeast. *J. Biol. Chem.* **270**: 29476—29482.

1897. **Roussel, M. F., R. A. Ashmun, C. J. Sherr, R. E. Eisenman, and D. E. Ayer.** 1996. Inhibition of cell proliferation by the Mad1 transcriptional repressor. *Mol. Cell. Biol.* **16**: 2796—2801.

1898. **Roy, B., J. Beamon, E. Balint, and D. Reisman.** 1994. Transactivation of the human p53 tumor suppressor gene by c-Myc/Max contributes to elevated mutant p53 expression in some tumors. *Mol. Cell Biol.* **14**: 7805—7815.

1899. **Ruiz Ruiz, M. C., F. J. Oliver, M. Izquierdo, and A. Lopez Rivas.** 1995. Activation-induced apoptosis in Jurkat cells through a myc-independent mechanism. *Mol. Immunol.* **32**: 947—955.

1900. **Rushforth, A. M. and P. Anderson.** 1996. Splicing removes the *Caenorhabditis elegans* transposon Tc1 from most mutant pre-mRNAs. *Mol. Cell Biol.* **16**: 422—429.

1901. **Safe, S. and V. Krishnan.** 1995. Cellular and molecular biology of aryl hydrocarbon (Ah) receptor-mediated gene expression. *Arch. Toxicol. Suppl.* **17**: 99—115.

1902. **Sagara, M., F. Sugiyama, H. Horiguchi, H. Kamma, T. Ogata, K. Yagami, K. Murakami, and A. Fukamizu.** 1995. Activation of the nuclear oncogenes N-myc and c-jun in carcinoid tumors of transgenic mice carrying the human adenovirus type 12 E1 region gene. *DNA Cell Biol.* **14**: 95—101.

1903. **Sakagami, T., K. Sakurada, Y. Sakai, T. Watanabe, S. Nakanishi, and R. Kageyama.** 1994. Structure and chromosomal locus of the mouse gene encoding a cerebellar Purkinje cell-specific helix—loop—helix factor Hes-3. *Biochem. Biophys. Res. Commun.* **203**: 594—601.

1904. **Sakamuro, D., V. Eviner, K. J. Elliott, L. Showe, E. White, and G. C. Prendergast.** 1995. c-Myc induces apoptosis in epithelial cells by both p53-dependent and p53-independent mechanisms. *Oncogene.* **11**: 2411—2418.

1905. **Sanchez, H. B., L. Yieh, and T. F. Osborne.** 1995. Cooperation by sterol regulatory element-binding protein and Sp1 in sterol regulation of low density lipoprotein receptor gene. *J. Biol. Chem.* **270**: 1161—1169.

1906. **Sandgren, E. P., J. A. Schroeder, T. H. Qui, R. D. Palmiter, R. L. Brinster, and D. C. Lee.** 1995. Inhibition of mammary gland involution is associated with transforming growth factor α but not c-myc-induced tumorigenesis in transgenic mice. *Cancer Res.* **55**: 3915—3927.

1907. **Saranath, D., R. G. Panchal, M. G. Deo, V. Sanghvi, and A. R. Mehta.** 1994. Restriction fragment length polymorphisms of the human N-myc gene in normal healthy individuals and oral cancer patients in India. *Indian J. Biochem. Biophys.* **31**: 177—183.

1908. **Sarbassov, D. D., R. Stefanova, V. G. Grigoriev, and C. A. Peterson.** 1995. Role of insulin-like growth factors and myogenin in the altered program of proliferation and differentiation in the NFB4 mutant muscle cell line. *Proc. Natl. Acad. Sci. U. S. A.* **92**: 10874—10878.

1909. **Sato, A., M. Bo, T. Maruo, S. Yoshida, and M. Mochizuki.** 1994. Stage-specific expression of c-myc messenger ribonucleic acid in porcine granulosa cells early in follicular growth. *Eur. J. Endocrinol.* **131**: 319—322.

1910. **Sato, K., M. Miyahara, T. Saito, and M. Kobayashi.** 1994. c-myc mRNA overexpression is associated with lymph node metastasis in colorectal cancer. *Eur. J. Cancer* **30A**: 1113—1117.

1911. **Sato, R., J. Yang, X. Wang, M. J. Evans, Y. K. Ho, J. L. Goldstein, and M. S. Brown.** 1994. Assignment of the membrane attachment, DNA binding, and transcriptional activation domains of sterol regulatory element-binding protein-1 (SREBP-1). *J. Biol. Chem.* **269**: 17267—17273.

1912. **Saunders, D. E., C. S. Zajac, and N. L. Wappler.** 1995. Alcohol inhibits neurite extension and increases N-myc and c-myc proteins. *Alcohol.* **12**: 475–483.

1913. **Sauter, G., P. Carroll, H. Moch, A. Kallioniemi, R. Kerschmann, P. Narayan, M. J. Mihatsch, and F. M. Waldman.** 1995. c-myc copy number gains in bladder cancer detected by fluorescence *in situ* hybridization. *Am. J. Pathol.* **146**: 1131–1139.

1914. **Schaeffer, B. K., P. G. Terhune, and D. S. Longnecker.** 1994. Pancreatic carcinomas of acinar and mixed acinar/ductal phenotypes in Ela-1-myc transgenic mice do not contain c-K-ras mutations. *Am. J. Pathol.* **145**: 696–701.

1915. **Schmidt, M. L., H. R. Salwen, C. F. Manohar, N. Ikegaki, and S. L. Cohn.** 1994. The biological effects of antisense N-myc expression in human neuroblastoma. *Cell Growth. Differ.* **5**: 171–178.

1916. **Schneider, K. R., R. L. Smith, and E. K. O'Shea.** 1994. Phosphate-regulated inactivation of the kinase PHO80–PHO85 by the CDK inhibitor PHO81. *Science* **266**: 122–126.

1916a. **Schreiber-Agus, N., Stein, D., Chen, K., Goltz, J. S., Stevens, L. and DePinho, R. A.** 1997. *Drosophila* Myc is oncogenic in mammalian cells and plays a role in the *diminutive* phenotype. *Proc. Natl. Acad. Sci. U.S.A.* **94**: 1235–1240.

1917. **Schuller, H. J., K. Richter, B. Hoffmann, R. Ebbert, and E. Schweizer.** 1995. DNA binding site of the yeast heteromeric Ino2p/Ino4p basic helix–loop–helix transcription factor: structural requirements as defined by saturation mutagenesis. *FEBS Lett.* **370**: 149–152.

1918. **Schuller, H. J., R. Schorr, B. Hoffmann, and E. Schweizer.** 1992. Regulatory gene INO4 of yeast phospholipid biosynthesis is positively autoregulated and functions as a transactivator of fatty acid synthase genes FAS1 and FAS2 from *Saccharomyces cerevisiae*. *Nucleic. Acids. Res.* **20**: 5955–5961.

1919. **Schwab, M.** 1994. Human neuroblastoma: amplification of the N-myc oncogene and loss of a putative cancer-preventing gene on chromosome 1p. *Recent. Results. Cancer Res.* **135**: 7–16.

1920. **Schwank, S., R. Ebbert, K. Rautenstrauss, E. Schweizer, and H. J. Schuller.** 1995. Yeast transcriptional activator INO2 interacts as an Ino2p/Ino4p basic helix–loop–helix heteromeric complex with the inositol/choline-responsive element necessary for expression of phospholipid biosynthetic genes in *Saccharomyces cerevisiae*. *Nucleic Acids Res.* **23**: 230–237.

1921. **Schwartz, B., D. Benharroch, I. Prinsloo, E. Cagnano, and S. A. Lamprecht.** 1995. Phosphotyrosine, p62 c-myc and p21 c-Ha-ras proteins in colonic epithelium of normal and dimethylhydrazine-treated rats: an immunohistochemical analysis. *Anticancer. Res.* **15**: 211–218.

1922. **Seckinger, P., M. Milili, C. Schiff, and M. Fougereau.** 1994. Interleukin-7 regulates c-myc expression in murine T cells and thymocytes: a role for tyrosine kinase(s) and calcium mobilization. *Eur. J. Immunol.* **24**: 716–722.

1923. **Serra, R., R. W. Pelton, and H. L. Moses.** 1994. TGF β_1 inhibits branching morphogenesis and N-myc expression in lung bud organ cultures. *Development.* **120**: 2153–2161.

1924. **Seruca, R., R. F. Suijkerbuijk, F. Gartner, B. Criado, I. Veiga, D. Olde Weghuis, L. David, S. Castedo, and M. Sobrinho Simoes.** 1995. Increasing levels of MYC and MET co-amplification during tumor progression of a case of gastric cancer. *Cancer Genet. Cytogenet.* **82**: 140–145.

1925. **Sethupathi, P., H. Spieker Polet, H. Polet, P. C. Yam, C. Tunyaplin, and K. L. Knight.** 1994. Lymphoid and non-lymphoid tumors in E κ-myc transgenic rabbits. *Leukemia* **8**: 2144–2155.

1926. **Shain, D. H., T. Neuman, and M. X. Zuber.** 1995. A novel initiator regulates expression of the nontissue-specific helix–loop–helix gene ME1. *Nucleic Acids Res.* **23**: 1696–1703.

1927. **Shain, D. H. and M. X. Zuber.** 1995. Identification of non-tissue-specific helix–loop–helix genes in *Xenopus laevis*. *Gene* **165**: 319–320.

1928. **Sharma, S., J. Leonard, S. Lee, H. D. Chapman, E. H. Leiter, and M. R. Montminy.** 1996. Pancreatic islet expression of the homeobox factor STF-1 relies on an E-box motif that binds USF. *J. Biol. Chem.* **271**: 2294–2299.

1929. **Sheng, Z., H. Otani, M. S. Brown, and J. L. Goldstein.** 1995. Independent regulation of sterol regulatory element-binding proteins 1 and 2 in hamster liver. *Proc. Natl. Acad. Sci. U. S. A.* **92**: 935–938.

1930. **Shi, Y., A. Fard, A. Galeo, H. G. Hutchinson, P. Vermani, G. R. Dodge, D. J. Hall, F. Shaheen, and A. Zalewski.** 1994. Transcatheter delivery of c-myc antisense oligomers reduces neointimal formation in a porcine model of coronary artery balloon injury. *Circulation.* **90**: 944–951.

1931. **Shimada, H., D. O. Stram, J. Chatten, V. V. Joshi, Y. Hachitanda, G. M. Brodeur, J. N. Lukens, K. K. Matthay, and R. C. Seeger.** 1995. Identification of subsets of neuroblastomas by combined histopathologic and N-myc analysis. *J. Natl. Cancer Inst.* **87**: 1470–1476.

1932. **Shimamoto, T., K. Ohyashiki, J. H. Ohyashiki, K. Kawakubo, T. Fujimura, H. Iwama, S. Nakazawa, and K. Toyama.** 1995. The expression pattern of erythrocyte/megakaryocyte-related transcription factors GATA-1 and the stem cell leukemia gene correlates with hematopoietic differentiation and is associated with outcome of acute myeloid leukemia. *Blood.* **86**: 3173–3180.

1933. Shimizu, C., C. Akazawa, S. Nakanishi, and R. Kageyama. 1995. MATH-2, a mammalian helix−loop−helix factor structurally related to the product of *Drosophila* proneural gene atonal, is specifically expressed in the nervous system. *Eur. J. Biochem.* **229**: 239−248.

1934. Shimizu, N., H. Nakamura, T. Kadota, K. Kitajima, T. Oda, T. Hirano, and H. Utiyama. 1994. Loss of amplified c-myc genes in the spontaneously differentiated HL-60 cells. *Cancer Res.* **54**: 3561−3567.

1935. Shivdasani, R. A., E. L. Mayer, and S. H. Orkin. 1995. Absence of blood formation in mice lacking the T-cell leukaemia oncoprotein tal-1/SCL. *Nature* **373**: 432−434.

1936. Shrivastava, A. and K. Calame. 1995. Association with c-Myc: an alternated mechanism for c-Myc function. *Curr. Top. Microbiol. Immunol.* **194**: 273−282.

1937. Shung, B., J. Miyakoshi, and H. Takebe. 1994. X-ray-induced transcriptional activation of c-myc and XRCC1 genes in ataxia telangiectasia cells. *Mutat. Res.* **307**: 43−51.

1938. Siderovski, D. P., S. P. Heximer, and D. R. Forsdyke. 1994. A human gene encoding a putative basic helix−loop−helix phosphoprotein whose mRNA increases rapidly in cycloheximide-treated blood mononuclear cells. *DNA Cell Biol.* **13**: 125−147.

1939. Sigvardsson, M., K. Johansson, L. G. Larsson, K. Nilsson, and T. Leanderson. 1994. Ectopic expression of myc or myn down-regulates immunoglobulin transcription. *Leukemia* **8**: 1157−1163.

1940. Simile, M. M., R. Pascale, M. R. De Miglio, A. Nufris, L. Daino, M. A. Seddaiu, L. Gaspa, and F. Feo. 1994. Correlation between *S*-adenosyl-L-methionine content and production of c-myc, c-Ha-ras, and c-Ki-ras mRNA transcripts in the early stages of rat liver carcinogenesis. *Cancer Lett.* **79**: 9−16.

1941. Simm, A., J. P. Halle, and G. Adam. 1994. Proliferative and metabolic capacity of rat embryo fibroblasts immortalized by c-myc depends on cellular age at oncogenic transfection. *Eur. J. Cell Biol.* **65**: 121−131.

1942. Simon, H. G., C. Nelson, D. Goff, E. Laufer, B. A. Morgan, and C. Tabin. 1995. Differential expression of myogenic regulatory genes and Msx-1 during dedifferentiation and redifferentiation of regenerating amphibian limbs. *Dev. Dyn.* **202**: 1−12.

1943. Singh, I. S., Z. Luo, M. T. Kozlowski, and J. Erlichman. 1994. Association of USF and c-Myc with a helix−loop−helix-consensus motif in the core promoter of the murine type II β regulatory subunit gene of cyclic adenosine 3',5'-monophosphate-dependent protein kinase. *Mol. Endocrinol.* **8**: 1163−1174.

1944. Skerjanc, I. S., R. S. Slack, and M. W. McBurney. 1994. Cellular aggregation enhances MyoD-directed skeletal myogenesis in embryonal carcinoma cells. *Mol. Cell Biol.* **14**: 8451−8459.

1945. Skerjanc, I. S., J. Truong, P. Filion, and M. W. McBurney. 1996. A splice variant of the ITF-2 transcript encodes a transcription factor that inhibits MyoD activity. *J. Biol. Chem.* **271**: 3555−3561.

1946. Skoda, R. C., S. F. Tsai, S. H. Orkin, and P. Leder. 1995. Expression of c-MYC under the control of GATA-1 regulatory sequences causes erythroleukemia in transgenic mice. *J. Exp. Med.* **181**: 1603−1613.

1947. Skorski, T., M. Nieborowska Skorska, K. Campbell, R. V. Iozzo, G. Zon, Z. Darzynkiewicz, and B. Calabretta. 1995. Leukemia treatment in severe combined immunodeficiency mice by antisense oligodeoxynucleotides targeting cooperating oncogenes. *J. Exp. Med.* **182**: 1645−1653.

1948. Sleight, B. J., S. Soukup, E. T. Ballard, and L. M. Parysek. 1993. S-cells from a highly N-myc-amplified neuroblastoma are tumorigenic in nude mice. *Anticancer. Res.* **13**: 2031−2036.

1949. Slovak, M. L., J. P. Ho, M. J. Pettenati, A. Khan, D. Douer, S. Lal, and S. T. Traweek. 1994. Localization of amplified MYC gene sequences to double minute chromosomes in acute myelogenous leukemia. *Genes. Chromosom. Cancer* **9**: 62−67.

1950. Smith, T. H., A. M. Kachinsky, and J. B. Miller. 1994. Somite subdomains, muscle cell origins, and the four muscle regulatory factor proteins. *J. Cell Biol.* **127**: 95−105.

1951. Smith-Sorensen, B., E. M. Hijmans, R. L. Beijersbergen, and R. Bernards. 1996. Functional analysis of Burkitt's lymphoma mutant c-Myc proteins. *J. Biol. Chem.* **271**: 5513−5518.

1952. Sogawa, K., K. Iwabuchi, H. Abe, and Y. Fujii Kuriyama. 1995. Transcriptional activation domains of the Ah receptor and Ah receptor nuclear translocator. *J. Cancer Res. Clin. Oncol.* **121**: 612−620.

1953. Sogawa, K., R. Nakano, A. Kobayashi, Y. Kikuchi, N. Ohe, N. Matsushita, and Y. Fujii Kuriyama. 1995. Possible function of Ah receptor nuclear translocator (Arnt) homodimer in transcriptional regulation. *Proc. Natl. Acad. Sci. U. S. A.* **92**: 1936−1940.

1954. Soini, Y., A. Mannermaa, R. Winqvist, D. Kamel, K. Poikonen, H. Kiviniemi, and P. Paakko. 1994. Application of fine-needle aspiration to the demonstration of ERBB2 and MYC expression by *in situ* hybridization in breast carcinoma. *J. Histochem. Cytochem.* **42**: 795−803.

1955. Solomon, D. L., A. Philipp, H. Land, and M. Eilers. 1995. Expression of cyclin D1 mRNA is not upregulated by Myc in rat fibroblasts. *Oncogene.* **11**: 1893−1897.

1956. **Spaventi, R., E. Kamenjicki, N. Pecina, S. Grazio, J. Pavelic, B. Kusic, D. Cvrtila, Z. Danilovic, S. Spaventi** *et al.* 1994. Immunohistochemical detection of TGF-α, EGF-R, c-erbB-2, c-H-ras, c-myc, estrogen and progesterone in benign and malignant human breast lesions: a concomitant expression. *In. Vivo.* **8**: 183−189.

1957. **Spicer, D. B., J. Rhee, W. L. Cheung, and A. B. Lassar.** 1996. Inhibition of myogenic bHLH and MEF2 transcription factors by the bHLH protein Twist. *Science* **272**: 1476−1480.

1958. **Srivastava, D., P. Cserjesi, and E. N. Olson.** 1995. A subclass of bHLH proteins required for cardiac morphogenesis. *Science* **270**: 1995−1999.

1959. **Stasiv, Y. Z., T. D. Mashkova, B. K. Chernov, I. V. Sokolova, A. V. Itkes, and L. L. Kisselev.** 1994. Cloning of a cDNA encoding a human protein which binds a sequence in the c-myc gene similar to the interferon-stimulated response element. *Gene* **145**: 267−272.

1960. **Steiner, P., A. Philipp, J. Lukas, D. Godden Kent, M. Pagano, S. Mittnacht, J. Bartek, and M. Eilers.** 1995. Identification of a Myc-dependent step during the formation of active G1 cyclin-cdk complexes. *EMBO J.* **14**: 4814−4826.

1961. **Steiner, S. M., Y. Hu, and M. R. Steiner.** 1995. Regulation of prostaglandin H synthase 1 and 2 in MyoD transfected cells. *Exp. Cell Res.* **218**: 389−393.

1962. **Steingrimsson, E., K. J. Moore, M. L. Lamoreux, D. A. Ferre, S. K. Burley, D. C. Zimring, L. C. Skow, C. A. Hodgkinson, H. Arnheiter, N. G. Copeland** *et al.* 1994. Molecular basis of mouse microphthalmia (mi) mutations helps explain their developmental and phenotypic consequences. *Nat. Genet.* **8**: 256−263.

1963. **Steingrimsson, E., M. Sawadogo, D. J. Gilbert, A. S. Zervos, R. Brent, M. A. Blanar, D. E. Fisher, N. G. Copeland, and N. A. Jenkins.** 1995. Murine chromosomal location of five bHLH-Zip transcription factor genes. *Genomics.* **28**: 179−183.

1964. **Stocker, U., A. Schaefer, and H. Marquardt.** 1995. DMSO-like rapid decrease in c-myc and c-myb mRNA levels and induction of differentiation in HL-60 cells by the anthracycline antitumor antibiotic aclarubicin. *Leukemia* **9**: 146−154.

1965. **Streicher, R., J. Kotzka, D. Muller-Wieland, G. Siemeister, M. Munck, H. Avci, and W. Krone.** 1996. SREBP-1 mediates activation of the low density lipoprotein receptor promoter by insulin and insulin-like growth factor-1. *J. Biol. Chem.* **271**: 7128−7133.

1966. **Suda, K., H. O. Nornes, and T. Neuman.** 1994. Class A basic helix−loop−helix transcription factors in early stages of chick neural tube development: evidence for functional redundancy. *Neurosci. Lett.* **177**: 87−90.

1967. **Sugimoto, T., F. Tsukamato, M. Fujita, and S. Takai.** 1994. Ki-ras and c-myc oncogene expression measured by coamplification polymerase chain reaction. *Biochem. Biophys. Res. Commun.* **201**: 574−580.

1968. **Sun, X. H.** 1994. Constitutive expression of the Id1 gene impairs mouse B cell development. *Cell* **79**: 893−900.

1969. **Svaren, J. and W. Horz.** 1995. Interplay between nucleosomes and transcription factors at the yeast PHO5 promoter. *Semin. Cell Biol.* **6**: 177−183.

1970. **Svaren, J., J. Schmitz, and W. Horz.** 1994. The transactivation domain of Pho4 is required for nucleosome disruption at the PHO5 promoter. *EMBO J.* **13**: 4856−4862.

1971. **Swanson, H. I. and C. A. Bradfield.** 1993. The AH-receptor: genetics, structure and function. *Pharmacogenetics.* **3**: 213−230.

1972. **Tabib, A. and U. Bachrach.** 1994. Activation of the proto-oncogene c-myc and c-fos by c-ras: involvement of polyamines. *Biochem. Biophys. Res. Commun.* **202**: 720−727.

1973. **Tachibana, M., L. A. Perez Jurado, A. Nakayama, C. A. Hodgkinson, X. Li, M. Schneider, T. Miki, J. Fex, U. Francke, and H. Arnheiter.** 1994. Cloning of MITF, the human homolog of the mouse microphthalmia gene and assignment to chromosome 3p14.1-p12.3. *Hum. Mol. Genet.* **3**: 553−557.

1974. **Tajbakhsh, S. and M. E. Buckingham.** 1995. Lineage restriction of the myogenic conversion factor myf-5 in the brain. *Development.* **121**: 4077−4083.

1975. **Takahashi, N., U. Harttig, D. E. Williams, and G. S. Bailey.** 1996. The model Ah-receptor agonist β-naphthoflavone inhibits aflatoxin B1-DNA binding *in vivo* in rainbow trout at dietary levels that do not induce CYP1A enzymes. *Carcinogenesis* **17**: 79−87.

1976. **Takai, T., Y. Nishita, S. M. Iguchi Ariga, and H. Ariga.** 1994. Molecular cloning of MSSP-2, a c-myc gene single-strand binding protein: characterization of binding specificity and DNA replication activity. *Nucleic Acids Res.* **22**: 5576−5581.

1977. **Takebayashi, K., C. Akazawa, S. Nakanishi, and R. Kageyama.** 1995. Structure and promoter analysis of the gene encoding the mouse helix−loop−helix factor HES-5. Identification of the neural precursor cell-specific promoter element. *J. Biol. Chem.* **270**: 1342−1349.

1978. **Tamura, M. and M. Noda.** 1994. Identification of a DNA sequence involved in osteoblast-specific gene expression via interaction with helix−loop−helix (HLH)-type transcription factors. *J. Cell Biol.* **126**: 773−782.

1979. **Tanaka, N., M. Ishihara, and T. Taniguchi.** 1994. Suppression of c-myc or fosB-induced cell transformation by the transcription factor IRF-1. *Cancer Lett.* **83**: 191−196.

1980. Tanaka, T., R. C. Seeger, M. Tanabe, E. Hiyama, H. Shimoda, and N. Ida. 1994. Prognostic prediction in neuroblastomas: clinical significance of combined analysis for Ha-ras p21 expression and N-myc gene amplification. *Cancer Detect. Prev.* **18**: 283–289.

1981. Tanigawa, T., N. Elwood, D. Metcalf, D. Cary, E. DeLuca, N. A. Nicola, and C. G. Begley. 1993. The SCL gene product is regulated by and differentially regulates cytokine responses during myeloid leukemic cell differentiation. *Proc. Natl. Acad. Sci. U. S. A.* **90**: 7864–7868.

1982. Tanji, K., S. Sancho, and A. F. Miranda. 1994. Innervation of MyoD-converted human amniocytes and fibroblasts by fetal rodent spinal cord neurons. *Neuromuscul. Disord.* **4**: 317–324.

1983. Tappero, G., G. Natoli, G. Anfossi, F. Rosina, F. Negro, A. Smedile, F. Bonino, A. Angeli, R. H. Purcell, M. Rizzetto *et al.* 1994. Expression of the c-myc protooncogene product in cells infected with the hepatitis delta virus. *Hepatology* **20**: 1109–1114.

1984. Tarakhovsky, A., M. Turner, S. Schaal, P. J. Mee, L. P. Duddy, K. Rajewsky, and V. L. Tybulewicz. 1995. Defective antigen receptor-mediated proliferation of B and T cells in the absence of Vav. *Nature* **374**: 467–470.

1985. Tate, J. E., G. L. Mutter, C. J. Prasad, R. Berkowitz, H. Goodman, and C. P. Crum. 1994. Analysis of HPV-positive and -negative vulvar carcinomas for alterations in c-myc, Ha-, Ki-, and N-ras genes. *Gynecol. Oncol.* **53**: 78–83.

1986. Tatsuta, M., H. Iishi, M. Baba, A. Nakaizumi, H. Uehara, and H. Taniguchi. 1994. Expression of c-myc mRNA as an aid in histologic differentiation of adenoma from well differentiated adenocarcinoma in the stomach. *Cancer* **73**: 1795–1799.

1987. Tavtigian, S. V., S. D. Zabludoff, and B. J. Wold. 1994. Cloning of mid-G1 serum response genes and identification of a subset regulated by conditional myc expression. *Mol. Biol. Cell* **5**: 375–388.

1988. Tedesco, D., M. Caruso, L. Fischer Fantuzzi, and C. Vesco. 1995. The inhibition of cultured myoblast differentiation by the simian virus 40 large T antigen occurs after myogenin expression and Rb up-regulation and is not exerted by transformation-competent cytoplasmic mutants. *J. Virol.* **69**: 6947–6957.

1989. Theopold, U., S. Ekengren, and D. Hultmark. 1996. HLH106, a *Drosophila* transcription factor with similarity to the vertebrate sterol responsive element binding protein. *Proc. Natl. Acad. Sci. U. S. A.* **93**: 1195–1199.

1990. Thompson, E. B., R. Thulasi, M. F. Saeed, and B. H. Johnson. 1995. Glucocorticoid antagonist RU 486 reverses agonist-induced apoptosis and c-myc repression in human leukemic CEM-C7 cells. *Ann. N. Y. Acad. Sci.* **761**: 261–275.

1991. Tikhonenko, A. T., D. J. Black, and M. L. Linial. 1995. v-Myc is invariably required to sustain rapid proliferation of infected cells but in stable cell lines becomes dispensable for other traits of the transformed phenotype. *Oncogene.* **11**: 1499–1508.

1992. Timchenko, N., D. R. Wilson, L. R. Taylor, S. Abdelsayed, M. Wilde, M. Sawadogo, and G. J. Darlington. 1995. Autoregulation of the human C/EBP α gene by stimulation of upstream stimulatory factor binding. *Mol. Cell Biol.* **15**: 1192–1202.

1993. Tobias, K. E., J. Shor, and C. Kahana. 1995. c-Myc and Max transregulate the mouse ornithine decarboxylase promoter through interaction with two downstream CACGTG motifs. *Oncogene.* **11**: 1721–1727.

1994. Toda, T., T. Tamamoto, S. Shimajiri, A. M. Sadi, Y. Nakashima, and H. Takei. 1995. Expression of PDGF and C-myc in atherosclerotic lesions in cholesterol-fed chicken. Immunohistochemical and *in situ* hybridization study. *Ann. N. Y. Acad. Sci.* **748**: 514–516.

1995. Tomonaga, T., H. Hayashi, M. Taira, K. Isono, and I. Kojima. 1994. Signaling pathway other than phosphatidylinositol turnover is responsible for constant expression of c-myc gene in primary cultures of rat hepatocytes. *Biochem. Mol. Biol. Int.* **33**: 429–437.

1996. Tonjes, R. R., J. Lohler, J. F. O'Sullivan, G. F. Kay, G. H. Schmidt, W. Dalemans, A. Pavirani, and D. Paul. 1995. Autocrine mitogen IgEGF cooperates with c-myc or with the Hcs locus during hepatocarcinogenesis in transgenic mice. *Oncogene.* **10**: 765–768.

1997. Toren, A. and G. Rechavi. 1994. The anti-apoptotic role of infectious agents in lymphoid malignancies characterized by c-myc deregulation. *Br. J. Haematol.* **87**: 675–677.

1998. Tournay, O. and R. Benezra. 1996. Transcription of the dominant-negative helix–loop–helix protein Id1 is regulated by a protein complex containing the immediate-early response gene *Egr-1. Mol. Cell. Biol.* **16**: 2418–2430.

1999. Troussard, X., R. Rimokh, F. Valensi, D. Leboeuf, O. Fenneteau, A. M. Guitard, A. M. Manel, F. Schillinger, C. Leglise, A. Brizard *et al.* 1995. Heterogeneity of t(1;19)(q23;p13) acute leukaemias. French Haematological Cytology Group. *Br. J. Haematol.* **89**: 516–526.

2000. Trudel, M., N. Chretien, and V. D'Agati. 1994. Disappearance of polycystic kidney disease in revertant c-myc transgenic mice. *Mamm. Genome.* **5**: 149–152.

2001. Uittenbogaard, M. N., A. P. Armstrong, A. Chiaramello, and J. K. Nyborg. 1994. Human T-cell leukemia virus type I Tax protein represses gene expression through the basic helix–loop–helix family of transcription factors. *J. Biol. Chem.* **269**: 22466–22469.

2002. **Uittenbogaard, M. N., H. A. Giebler, D. Reisman, and J. K. Nyborg.** 1995. Transcriptional repression of p53 by human T-cell leukemia virus type I Tax protein. *J. Biol. Chem.* **270**: 28503−28506.

2003. **Umbhauer, M., J. F. Riou, J. C. Smith, and J. C. Boucaut.** 1994. Control of somitic expression of tenascin in *Xenopus* embryos by myogenic factors and Brachyury. *Dev. Dyn.* **200**: 269−277.

2004. **Usa, T., T. Tsukazaki, H. Namba, A. Ohtsuru, H. Kimura, M. C. Villadolid, S. Nagataki, and S. Yamashita.** 1994. Correlation between suppression of c-myc and antiproliferative effect of transforming growth factor-β_1 in thyroid carcinoma cell growth. *Endocrinology* **135**: 1378−1384.

2005. **Vairo, G., P. K. Vadiveloo, A. K. Royston, S. P. Rockman, C. O. Rock, S. Jackowski, and J. A. Hamilton.** 1995. Deregulated c-myc expression overrides IFNγ-induced macrophage growth arrest. *Oncogene.* **10**: 1969−1976.

2006. **Valera, A., A. Pujol, X. Gregori, E. Riu, J. Visa, and F. Bosch.** 1995. Evidence from transgenic mice that myc regulates hepatic glycolysis. *FASEB. J.* **9**: 1067−1078.

2007. **van Dam, P. A., I. B. Vergote, D. G. Lowe, J. V. Watson, P. van Damme, J. C. van der Auwera, and J. H. Shepherd.** 1994. Expression of c-erbB-2, c-myc, and c-ras oncoproteins, insulin-like growth factor receptor I, and epidermal growth factor receptor in ovarian carcinoma. *J. Clin. Pathol.* **47**: 914−919.

2008. **van der Lugt, N. M., J. Domen, E. Verhoeven, K. Linders, H. van der Gulden, J. Allen, and A. Berns.** 1995. Proviral tagging in E μ-myc transgenic mice lacking the Pim-1 proto-oncogene leads to compensatory activation of Pim-2. *EMBO J.* **14**: 2536−2544.

2009. **Vandromme, M., J. C. Cavadore, A. Bonnieu, A. Froeschle, N. Lamb, and A. Fernandez.** 1995. Two nuclear localization signals present in the basic-helix 1 domains of MyoD promote its active nuclear translocation and can function independently. *Proc. Natl. Acad. Sci. U. S. A.* **92**: 4646−4650.

2010. **Vastrik, I., A. Kaipainen, T-L. Penttila, A. Lymboussakis, R. Alitalo, M. Parninen, and K. Alitalo.** 1995. Expression of the *mad* gene during cell differentiation *in vivo* and its inhibition of cell growth *in vitro. J. Cell Biol.* **128**: 1197−1208.

2011. **Vastrik, I., T. P. Makela, P. J. Koskinen, and K. Alitalo.** 1995. Determination of sequences responsible for the differential regulation of Myc function by δ Max and Max. *Oncogene.* **11**: 553−560.

2012. **Vaulont, S. and A. Kahn.** 1994. Transcriptional control of metabolic regulation genes by carbohydrates. *FASEB. J.* **8**: 28−35.

2013. **Veal, E. A. and M. J. Jackson.** 1995. Expression of c-fos and c-myc in satellite cell cultures from dystrophic mdx and control mouse muscle. *Biochem. Soc. Trans.* **23**: 456S.

2014. **Veal, E. A. and M. J. Jackson.** 1995. Expression of the proto-oncogenes c-fos and c-myc in mdx dystrophic mouse muscle. *Biochem. Soc. Trans.* **23**: 131S.

2015. **Veronese, M. L., M. Ohta, J. Finan, P. C. Nowell, and C. M. Croce.** 1995. Detection of myc translocations in lymphoma cells by fluorescence *in situ* hybridization with yeast artificial chromosomes. *Blood.* **85**: 2132−2138.

2016. **Vierra, C. A. and C. Nelson.** 1995. The Pan basic helix−loop−helix proteins are required for insulin gene expression. *Mol. Endocrinol.* **9**: 64−71.

2017. **Vierra, C. A., X. Q. Xin, Y. T. Jacobs, J. M. Campbell, L. P. Shen, W. J. Rutter, and C. Nelson.** 1994. Purification of *E. coli*-synthesized Pan proteins and development of a Pan-specific monoclonal antibody. *Hybridoma.* **13**: 191−197.

2018. **Vostrov, A. A., W. W. Quitschke, F. Vidal, A. L. Schwarzman, and D. Goldgaber.** 1995. USF binds to the APB α sequence in the promoter of the amyloid β-protein precursor gene. *Nucleic Acids Res.* **23**: 2734−2741.

2019. **Wagner, A. J., J. M. Kokontis, and N. Hay.** 1994. Myc-mediated apoptosis requires wild-type p53 in a manner independent of cell cycle arrest and the ability of p53 to induce p21waf1/cip1. *Genes. Dev.* **8**: 2817−2830.

2020. **Waller, C. L. and J. D. McKinney.** 1995. Three-dimensional quantitative structure-activity relationships of dioxins and dioxin-like compounds: model validation and Ah receptor characterization. *Chem. Res. Toxicol.* **8**: 847−858.

2021. **Wang, A., N. Yoshimi, T. Tanaka, and H. Mori.** 1993. Inhibitory effects of magnesium hydroxide on c-myc expression and cell proliferation induced by methylazoxymethanol acetate in rat colon. *Cancer Lett.* **75**: 73−78.

2022. **Wang, D. and H. S. Sul.** 1995. Upstream stimulatory factors bind to insulin response sequence of the fatty acid synthase promoter. USF1 is regulated. *J. Biol. Chem.* **270**: 28716−28722.

2023. **Wang, E. and S. Pandey.** 1995. Down-regulation of statin, a nonproliferation-specific nuclear protein, and up-regulation of c-myc after initiation of programmed cell death in mouse fibroblasts. *J. Cell Physiol.* **163**: 155−163.

2024. **Wang, G. L., B. H. Jiang, E. A. Rue, and G. L. Semenza.** 1995. Hypoxia-inducible factor 1 is a basic-helix−loop−helix-PAS heterodimer regulated by cellular O_2 tension. *Proc. Natl. Acad. Sci. U. S. A.* **92**: 5510−5514.

2025. **Wang, G. L. and G. L. Semenza.** 1993. Characterization of hypoxia-inducible factor 1 and regulation of DNA binding activity by hypoxia. *J. Biol. Chem.* **268**: 21513−21518.

2026. **Wang, G. L. and G. L. Semenza.** 1995. Purification and characterization of hypoxia-inducible factor 1. *J. Biol. Chem.* **270**: 1230–1237.

2027. **Wang, J., K. Helin, P. Jin, and B. Nadal-Ginard.** 1996. Inhibition of *in vitro* myogenic differentiation by cellular transcription factor E2F1. *Cell Growth. Differ.* **6**: 1299–1306.

2028. **Wang, J., L. Li, S. Li, H. Cui, and G. Shen.** 1994. A study of c-myc oncogene expression and amplification in colorectal cancer. *Chin. Med. Sci. J.* **9**: 24–28.

2029. **Wang, J. Y. and L. R. Johnson.** 1994. Expression of protooncogenes c-fos and c-myc in healing of gastric mucosal stress ulcers. *Am. J. Physiol.* **266**:G878-G886.

2030. **Wang, N. P., J. Marx, M. A. McNutt, J. C. Rutledge, and A. M. Gown.** 1995. Expression of myogenic regulatory proteins (myogenin and MyoD1) in small blue round cell tumors of childhood. *Am. J. Pathol.* **147**: 1799–1810.

2031. **Wang, S., J. V. Bartolome, and S. M. Schanberg.** 1996. Neonatal deprivation of maternal touch may suppress ornithine decarboxylase via downregulation of the proto-oncogenes c-myc and max. *J. Neurosci.* **16**: 836–842.

2032. **Wang, X., J. T. Pai, E. A. Wiedenfeld, J. C. Medina, C. A. Slaughter, J. L. Goldstein, and M. S. Brown.** 1995. Purification of an interleukin-1 β converting enzyme-related cysteine protease that cleaves sterol regulatory element-binding proteins between the leucine zipper and transmembrane domains. *J. Biol. Chem.* **270**: 18044–18050.

2033. **Wang, X. and S. Safe.** 1994. Development of an *in vitro* model for investigating the formation of the nuclear Ah receptor complex in mouse Hepa 1c1c7 cells. *Arch. Biochem. Biophys.* **315**: 285–292.

2034. **Wang, X. H., C. A. Whyzmuzis, S. An, Y. Chen, J. M. Wu, T. A. Schneidau, C. Mallouh, and H. Tazaki.** 1994. Regulation of cell growth and the c-myc proto-oncogene expression by phorbol ester 12-O-tetradecanoyl phorbol-13-acetate (TPA) in the androgen-independent human prostatic JCA-1 cells. *Biochem. Mol. Biol. Int.* **34**: 47–53.

2035. **Wang, Y., P. N. Schnegelsberg, J. Dausman, and R. Jaenisch.** 1996. Functional redundancy of the muscle-specific transcription factors Myf5 and myogenin. *Nature.* **379**: 823–825.

2036. **Wang, Z., D. L. Morris, and T. L. Rothstein.** 1995. Constitutive and inducible levels of egr-1 and c-myc early growth response gene expression in self-renewing B-1 lymphocytes. *Cell Immunol.* **162**: 309–314.

2037. **Wassermann, K., P. M. O'Connor, J. Jackman, A. May, and V. A. Bohr.** 1994. Transcription-independent repair of nitrogen mustard-induced N-alkylpurines in the c-myc gene in Burkitt's lymphoma CA46 cells. *Carcinogenesis* **15**: 1779–1783.

2038. **Watada, H., Y. Kajimoto, Y. Umayahara, T. Matsuoka, T. Morishima, Y. Yamasaki, R. Kawamori, and T. Kamada.** 1995. Ubiquitous, but variable, expression of two alternatively spliced mRNAs encoding mouse homologues of transcription factors E47 and E12. *Gene* **153**: 255–259.

2039. **Watanabe, S., S. Ishida, K. Koike, and K. Arai.** 1995. Characterization of cis-regulatory elements of the c-myc promoter responding to human GM-CSF or mouse interleukin 3 in mouse proB cell line BA/F3 cells expressing the human GM-CSF receptor. *Mol. Biol. Cell* **6**: 627–636.

2040. **Watanabe, Y., K. Kawakami, Y. Hirayama, and K. Nagano.** 1993. Transcription factors positively and negatively regulating the Na,K-ATPase α_1 subunit gene. *J. Biochem. Tokyo.* **114**: 849–855.

2041. **Watt, F. and P. L. Molloy.** 1993. Specific cleavage of transcription factors by the thiol protease, m-calpain. *Nucleic Acids Res.* **21**: 5092–5100.

2042. **Weinberg, E. S., M. L. Allende, C. S. Kelly, A. Abdelhamid, T. Murakami, P. Andermann, O. G. Doerre, D. J. Grunwald, and B. Riggleman.** 1996. Developmental regulation of zebrafish MyoD in wild-type, no tail and spadetail embryos. *Development.* **122**: 271–280.

2043. **West, M. J., N. F. Sullivan, and A. E. Willis.** 1995. Translational upregulation of the c-myc oncogene in Bloom's syndrome cell lines. *Oncogene.* **11**: 2515–2524.

2044. **Weston, A., H. M. Ling Cawley, N. E. Caporaso, E. D. Bowman, R. N. Hoover, B. F. Trump, and C. C. Harris.** 1994. Determination of the allelic frequencies of an L-myc and a p53 polymorphism in human lung cancer. *Carcinogenesis* **15**: 583–587.

2045. **Whitelaw, M. L., J. A. Gustafsson, and L. Poellinger.** 1994. Identification of transactivation and repression functions of the dioxin receptor and its basic helix–loop–helix/PAS partner factor **Arnt**:inducible versus constitutive modes of regulation. *Mol. Cell Biol.* **14**: 8343–8355.

2046. **Wiener, F., A. Coleman, B. A. Mock, and M. Potter.** 1995. Nonrandom chromosomal change (trisomy 11) in murine plasmacytomas induced by an ABL-MYC retrovirus. *Cancer Res.* **55**: 1181–1188.

2047. **Wilhelmsson, A., M. L. Whitelaw, J. A. Gustafsson, and L. Poellinger.** 1994. Agonistic and antagonistic effects of α-naphthoflavone on dioxin receptor function. Role of the basic region helix–loop–helix dioxin receptor partner factor Arnt. *J. Biol. Chem.* **269**: 19028–19033.

2048. **Wilk, R., I. Weizman, and B. Z. Shilo.** 1996. trachealess encodes a bHLH-PAS protein that is an inducer of tracheal cell fates in *Drosophila*. *Genes. Dev.* **10**: 93–102.

2049. **Wolberger, C.** 1994. b/HLH without the zip. *Nat. Struct. Biol.* **1**: 413−416. [Published erratum appears in 1994. *Nat. Struct. Biol.* **1**:829.]

2050. **Wolfl, S., B. Wittig, and A. Rich.** 1995. Identification of transcriptionally induced Z-DNA segments in the human c-myc gene. *Biochim. Biophys. Acta* **1264**: 294−302.

2051. **Woloschak, M., J. L. Roberts, and K. Post.** 1994. c-myc, c-fos, and c-myb gene expression in human pituitary adenomas. *J. Clin. Endocrinol. Metab.* **79**: 253−257.

2052. **Wong, K. K., J. D. Hardin, S. Boast, C. L. Cooper, K. T. Merrell, T. G. Doyle, S. P. Goff, and K. L. Calame.** 1995. A role for c-Abl in c-myc regulation. *Oncogene.* **10**: 705−711.

2053. **Wong, K. K., X. Zou, K. T. Merrell, A. J. Patel, K. B. Marcu, S. Chellappan, and K. Calame.** 1995. v-Abl activates c-myc transcription through the E2F site. *Mol. Cell Biol.* **15**: 6535−6544.

2054. **Wong, M. W., M. Pisegna, M. F. Lu, D. Leibham, and M. Perry.** 1994. Activation of *Xenopus* MyoD transcription by members of the MEF2 protein family. *Dev. Biol.* **166**: 683−695.

2055. **Wood, A. C., P. Elvin, and J. A. Hickman.** 1995. Induction of apoptosis by anti-cancer drugs with disparate modes of action: kinetics of cell death and changes in c-myc expression. *Br. J. Cancer* **71**: 937−941.

2056. **Woodruff, K. A., J. D. Rosenblatt, T. B. Moore, R. H. Medzoyan, D. S. Pai, J. L. Noland, J. M. Yamashiro, and R. K. Wada.** 1995. Cell type-specific activity of the N-myc promoter in human neuroblastoma cells is mediated by a downstream silencer. *Oncogene.* **10**: 1335−1341.

2057. **Wright, S., X. Lu, and B. M. Peterlin.** 1994. Human immunodeficiency virus type 1 tat directs transcription through attenuation sites within the mouse c-myc gene. *J. Mol. Biol.* **243**: 568−573.

2058. **Wu Pong, S., T. L. Weiss, and C. A. Hunt.** 1994. Antisense c-myc oligonucleotide cellular uptake and activity. *Antisense. Res. Dev.* **4**: 155−163.

2059. **Wu, H. K., H. H. Heng, X. M. Shi, D. R. Forsdyke, L. C. Tsui, T. W. Mak, M. D. Minden, and D. P. Siderovski.** 1995. Differential expression of a basic helix−loop−helix phosphoprotein gene, G0S8, in acute leukemia and localization to human chromosome 1q31. *Leukemia* **9**: 1291−1298.

2060. **Wu, J., S. Katzav, and A. Weiss.** 1995. A functional T-cell receptor signaling pathway is required for p95vav activity. *Mol. Cell Biol.* **15**: 4337−4346.

2061. **Wu, S., A. Pena, A. Korcz, D. Robert-Soprano, and K. J. Soprano.** 1996. Overexpression of Mxi1 inhibits the induction of the human ornithine decarboxylase gene by the Myc/Max protein complex. *Oncogene.* **12**: 621−629.

2062. **Wulbeck, C., C. Fromental Ramain, and J. A. Campos Ortega.** 1994. The HLH domain of a zebrafish HE12 homologue can partially substitute for functions of the HLH domain of *Drosophila* DAUGHTERLESS. *Mech. Dev.* **46**: 73−85.

2063. **Wulf, G. M., C. N. Adra, and B. Lim.** 1993. Inhibition of hematopoietic development from embryonic stem cells by antisense vav RNA. *EMBO J.* **12**: 5065−5074.

2064. **Xiao, G. H., J. A. Pinaire, A. D. Rodrigues, and R. A. Prough.** 1995. Regulation of the Ah gene battery via Ah receptor-dependent and independent processes in cultured adult rat hepatocytes. *Drug. Metab. Dispos.* **23**: 642−650.

2065. **Xu, L., Y. Meng, R. Wallen, and R. A. DePinho.** 1995. Loss of transcriptional attenuation in N-myc is associated with progression towards a more malignant phenotype. *Oncogene.* **11**: 1865−1872.

2066. **Xu, L., D. Rungger, O. Georgiev, K. Seipel, and W. Schaffner.** 1994. Different potential of cellular and viral activators of transcription revealed in oocytes and early embryos of *Xenopus laevis. Biol. Chem. Hoppe. Seyler.* **375**: 105−112.

2067. **Yang, J., M. S. Brown, Y. K. Ho, and J. L. Goldstein.** 1995. Three different rearrangements in a single intron truncate sterol regulatory element binding protein-2 and produce sterol-resistant phenotype in three cell lines. Role of introns in protein evolution. *J. Biol. Chem.* **270**: 12152−12161.

2068. **Yasumoto, K., K. Yokoyama, K. Shibata, Y. Tomita, and S. Shibahara.** 1994. Microphthalmia-associated transcription factor as a regulator for melanocyte-specific transcription of the human tyrosinase gene. *Mol. Cell Biol.* **14**: 8058−8070. [Published erratum appears in 1995. *Mol. Cell Biol.* 15:1833.]

2069. **Yen, A. and S. Varvayanis.** 1995. The ratio of retinoblastoma (RB) to fos and RB to myc expression during the cell cycle. *Proc. Soc. Exp. Biol. Med.* **210**: 205−212.

2070. **Yieh, L., H. B. Sanchez, and T. F. Osborne.** 1995. Domains of transcription factor Sp1 required for synergistic activation with sterol regulatory element binding protein 1 of low density lipoprotein receptor promoter. *Proc. Natl. Acad. Sci. U. S. A.* **92**: 6102−6106.

2071. **Yoon, S. O. and D. M. Chikaraishi.** 1994. Isolation of two E-box binding factors that interact with the rat tyrosine hydroxylase enhancer. *J. Biol. Chem.* **269**: 18453−18462.

2072. **Yoshida, S., A. Fujisawa Sehara, T. Taki, K. Arai, and Y. Nabeshima.** 1996. Lysophosphatidic acid and bFGF control different modes in proliferating myoblasts. *J. Cell Biol.* **132**: 181−193.

2073. **Yoshimura, I., J. M. Wu, Y. Chen, C. Ng, C. Mallouh, J. M. Backer, C. E. Mendola, and H. Tazaki.** 1995. Effects of 5α-dihydrotesto-sterone (DHT) on the transcription of nm23 and c-myc genes in human prostatic LNCaP cells. *Biochem. Biophys. Res. Commun.* **208**: 603–609.

2074. **Young, J., R. Buttenshaw, L. Butterworth, M. Ward, J. Searle, B. Leggett, and G. Chenevix Trench.** 1994. Association of the SS genotype of the L-myc gene and loss of 18q sequences with a worse clinical prognosis in colorectal cancers. *Oncogene.* **9**: 1053–1056.

2075. **Yu, K., Q. Chen, H. Liu, Y. Zhan, and J. L. Stevens.** 1994. Signalling the molecular stress response to nephrotoxic and mutagenic cysteine conjugates: differential roles for protein synthesis and calcium in the induction of c-fos and c-myc mRNA in LLC-PK1 cells. *J. Cell Physiol.* **161**: 303–311.

2076. **Zhang, H., N. Okamoto, and Y. Ikeda.** 1995. Two c-myc genes from a tetraploid fish, the common carp (*Cyprinus carpio*). *Gene* **153**: 231–236.

2077. **Zhang, R., F. W. Alt, L. Davidson, S. H. Orkin, and W. Swat.** 1995. Defective signalling through the T- and B-cell antigen receptors in lymphoid cells lacking the vav proto-oncogene. *Nature* **374**: 470–473.

2078. **Zhang, R., F. Y. Tsai, and S. H. Orkin.** 1994. Hematopoietic development of vav-/- mouse embryonic stem cells. *Proc. Natl. Acad. Sci. U. S. A.* **91**: 12755–12759.

2079. **Zhuang, Y., P. Cheng, and H. Weintraub.** 1996. B-lymphocyte development is regulated by the combined dosage of three basic helix–loop–helix genes, *E2A, E2-2,* and *HEB. Mol. Cell. Biol.* **16**: 2898–2905.

2080. **Zhuang, Y., P. Soriano, and H. Weintraub.** 1994. The helix–loop–helix gene E2A is required for B cell formation. *Cell* **79**: 875–884.

2081. **Zijderveld, D. C., F. d'Adda di Fagagna, M. Giacca, H. T. Timmers, and P. C. van der Vliet.** 1994. Stimulation of the adenovirus major late promoter *in vitro* by transcription factor USF is enhanced by the adenovirus DNA binding protein. *J. Virol.* **68**: 8288–8295.

2082. **Zmuidzinas, A., K. D. Fischer, S. A. Lira, L. Forrester, S. Bryant, A. Bernstein, and M. Barbacid.** 1995. The vav proto-oncogene is required early in embryogenesis but not for hematopoietic development *in vitro. EMBO J.* **14**: 1–11.

2083. **Zornig, M., G. Busch, R. Beneke, E. Gulbins, F. Lang, A. Ma, S. Korsmeyer, and T. Moroy.** 1995. Survival and death of prelymphomatous B-cells from N-myc/bcl-2 double transgenic mice correlates with the regulation of intracellular Ca^{2+} fluxes. *Oncogene.* **11**: 2165–2174.

2084. **Zornig, M., A. Grzeschiczek, M. B. Kowalski, K. U. Hartmann, and T. Moroy.** 1995. Loss of Fas/Apo-1 receptor accelerates lymphomagenesis in Eμ L-MYC transgenic mice but not in animals infected with MoMuLV. *Oncogene.* **10**: 2397–2401.

Structure/function relationships of HLH proteins

2085. **Hakoshima, T., Y. Teranishi, T. Ohira, K. Suzuki, M. Shimizu, M. Shirakawa, Y. Kyogoku, N. Ogawa, and Y. Oshima.** 1993. Crystallographic characterization of a PHO4–DNA complex. *J. Mol. Biol.* **229**: 566–569.

2086. **Horimoto, K., H. Yamamoto, K. Yanagi, K. Ohshima, and J. Otsuka.** 1994. A simple procedure for assigning a sequence motif with an obscure pattern: application to the basic/helix–loop–helix motif. *Protein. Eng.* **7**: 1433–1440.

2087. **Hua, X., J. Sakai, Y. K. Ho, J. L. Goldstein, and M. S. Brown.** 1995. Hairpin orientation of sterol regulatory element-binding protein-2 in cell membranes as determined by protease protection. *J. Biol. Chem.* **270**: 29422–29427.

2088. **Johnson, N. P., J. Lindstrom, W. A. Baase, and P. H. von Hippel.** 1994. Double-stranded DNA templates can induce α-helical conformation in peptides containing lysine and alanine: functional implications for leucine zipper and helix–loop–helix transcription factors. *Proc. Natl. Acad. Sci. U. S. A.* **91**: 4840–4844.

2089. **Lavigne, P., L. H. Kondejewski, M. E. J. Houston, F. D. Sonnichsen, B. Lix, B. D. Skyes, R. S. Hodges, and C. M. Kay.** 1995. Preferential heterodimeric parallel coiled-coil formation by synthetic Max and c-Myc leucine zippers: a description of putative electrostatic interactions responsible for the specificity of heterodimerization. *J. Mol. Biol.* **254**: 505–520.

2090. **Muhle Goll, C., T. Gibson, P. Schuck, D. Schubert, D. Nalis, M. Nilges, and A. Pastore.** 1994. The dimerization stability of the HLH-LZ transcription protein family is modulated by the leucine zippers: a CD and NMR study of TFEB and c-Myc. *Biochemistry* **33**: 11296–11306.

2091. **Takemoto, C. and D. E. Fisher.** 1995. Structural constraints for DNA recognition by Myc and other b-HLH-ZIP proteins: design of oncoprotein analogues. *Gene Expr.* **4**: 311–317.

2092. **Wolberger, C.** 1994. b/HLH without the zip. *Nat. Struct. Biol.* **1**: 413–416.

Sequence-specific DNA binding by HLH proteins

2093. **Bacsi, S. G., S. Reisz Porszasz, and O. Hankinson.** 1995. Orientation of the heterodimeric aryl hydrocarbon (dioxin) receptor complex on its asymmetric DNA recognition sequence. *Mol. Pharmacol.* **47**: 432–438.

2094. **Barbaric, S., K. D. Fascher, and W. Horz.** 1992. Activation of the weakly regulated PHO8 promoter in *S. cerevisiae*:chromatin transition and binding sites for the positive regulatory protein PHO4. *Nucleic Acids Res.* **20**: 1031–1038. [Published erratum appears in 1992. *Nucleic Acids Res.* **20**:1450.]

2095. **Bishop, P., C. Jones, I. Ghosh, and J. Chmielewski.** 1995. Synthesis of the basic-helix–loop–helix region of the immunoglobulin enhancer binding protein E47 and evaluation of its structural and DNA binding properties. *Int. J. Pept. Protein. Res.* **46**: 149–154.

2096. **Briggs, M. R., C. Yokoyama, X. Wang, M. S. Brown, and J. L. Goldstein.** 1993. Nuclear protein that binds sterol regulatory element of low density lipoprotein receptor promoter. I. Identification of the protein and delineation of its target nucleotide sequence. *J. Biol. Chem.* **268**: 14490–14496.

2097. **Buckle, R. S. and M. Mechali.** 1995. Analysis of c-Myc and Max binding to the c-myc promoter: evidence that autosuppression occurs via an indirect mechanism. *Oncogene.* **10**: 1249–1255.

2098. **Czernik, P. J., C. A. Peterson, and B. K. Hurlburt.** 1996. Preferential binding of MyoD–E12 *versus* myogenin–E12 to the murine sarcoma virus enhancer *in vitro*. *J. Biol. Chem.* **271**: 9141–9149.

2099. **1. Dong, L., Q. Ma, and J. P. Whitlock.** 1996. DNA binding by the heterodimeric Ah receptor. Relationship to dioxin-induced *CYP1A1* transcription *in vivo*. *J. Biol. Chem.* **271**: 7942–7948.

2100. **Huang, J., T. K. Blackwell, L. Kedes, and H. Weintraub.** 1996. Differences between MyoD DNA binding and activation site requirements revealed by functional random sequence selection. *Mol. Cell. Biol.* **16**: 3893–3900.

2101. **Ireland, R. C., S. Y. Li, and J. J. Dougherty.** 1995. The DNA binding of purified Ah receptor heterodimer is regulated by redox conditions. *Arch. Biochem. Biophys.* **319**: 470–480.

2102. **Kim, J. B., G. D. Spotts, Y. D. Halvorsen, H. M. Shih, T. Ellenberger, H. C. Towle, and B. M. Spiegelman.** 1995. Dual DNA binding specificity of ADD1/SREBP1 controlled by a single amino acid in the basic helix–loop–helix domain. *Mol. Cell Biol.* **15**: 2582–2588.

2103. **Lecointe, N., O. Bernard, K. Naert, V. Joulin, C. J. Larsen, P. H. Romeo, and D. Mathieu Mahul.** 1994. GATA-and SP1-binding sites are required for the full activity of the tissue-specific promoter of the tal-1 gene. *Oncogene.* **9**: 2623–2632.

2104. **Lu, T. and M. Sawadogo.** 1994. Role of the leucine zipper in the kinetics of DNA binding by transcription factor USF. *J. Biol. Chem.* **269**: 30694–30700.

2105. **McLane, K. E., D. R. Burton, and P. Ghazal.** 1995. Transplantation of a 17-amino acid α-helical DNA-binding domain into an antibody molecule confers sequence-dependent DNA recognition. *Proc. Natl. Acad. Sci. U. S. A.* **92**: 5214–5218.

2106. **McLane, K. E. and J. P. J. Whitlock.** 1994. DNA sequence requirements for Ah receptor/Arnt recognition determined by *in vitro* transcription. *Receptor.* **4**: 209–222.

2107. **Meierhan, D., C. el Ariss, M. Neuenschwander, M. Sieber, J. F. Stackhouse, and R. K. Allemann.** 1995. DNA binding specificity of the basic-helix–loop–helix protein MASH-1. *Biochemistry* **34**: 11026–11036.

2108. **Mellor, J., J. Rathjen, W. Jiang, C. A. Barnes, and S. J. Dowell.** 1991. DNA binding of CPF1 is required for optimal centromere function but not for maintaining methionine prototrophy in yeast. *Nucleic Acids Res.* **19**: 2961–2969. [Published erratum appears in 1991. *Nucleic Acids Res.* **19**:5112.]

2109. **Niedenthal, R. K., M. Sen Gupta, A. Wilmen, and J. H. Hegemann.** 1993. Cpf1 protein induced bending of yeast centromere DNA element I. *Nucleic Acids Res.* **21**: 4726–4733.

2110. **Nielsen, A. L., N. Pallisgaard, F. S. Pedersen, and P. Jorgensen.** 1994. Basic helix–loop–helix proteins in murine type C retrovirus transcriptional regulation. *J. Virol.* **68**: 5638–5647.

2111. **Okino, S. T. and J. P. J. Whitlock.** 1995. Dioxin induces localized, graded changes in chromatin structure: implications for Cyp1A1 gene transcription. *Mol. Cell Biol.* **15**: 3714–3721.

2112. **Peyton, M., L. G. Moss, and M. J. Tsai.** 1994. Two distinct class A helix–loop–helix transcription factors, E2A and BETA1, form separate DNA binding complexes on the insulin gene E box. *J. Biol. Chem.* **269**: 25936–25941.

2113. **Sha, M., D. A. Ferre, S. K. Burley, and D. J. Goss.** 1995. Anti-cooperative biphasic equilibrium binding of transcription factor upstream stimulatory factor to its cognate DNA monitored by protein fluorescence changes. *J. Biol. Chem.* **270**: 19325–19329.

2114. **Swanson, H. I., W. K. Chan, and C. A. Bradfield.** 1995. DNA binding specificities and pairing rules of the Ah receptor, ARNT, and SIM proteins. *J. Biol. Chem.* **270**: 26292–26302.

2115. **Trepicchio, W. L. and T. G. Krontiris.** 1993. IGH minisatellite suppression of USF-binding-site- and Eμ-mediated transcriptional activation of the adenovirus major late promoter. *Nucleic Acids Res.* **21**: 977–985.

2116. **Venter, U., J. Svaren, J. Schmitz, A. Schmid, and W. Horz.** 1994. A nucleosome precludes binding of the transcription factor Pho4 *in vivo* to a critical target site in the PHO5 promoter. *EMBO J.* **13**: 4848–4855.

2117. **Wechsler, D. S., O. Papoulas, C. V. Dang, and R. E. Kingston.** 1994. Differential binding of c-Myc and Max to nucleosomal DNA. *Mol. Cell Biol.* **14**: 4097–4107.

2118. **Weintraub, H., T. Genetta, and T. Kadesch.** 1994. Tissue-specific gene activation by **MyoD**:determination of specificity by cis-acting repression elements. *Genes. Dev.* **8**: 2203–2211.

2119. **Wilmen, A., H. Pick, R. K. Niedenthal, M. Sen Gupta, and J. H. Hegemann.** 1994. The yeast centromere CDEI/Cpf1 complex: differences between *in vitro* binding and *in vivo* function. *Nucleic Acids Res.* **22**: 2791–2800.

Dimerization partners

2120. **Alexandrova, N., J. Niklinski, V. Bliskovsky, G. A. Otterson, M. Blake, F. J. Kaye, and M. Zajac Kaye.** 1995. The N-terminal domain of c-Myc associates with α-tubulin and microtubules *in vivo* and *in vitro*. *Mol. Cell Biol.* **15**: 5188–5195.

2120a. **Bao, J. and A. S. Zervos.** 1996. Isolation and characterization Nmi1, a novel partner of Myc proteins. *Oncogene* **12**: 2171–2176.

2121. **Bissonnette, R. P., A. McGahon, A. Mahboubi, and D. R. Green.** 1994. Functional Myc—Max heterodimer is required for activation-induced apoptosis in T cell hybridomas. *J. Exp. Med.* **180**: 2413–2418.

2122. **Bresnick, E. H. and G. Felsenfeld.** 1994. The leucine zipper is necessary for stabilizing a dimer of the helix—loop—helix transcription factor USF but not for maintenance of an elongated conformation. *J. Biol. Chem.* **269**: 21110–21116.

2123. **Bunker, C. A. and R. E. Kingston.** 1995. Identification of a cDNA for SSRP1, an HMG-box protein, by interaction with the c-Myc oncoprotein in a novel bacterial expression screen. *Nucleic Acids Res.* **23**: 269–276.

2124. **Bustelo, X. R., K. L. Suen, W. M. Michael, G. Dreyfuss, and M. Barbacid.** 1995. Association of the vav proto-oncogene product with poly(rC)-specific RNA-binding proteins. *Mol. Cell Biol.* **15**: 1324–1332.

2125. **Castresana, J. and M. Saraste.** 1995. Does Vav bind to F-actin through a CH domain? *FEBS Lett.* **374**: 149–151.

2126. **Fields, S. and O. Song.** 1989. A novel genetic system to detect protein—protein interactions. *Nature* **340**: 245–246.

2127. **Goldfarb, A. N. and K. Lewandowska.** 1994. Nuclear redirection of a cytoplasmic helix—loop—helix protein via heterodimerization with a nuclear localizing partner. *Exp. Cell Res.* **214**: 481–485.

2128. **Goldfarb, A. N., K. Lewandowska, and M. Shoham.** 1996. Determinants of helix—loop—helix dimerization affinity. Random mutational analysis of SCL/tal. *J. Biol. Chem.* **271**: 2683–2688.

2129. **Hemesath, T. J., E. Steingrimsson, G. McGill, M. J. Hansen, J. Vaught, C. A. Hodgkinson, H. Arnheiter, N. G. Copeland, N. A. Jenkins, and D. E. Fisher.** 1994. microphthalmia, a critical factor in melanocyte development, defines a discrete transcription factor family. *Genes. Dev.* **8**: 2770–2780.

2130. **Hobert, O., B. Jallal, J. Schlessinger, and A. Ullrich.** 1994. Novel signaling pathway suggested by SH3 domain-mediated p95vav/heterogeneous ribonucleoprotein K interaction. *J. Biol. Chem.* **269**: 20225–20228.

2131. **Hossain, A., H. Kikuchi, S. Ikawa, I. Sagami, and M. Watanabe.** 1995. Identification of a 120-kDa protein associated with aromatic hydrocarbon receptor nuclear translocator. *Biochem. Biophys. Res. Commun.* **212**: 144–150.

2132. **Katzav, S., M. Sutherland, G. Packham, T. Yi, and A. Weiss.** 1994. The protein tyrosine kinase ZAP-70 can associate with the SH2 domain of proto-Vav. *J. Biol. Chem.* **269**: 32579–32585.

2133. **Laue, T. M., M. A. Starovasnik, H. Weintraub, X. H. Sun, L. Snider, and R. E. Klevit.** 1995. MyoD forms micelles which can dissociate to form heterodimers with E47: implications of micellization on function. *Proc. Natl. Acad. Sci. U. S. A.* **92**: 11824–11828.

2134. **Lindebro, M. C., L. Poellinger, and M. L. Whitelaw.** 1995. Protein—protein interaction via PAS domains: role of the PAS domain in positive and negative regulation of the bHLH/PAS dioxin receptor—Arnt transcription factor complex. *EMBO J.* **14**: 3528–3539.

2135. **Lu, T., M. Van Dyke, and M. Sawadogo.** 1993. Protein—protein interaction studies using immobilized oligohistidine fusion proteins. *Anal. Biochem.* **213**: 318–322.

2136. **Machide, M., H. Mano, and K. Todokoro.** 1995. Interleukin 3 and erythropoietin induce association of Vav with Tec kinase through Tec homology domain. *Oncogene.* **11**: 619–625.

2137. **Mak, K. L., L. C. Longcor, S. E. Johnson, C. Lemercier, R. Q. To, and S. F. Konieczny.** 1996. Examination of mammalian basic helix—loop—helix transcription factors using a yeast one-hybrid system. *DNA Cell Biol.* **15**: 1–8.

2138. **Mao, Z. and B. Nadal-Ginard.** 1996. Functional and physical interactions between mammalian achaete—scute homolog 1 and myocyte enhancer factor 2A. *J. Biol. Chem.* **271**: 14371–14375.

2139. **Marchetti, A., M. Abril Marti, B. Illi, G. Cesareni, and S. Nasi.** 1995. Analysis of the Myc and Max interaction specificity with λ repressor-HLH domain fusions. *J. Mol. Biol.* **248**: 541–550.

2140. **McGuire, J., P. Coumailleau, M. L. Whitelaw, J. A. Gustafsson, and L. Poellinger.** 1995. The basic helix—loop—helix/PAS factor Sim is associated with hsp90. Implications for regulation by interaction with partner factors. *J. Biol. Chem.* **270**: 31353–31357.

2141. **Muhle Goll, C., M. Nilges, and A. Pastore.** 1995. The leucine zippers of the HLH-LZ proteins Max and c-Myc preferentially form heterodimers. *Biochemistry* **34**: 13554–13564.

2142. **Ramos Morales, F., B. J. Druker, and S. Fischer.** 1994. Vav binds to several SH2/SH3 containing proteins in activated lymphocytes. *Oncogene.* **9**: 1917–1923.

2143. **Ramos Morales, F., F. Romero, F. Schweighoffer, G. Bismuth, J. Camonis, M. Tortolero, and S. Fischer.** 1995. The proline-rich region of Vav binds to Grb2 and Grb3–3. *Oncogene.* **11**: 1665–1669.

2144. **Ribon, V., T. Leff, and A. R. Saltiel.** 1994. c-Myc does not require max for transcriptional activity in PC-12 cells. *Mol. Cell Neurosci.* **5**: 277–282.

2145. **Romero, F., C. Dargemont, F. Pozo, W. H. Reeves, J. Camonis, S. Gisselbrecht, and S. Fischer.** 1996. p95vav associates with the nuclear protein Ku-70. *Mol. Cell Biol.* **16**: 37–44.

2146. **Schreiber Agus, N., L. Chin, K. Chen, R. Torres, G. Rao, P. Guida, A. I. Skoultchi, and R. A. DePinho.** 1995. An amino-terminal domain of Mxi1 mediates anti-Myc oncogenic activity and interacts with a homolog of the yeast transcriptional repressor SIN3. *Cell.* **80**: 777–786.

2147. **Shirakata, M. and B. M. Paterson.** 1995. The E12 inhibitory domain prevents homodimer formation and facilitates selective heterodimerization with the MyoD family of gene regulatory factors. *EMBO J.* **14**: 1766–1772.

2148. **Songyang, Z., S. E. Shoelson, J. McGlade, P. Olivier, T. Pawson, X. R. Bustelo, M. Barbacid, H. Sabe, H. Hanafusa, T. Yi** *et al.* 1994. Specific motifs recognized by the SH2 domains of Csk, 3BP2, fps/fes, GRB-2, HCP, SHC, Syk, and Vav. *Mol. Cell Biol.* **14**: 2777–2785.

2149. **Valge Archer, V. E., H. Osada, A. J. Warren, A. Forster, J. Li, R. Baer, and T. H. Rabbitts.** 1994. The LIM protein RBTN2 and the basic helix–loop–helix protein TAL1 are present in a complex in erythroid cells. *Proc. Natl. Acad. Sci. U. S. A.* **91**: 8617–8621.

2150. **Van Seuningen, I., J. Ostrowski, X. R. Bustelo, P. R. Sleath, and K. Bomsztyk.** 1995. The K protein domain that recruits the interleukin 1-responsive K protein kinase lies adjacent to a cluster of c-Src and Vav SH3-binding sites. Implications that K protein acts as a docking platform. *J. Biol. Chem.* **270**: 26976–26985.

2151. **Wadman, I., J. Li, R. O. Bash, A. Forster, H. Osada, T. H. Rabbitts, and R. Baer.** 1994. Specific *in vivo* association between the bHLH and LIM proteins implicated in human T cell leukemia. *EMBO J.* **13**: 4831–4839.

2152. **Weng, W. K., L. Jarvis, and T. W. LeBien.** 1994. Signaling through CD19 activates Vav/mitogen-activated protein kinase pathway and induces formation of a CD19/Vav/phosphati-dylinositol 3-kinase complex in human B cell precursors. *J. Biol. Chem.* **269**: 32514–32521.

2153. **Wenzel, A., C. Cziepluch, J. Schurmann, and M. Schwab.** 1994. The N-myc oncoprotein is a transcriptional activator and associates with max and RB1 proteins. *Prog. Clin. Biol. Res.* **385**: 59–66.

2154. **Whitelaw, M. L., J. McGuire, D. Picard, J. A. Gustafsson, and L. Poellinger.** 1995. Heat shock protein hsp90 regulates dioxin receptor function *in vivo*. *Proc. Natl. Acad. Sci. U. S. A.* **92**: 4437–4441.

2155. **Yamaguchi, Y. and M. T. Kuo.** 1995. Functional analysis of aryl hydrocarbon receptor nuclear translocator interactions with aryl hydrocarbon receptor in the yeast two-hybrid system. *Biochem. Pharmacol.* **50**: 1295–1302.

2156. **Yavuzer, U. and C. R. Goding.** 1994. Melanocyte-specific gene expression: role of repression and identification of a melanocyte-specific factor, MSF. *Mol. Cell Biol.* **14**: 3494–3503.

2157. **Yavuzer, U., E. Keenan, P. Lowings, J. Vachtenheim, G. Currie, and C. R. Goding.** 1995. The Microphthalmia gene product interacts with the retinoblastoma protein *in vitro* and is a target for deregulation of melanocyte-specific transcription. *Oncogene.* **10**: 123–134.

2158. **Ye, Z. S. and D. Baltimore.** 1994. Binding of Vav to Grb2 through dimerization of Src homology 3 domains. *Proc. Natl. Acad. Sci. U. S. A.* **91**: 12629–12633.

2159. **Zervos**, 1994. Mxi1, a protein that specifically interacts with Max to bind Myc–Max recognition sites. *Cell* **79**:389.

Post-transcriptional regulation of the activity of HLH proteins

2160. **Alai, M., A. L. Mui, R. L. Cutler, X. R. Bustelo, M. Barbacid, and G. Krystal.** 1992. Steel factor stimulates the tyrosine phosphorylation of the proto-oncogene product, p95vav, in human hemopoietic cells. *J. Biol. Chem.* **267**: 18021–18025.

2161. **Bousset, K., M. H. Oelgeschlager, M. Henriksson, S. Schreek, H. Burkhardt, D. W. Litchfield, J. M. Luscher Firzlaff, and B. Luscher.** 1994. Regulation of transcription factors c-Myc, Max, and c-Myb by casein kinase II. *Cell Mol. Biol. Res.* **40**: 501–511.

2162. **Cheng, J. T., M. H. Cobb, and R. Baer.** 1993. Phosphorylation of the TAL1 oncoprotein by the extracellular-signal-regulated protein kinase ERK1. *Mol. Cell Biol.* **13**: 801–808.

2163. **Chou, T. Y., C. V. Dang, and G. W. Hart.** 1995. Glycosylation of the c-Myc transactivation domain. *Proc. Natl. Acad. Sci. U. S. A.* **92**: 4417−4421.

2164. **Darby, C., R. L. Geahlen, and A. D. Schreiber.** 1994. Stimulation of macrophage Fcγ RIIIA activates the receptor-associated protein tyrosine kinase Syk and induces phosphorylation of multiple proteins including p95Vav and p62/GAP-associated protein. *J. Immunol.* **152**: 5429−5437.

2165. **Evans, G. A., O. M. Howard, R. Erwin, and W. L. Farrar.** 1993. Interleukin-2 induces tyrosine phosphorylation of the vav proto-oncogene product in human T cells: lack of requirement for the tyrosine kinase lck. *Biochem. J.* **294**: 339−342.

2166. **Gouy, H., P. Debre, and G. Bismuth.** 1995. The proto-oncogene Vav product is constitutively tyrosine-phosphorylated in normal human immature T cells. *Eur. J. Immunol.* **25**: 3030−3034.

2167. **Gupta, S. and R. J. Davis.** 1994. MAP kinase binds to the NH2-terminal activation domain of c-Myc. *FEBS Lett.* **353**: 281−285.

2168. **Hanazono, Y., K. Sasaki, H. Odai, T. Mimura, K. Mitani, Y. Yazaki, and H. Hirai.** 1995. Tyrosine phosphorylation of the proto-oncogene product Vav and its association with the adapter Grb2/Ash in a human leukemia cell line UT-7. *Jpn. J. Cancer Res.* **86**: 336−341.

2169. **Johnson, S. E., X. Wang, S. Hardy, E. J. Taparowsky, and S. F. Konieczny.** 1996. Casein kinase II increases the transcriptional activities of MRF4 and MyoD independently of their direct phosphorylation. *Mol. Cell. Biol.* **16**: 1604−1613.

2170. **Mahon, M. J. and T. A. Gasiewicz.** 1995. Ah receptor phosphorylation: localization of phosphorylation sites to the C-terminal half of the protein. *Arch. Biochem. Biophys.* **318**: 166−174.

2171. **Matsuguchi, T., R. C. Inhorn, N. Carlesso, G. Xu, B. Druker, and J. D. Griffin.** 1995. Tyrosine phosphorylation of p95Vav in myeloid cells is regulated by GM-CSF, IL-3 and steel factor and is constitutively increased by p210BCR/ABL. *EMBO J.* **14**: 257−265.

2172. **Miura, O., Y. Miura, N. Nakamura, F. W. Quelle, B. A. Witthuhn, J. N. Ihle, and N. Aoki.** 1994. Induction of tyrosine phosphorylation of Vav and expression of Pim-1 correlates with Jak2-mediated growth signaling from the erythropoietin receptor. *Blood.* **84**: 4135−4141.

2173. **Nagata, Y., W. Shoji, M. Obinata, and K. Todokoro.** 1995. Phosphorylation of helix−loop−helix proteins ID1, ID2 and ID3. *Biochem. Biophys. Res. Commun.* **207**: 916−926.

2174. **O'Neill, E. M., A. Kaffman, E. R. Jolly, and E. K. O'Shea.** 1996. Regulation of PHO4 nuclear localization by the PHO80-PHO85 cyclin-CDK complex. *Science* **271**: 209−212.

2175. **Platanias, L. C. and M. E. Sweet.** 1994. Interferon α induces rapid tyrosine phosphorylation of the vav proto-oncogene product in hematopoietic cells. *J. Biol. Chem.* **269**: 3143−3146.

2176. **Sasaki, K., H. Odai, Y. Hanazono, H. Ueno, S. Ogawa, W. Y. Langdon, T. Tanaka, K. Miyagawa, K. Mitani, Y. Yazaki** *et al.* 1995. TPO/c-mpl ligand induces tyrosine phosphorylation of multiple cellular proteins including proto-oncogene products, Vav and c-Cbl, and Ras signaling molecules. *Biochem. Biophys. Res. Commun.* **216**: 338−347.

2177. **Uddin, S., S. Katzav, M. F. White, and L. C. Platanias.** 1995. Insulin-dependent tyrosine phosphorylation of the vav protooncogene product in cells of hematopoietic origin. *J. Biol. Chem.* **270**: 7712−7716.

2178. **Yuo, A., S. Kitagawa, S. Iki, M. Yagisawa, E. K. Inuo, T. Mimura, S. Minoda, Y. Hanazono, H. Hirai, A. Urabe** *et al.* 1995. Tyrosine phosphorylation of vav protooncogene product in primary human myelogenous leukemic cells stimulated by granulocyte colony-stimulating factor. *Biochem. Biophys. Res. Commun.* **211**: 677−685.

2179. **Zervos, A. S., L. Faccio, J. P. Gatto, J. M. Kyriakis, and R. Brent.** 1995. Mxi2, a mitogen-activated protein kinase that recognizes and phosphorylates Max protein. *Proc. Natl. Acad. Sci. U. S. A.* **92**: 10531−10534.

Appendix
Sequence alignment of
75 HLH protein sequences

Protein sequences were aligned using the GCG program 'Pileup'. Mammalian-derived proteins are either human (c, N and L-Myc, Max, Mad1, Mxi1, AP4, USF1, USF2, TFE3, TFEB, SREBP1, E12, ITF2, HEB, NeuroD, MyoD, Myogenin, Myf5, MRF4, Tal1, Tal2, Hen1, Hen2, Arnt1 and Scleraxis), rat (S-Myc, TFEC, Mash1, Mash2 and Hes proteins), mouse (Mi, AhR, MATH1, MATH2, Lyl1 and Lyl2, Thing1, Thing2 and Id proteins), hamster (BETA3) or chicken (GbHLH1.4). Drosophila proteins (Da, Twist, Sim, L-Sc, Scute, Achaete, Asense, Atonal, Trh, E(spl) proteins, Hairy, Dpn and Emc) are from D. melanogaster. Yeast proteins (Cbf1, Pho4, Ino2p and Ino4p) are from S. cerevisiae. Plant proteins are either from Maize (R-Lc, R-S and B-Peru) or Antirrhinum (Del). The v-Myc sequence is derived from the gag–v-myc *fusion*

encoded by the avian myelocytamotosis virus MC29. The source of sequences is listed in Table 1.

Sequences are divided into broad phylogenetic and functional groups. The first block is bHLHZ proteins; the second block, bHLH proteins; the third block, HLH proteins lacking a functional DNA-binding domain; the fourth block, yeast proteins; and the fifth block, plant proteins.

The basic, helix–loop–helix and leucine zipper regions are indicated on the header line. Dashes have been introduced to maximize the alignment. In some cases (AP4, TFE3, TFEB, USF2, ITF2 and Id1) the N and C termini are uncertain and the extent of the sequence has not been completely determined.

Main section

bHLHZ proteins

```
c-Myc      251 DSEE------ -----EQEDE EEIDVVSVEK RQAPGKRSES GSPSAGGHSK --------PP HSPLVLKRCH VS--THQHNY
N-Myc      255 SGEDTLSDSD DEDDEEEDEE EEIDVVTVEK RRSSSNTKAV TTFTITVRPK NAALGPGRAQ SSELILKRCL PI--HQQHNY
L-Myc      157 SGSESPSDS- --------EN EEIDVVTVEK RQSLGIRKPV TI-------- -----TVRAD PLDPCMKHFH ISIHQQQHNY
v-Myc      234 DSEE------ -----EQEED EEIDVVTLAE ANESESSTES STEASEEHCK --------PH HSPLVLKRCH VN--IHQHNY
S-Myc      227 SLEDFLSNS- ---GYVEEGG EEIYVVMLGE TQFS---KTV TKLPTAAHSE NAALTPECAQ SGELILKRSD LI--QEQHNY
Max          1
Mad1         1
Mxi1         1
AP4          1
USF1        51 FRTENGGQVM YRVIQVSEGQ LDGQTEGTGA ISGYPATQSM TQAVIQGAFT SDDAVDTEGT AAETHYTYFP S--------T
USF2        10 VSTAAFAGGQ QAVTQVGVDG VAQRPGPAAA SVPPGPAAPF PLAVIQNPFS NGGSPAAEAV SGEARFAYFP A--------S
TFE3         1 EFGRASQAL TPP----PGK ASAQPLPAPE AAHTT----- ---------- ---GPTGSAP NSPMALLTIG SSSEKEIDDV
TFEB       196 YGNKFAAAHI SPA---QALR NPHQPPPPQGC ELDTC----- ---------- CPPPLATVLP ISPMAMLHIG SNPERELDDV
TFEC         3 LDHRLFSQTL KRA------- ---QPLAASC MP-------- ---------L AEHGPRSPDS DAGCAGNPFT NPLALGKEDG
Mi          40 LANKHASQVL SSPCPNQPGD HAMPPVPGSS APNSPMAMLT LNSNCEKEAF YKFEEQSRAE SECPGMNTHS RASCMQMDDV
SREBP1a    172 FSTGSPPGNT QQPLPGLPLA SPPGVPPVSL HTQVQVSVVPQ QLLTVTAAPT AAPVTTTVTS QIQQVPVLLQ P--------H
```

bHLH proteins

```
E12        420 PGH----GAL ASGFTGPMSL GGRHAGLVGG SHPEDGLAGS TSLMHNHAAL PS-------- -QPG---TLP DLS-RPPDSY
ITF2       379 PSHNGAMGGL GSGYGT-GLL SANRHSLMVG THREDGV--- -ALRGSHSLL PNQVPVPQLP VQSA---TSP DLNP-PQDPY
HEB        437 PSHNAPIGSL NSNYGGSSLV ASSRSASMVG THREDSV--- -SLNGNHSVL SSTV------ --TT---SST DLNHKTQENY
Da         410 NSP----SHL GSGGNSGSVS NTSNAALVHE VLALGAAAAA GTSGQSVGGA GSLASLKLDR SAST---SLP KQTKKRKEHT
Sim          1
NeuroD       1                                                                M TKSYSESGLM GEPQPQGPPS
Hen1         1                                                          MMLNSD-T MELDLP----
Hen2         1                                                           MMLSPDQA ADSDHPS---
MATH1       17 GDHHRHPQPH HVPPLTPQPP ATLQARDLPV YPAELSLLDS TDPRAWLTPT LQGLCTARAA QYLLHSPELG ASEAAAPRDE
MATH2        1                                                               ML TLPFDESVVM PESQ----MC
L-Sc         1
Scute        1                                                  MKNNN NTTKSTTMSS SVLSTNETFP
Achaete      1
Asense       1       MAALSF SPSPPPKENP KENPNPGIKT TLKPFGKITV HNVLSESGAN ALQQHIANQN TIIRKIRDFG MLGAVQSAAA
Atonal     125 ---------- -ASPPAVEVM GSSNVGTCKT IPASAAPKPK RSYTKKNQPS TTATSTPTAA AESS---ASV NLYTEEFQNF
Mash1        1                                                    MES-- ----SGKMES GAGQQPQPPQ PFLPPAACFE
Mash2        1                                               MESHF NWYGVPRLQK ASDACPRESC SSALPEAREG
MyoD         1                                              MELLSPPL RDVDLTAPDG SLCSFATTDD
Myogenin     1                                                       MELYET SPYFYQEEPRF
Myf5         1                                                       MDVMDG --CQFSPSEY
MRF4         1                                                       MMMDLFET GSYFF----Y
Lyl1         1       MCPPQAGAEV GSAMTEKTEM VCASSPAPAP PSKLASPGPL STEEVDHRNT CTPWLPPGVP VINLGHTRPI
Lyl2         1       MCPPQAGAE- ---------- ---------- ---------- --EEVDHRNT CTPWLPPGVP VINLGHTRPI
Tal1        30 HLVLLNGVAK ETSRAAAAEP PVIELGARGG PGGGPAGGGG AARDLKGRDA ATAEARHRVP TTELCRPPGP APAPAPASVT
Tal2         1
Arnt1        1                                                                                     M
AhR          1
Twist      203 ASAQSCPGVQ STCTSPQSHF DFPDEELPEH KAQVFLPLYN NQQQQSQQQQ QQQPHQQSHA QMHFQNAYRQ SFEGYEPANS
Delilah      1                                                                           MKSNT
bHLH-EC2     1                                                         MA FALLR--PVG AHVLYPPDVRL
Scleraxis    1                                                         MS FAMLRSAPPP GRYLYPEVSP
GbHLH1.4   243 PSHNGPIGSL NSSYGASSLV AANRQASMVA AHREESV--- -SLNSNHAVL PSTV------ --SA---QST ELNHKTQESY
Trh          1
BETA3       60 SSSPLGCFEP ADPEGAGLLL PPPGGGGGAG GGGGGGGGGG VSVPGLLVGS AGVGGDPNLS SLPAGAALCL KYGESAGRGS
Thing1       1                                               MNLVGS YAHHH-HHHH SHPPHPMLHE PFLFGPASRC
Thing2       1                                               MSLVGG FPHHHPVVHHE GYPLRRSRHH RFHHHHQPLH
```

HLH proteins (no functional DNA-binding domain)

```
Hes1         1
Hes2         1
Hes3         1
Hes5         1
E(spl)M5     1
E(spl)M7     1
E(spl)M8     1
Hairy        1
Dpn          1
Emc          1
Id1          1
Id2          1
Id3          1
Id4          1
```

Yeast proteins

```
Cbf1        63 TLKGTQSQYE SGLTSNKDEK GSDDEDASVA EAAVAATVNY TDLIQGQEDS SDAHTSNQTN ANGEHKDSLN GERAITPSNE
Pho4        82 ELVEGMDMDW MMPSHAHHSP ATTATIKPRL LYSPLIHTQS AVPVTISPNL VATATSTTSA NKVTKNKSNS SPYLNKRRGK
Ino2p       68 PSHVETIPAD NQTHHAPLHT HAHYLNHNPH QPSMGFDQAL GLKLSPSSSG LLSTNESNAI EQFLDNLISQ DMMSSNASMN
Ino4p        1
Esc1       166 SSSDSVSTSA SSSNASNTVS VTSPASSSAT PLPNQPSQQQ FLVSKNDAFT TFVHSVHNTP MQQSMYVPQQ QTSHSSGASY
```

Plant proteins

```
R-Lc       259 HGQEEELRLR EAEALSDDAS LEHITKEIEE FYSLCDEMDL QALPLPLEDG WTVDASNFEV PCS--SPQPA PPPVDRATAN
R-S        264 HGQEEELRLR EAEALSDDAS LEHITKEIEE FYSLCDEMDL QALPLPLEDG WTVDASNFEV PCS--SPQPA PPPVDRATAN
B-Peru     254 HGTGQELGEV ES---PSNAS LEHITKGIDE FYSLCEEMDV Q----PLEDA WIMDGSNFEV PSS--A---- ----------
Del        271 EGINGEVPQT QSWPFMDDAI SNCLNSSMNS SDCISQTHEN LESFAPLSDG KGPPETNNCM HSTQKCNQQI ENTGVQGDEV
```

```
AAPPS-----  ----------  --TRKDYPAA  KRVKLDSRV   LRQI-----S  NNRKCTSPRS  SDTEENV---  ----------  --------K  RRTHNVLERQ  RRNELKRSFF
AAPSP-----  ----------  --YVESEDAP  PQKKIKSEAS  PRPLKSVIPP  KAKSLSPR-N  SDSEDSE---  ----------  --------R  RRNHNILERQ  RRNDLRSSFL
AARFPPESCS  QEEASERGPQ  EEVLERDAAG  EKEDEEDEEI  VSPPPVESEA  AQSCHPKPVS  SDTEDVT---  ----------  --------R  RKNHNFLERK  RRNDLRSRFL
AAPPS-----  ----------  --TKVEYPAA  KRLKLDSGRV  LKQI-----S  NNRKCSSPRT  LDSEEND---  ----------  --------K  RRTHNVLERQ  RRNELKLRFF
AAP-P-----  ----------  --LPYAEDAR  PLKKPRSQDP  LGPLKCVLRP  KAPRLRSRSN  SDLEDIE---  ----------  --------R  RRNHNRMERD  RRDIMRSSFL
                                                           MSDNNDDI    EVE-------  ------SDEE  QPRFQSAADK  RAHHNALERK  RRDHIKDSFH
            --MAAAVRMN  IQMLLEAADY  LERREREAEH  GYASMLPYNN  KDR-------  ----DALKRR  NKSKKNNSSS  RSTHNEMEKN  RRAHLRLCLE
            --MERVKMIN  VQRLLEAAEF  LERRERECEH  GYASSFPSMP  SPRLQHSKPP  RRLSRAQKHS  SGTSNTSTAN  RSTHNELEKN  RRAHLRLCLE
                                               RK          TEKEVIGGLC  SLANIPLTPE  TQRDQERRIR  REIANSNERR  RMQSINAGFQ
AVGDGAGGTT  SGSTAAVVTT  QGSEALLGQA  TPPGTGQFFV  MMSPQEVLQG  GSQRSIA---  PRTHPYS---  ------PKSE  APRTTRDEKR  RAQHNEVERR  RRDKINNWIV
SVGDTTA---  ----VSVQTT  DQS-------  -LQAGGQFYV  MMTPQDVLQT  GTQRTIA---  PRTHPYS---  ----PKID   GTRTPRDERR  RAQHNEVERR  RRDKINNWIV
IDEIISLESS  YNDEMLSYLP  GGTTGLQLPS  TLPVSGNLLD  VYSS-QGVAT  PAITVSNSCP  AELPNIKREI  ------SETE  AKALLKERQK  KDNHNLIERR  RRFNINDRIK
IDNIMRLTMS  --------LG  YINPEMQMPN  TLPLSSSHLN  VYSSDPQVTA  SLVGVTSSSC  PADLTQKREL  ------TDAE  SRALAKERQK  KDNHNLIERR  RRFNINDRIK
VVE-------  ----------  ----------  -WRLSGSILD  VYSGEQGISP  VNTGLMNASC  PSILPMKKEI  ------AETD  TRALAKERQK  KDNHNLIERR  RRYNINYRIK
IDDIISLESS  YNEEILGLM-  --DPALQMAN  TLPVSGNLID  LYS-NQGLPP  PGLTISNSCP  ANLPNIKREL  TACIFPTESE  ARALAKERQK  KDNHNLIERR  RRFNINDRIK
FIKADSLLLT  AMKTDGATVK  AAGLSPLVSG  TTVQTGPLPT  LVSGGTILAT  VPLVVDAEKL  PINRLAA---  ------GSKA  PASAQSRGEK  RTAHNAIEKR  YRSSINDKII

----SGLGRA  GA---TAAAS  EIKREEKEDE  ENTSAADHSE  EEK-------  KELKAPRART  SPDEDEDDLL  PPEQKAEREK  E--------R  RVANNARERL  RVRDINEAFK
RGMPPGLQGQ  SV---SSGSS  EIKSDD-EGD  ENLQDTKSSE  DKKLDDD--K  KDIK-----S  ITSNNDDEDL  TPEQKAEREK  E--------R  RMANNARERL  RVRDINEAFK
R---GGLQSQ  SG---TVVTT  EIKTENEKED  ENLHEPPSSD  DMKSDDSESSQ  KDIKVSSRGR  TSSTNEDEDL  NPEQKIEREK  E--------R  RMANNARERL  RVRDINEAFK
AISNSVPAGV  ST---TSSLT  SLDISDTKPT  SSIESSNSGL  QQHSQGKGTK  R-----PRRY  CSSADEDDDA  EPAVKAIREK  E--------R  RQANNAARET  RREKENTEFC
                                               M           KEKSKNAART  RREKENTEFC

WTDECLSSQD  EDHEADKKED  EL-EAMNAEE  DSLRNGGDEE  DE--------  -DEDLEEEDE  EEEEDDQKPK  RRGPKKKKMT  KARLERFKLR  RMKANARERN  RMHGLNAALD
- -PTHSE----  -TES-GFSDCG  GGAGPDGAGP  GGPGGGQARG  PEPG------  ---EPGRKDL  QHLSREERRR  R---------  ---RRATAKY  RTAHATRERI  RVEAFNLAFA
- -SAHSD----  -PESLGGTDTK  VLGSVSDLEP  VEEAEGDKG   GSRA------  ---ALYPHP-  QQLSREEKRR  R---------  ---RRATAKY  RSAHATRERI  RVEAFNLAFA
ADSQGELVRR  SGCGGLSKSP  GPVKVREQLC  KLKGGVVVDE  LGCS------  ---RQRAPSS  KQVNGVQKQR  R---------  ---LAANA--  ------RERR  RMHGLNHAFD
RK---FARQC  EDQKQIKKSE  SFPKQVVLRG  KSIKRAPGEE  TE--------  -KEE-EEEDR  EEEDENGLSR  RRGLRKKKTT  KLRLERVKFR  RQEANARERN  RMHGLNDALD
MTSICSSKFQ  QQHYQLTNSN  IFLLQHQHHH  QTQQHQLIAP  KIPLGTSSQLQ  NMQQSQQSNV  GPMLSSQKKK  FNYNNMPYG-  --EQLPSVAR  R---NARERN  RVKQVNNGFV
TTINSATKIF  RYQHIMPAPS  PLI---PGGN  QNQPAGTMPI  KTRKYTPRGM  ALTRCSESVS  SLSPGSSPAP  YN------V-  --DQSQSVQR  R---NARERN  RVKQVNNSFA
                                    M           ALGSENHSVF  NDDEESSSA-  FN--------  ----GPSVIR  R---NARERN  RVKQVNNGFS
STTNTTPISS  QRKRPLGESQ  KQNRRHNQQNQ  QLSKTSVPAK  KCKTNKKLAV  ERPPKAGTIS  HPHKSQSDQS  FGTPGRKGL-  --PLPQAVAR  R---NARERN  RVKQVNNGFA
DFDNSALFDD  SV--------  -------EDD  EDLMLFSGGE  DFDGNDGSFD  ---------L  ADGENQDAAA  GGSGKKRRGK  QITPVVKRKR  RLAANARERR  RMQNLNQAFD
ATAAAAAAAA  AAAAAQSAQQ  QQQQQAPQQQ  APQLSPVADG  QPSGGGHKSA  AKQVKRQRSS  SPELMRCKRR  LNFSGFGYSL  PQQQPAAVAR  R----NERERN  RVKLVNLGFA
ANVHFPPHPV  PREHFSCGAP  KPVAGAPALN  ASLMDGGALP  RLVPTSSGVA  GACTARRRPP  SPELLRCSRR  RRSGATEASS  S---SAAVAR  R----NERERN  RVKLVNLGFQ
FYDDPCFDSP  DLRFFEDLDP  RLMHVGALLK  PEEHSHFPAA  VHPAPGARED  EHVRAPSG--  -H---HQAGR  CLLWACKACK  RKTTNAD--R  RKAATMRERR  RLSKVNEAFE
YDGENYLPVH  LQGFE----P  PGYERTELTL  SP--------  ---EAPGPLE  DKGLGTPE--  -----HCPGQ  CLPWACKVCK  RKSVSVD--R  RRAATLREKR  RLKKVNEAFE
FYDGSCIPSP  EGEFGDEFVP  RVAAFGA-HK  AELQ------  -----GSDED  EHVRAPTG--  -H---HQAGH  CLMWACKACK  RKSTTMD--R  RKAATMRERR  RLKKVNQAFE
LDGEN---VT  LQPLEVAEGS  PLYPGSDGTL  SPCQDQMPP-  -EAGSDSSGE  EHVLAPPGLQ  PP---HCPGQ  CLIWACKTCK  RKSAPTD--R  RKAATLRERR  RLKKINEAFE
GAAMPTTELS  AFRPSLLQLT  ALGRAPPTLA  VHYHPHPFLN  SVYI------  ---GPAGPFS  IF-PNSRLKR  RPSHSELDLA  DGHQPQKVAR  RVFTNSRERW  RQQHVNGAFA
GAAMPTTELS  AFRPSLLQLT  ALGRAPPTLA  VHYHPHPFLN  SVYI------  ---GPAGPFS  IF-PNSRLKR  RPSHSELDLA  DGHQPQKVAR  RVFTNSRERW  RQQHVNGAFA
AELPGDGRMV  QLSPPALAAP  A-APGRALLY  SLSQPLASLG  SGFF------  ---GEPDAFP  MFTTNNRVKR  RPSPYEMEIT  DGPHT-KVVR  RIFTNSRERW  RQQHVNSAFA
                                                                      MTR         KIFTNTRERW  RQQHVNSAFA

AATTANPEMT  SDVPSLGPAI  ASGNSGPGIQ  KRRPGLDFDD  DGEGNSKFLR  CDDDQMSNDK  ERFARSDDEQ  SSADKERLA-  RENHSEIERR  RRNKMTAYIT
                                               MSSGANI     TYASRKRRKP  VQKTVKPIPA  EGIKSNPSKR  HRDRLNTELD
LNGSAYSSSD  RDDMEYARHN  ALSSVSDLNG  GVMSPACLAD  DGSA------  ---GSLLDGS  DAGGKAFRKP  RRRLKRKSK  TEETDEFSNQ  RVMANVRERQ  RTQSLNDAFT
YELHNYADLN  DMARATDSKD  SRKRKTASAR  GEKYSLRQKR  QKRGSNEDGE  SANLADFQLE  LDPIAEPASK  SRKNAPTKSK  TKAPPLSKYR  RKTANARERT  RMREINTAFE
LSEDEE----  NRSESDASDQ  SFGCCEGPEA  ARRGP-GPGG  GRRA------  ---GGGG---  GAGPVVVVRQ  R---------  --QAANA--  ------RERD  RTQSVNTAFT
LSEDED----  RGSESSGSDE  KPCRVHAARC  GLQGARRRAG  GRRA------  ---AGSGPGP  GGRPGREPRQ  R---------  ---HTANA--  ------RERD  RTNSVNTAFT
RALSGGLQSQ  SV---AIGPT  EIKSEHKEKD  ENIHEPPSSD  DMKSDDESSQ  KDIKVSSRGR  TSSTNEDEDL  NPEQKIEREK  E--------R  RMANNARERL  RVRDINEAFK
                                    MP          AVPFTHSWMV  PTQDLCAMPP  YNKMTGHQQP  PGAGMHAQQQ  PLEPGILELR  KEKSRDAARS  RRGKENYEFY
VAESSGGEQS  PDDDSDGRCE  LVLRAGGADP  RASPGAGGGG  TKVVKQCSNA  HLHGGAGLPP  GGSTGSGGGG  SKKSKEQKAL  RLNINARERR  RMHDLNDALD
HQERPYFQSW  LLSPAD-AAP  DFP-AGGPPP  TTAVAAAAYG  ----------  ---PDARPSQ  SPGRLEALGS  RL--------  ------PKR  KGSGPKKERR  RTEISINSAFA
PRGEPLLHGW  LIGHPEMSPP  DYSMALSYSP  EYASGAAGLD  HSHY------  ---GGVPPGA  GPPGLG--GP  RP--------  ------VKR  RGTANRKERR  RTQSINSAFA

                                   MPADI       MEKNSSSPVA  ATPASVNTTP  DKPKTASEHR  KSSKPIMEKR  RRARINESLS
                                   MRLP        RGVGDAAELR  KSLKPLLEKR  RRARINESLS
                                                                      MEKK        RRARINLSLE
                                   MAPSTVA     VEMLSPKEKN  RLRKPVVEKM  RRDRINSSIE
                                   MAPQSNNSTT  F-VSKTQHYL  KVKKPLLERQ  RRARMNKCLD
                                   MATK        YEMSKTYQYR  KVMKPLLERR  RRARINKCLD
                                   ME          Y-TTKTQIYQ  KVKKPMLERQ  RRARMNKCLD
                                   MV          TGVTAANMTN  VLGTAVVPAQ  LKETPLKSDR  RSNKPIMEKR  RRARINNCLN
                                   MD          YKNDINSDDD  FDCSNGYSDS  YGSNGRMSNP  NGLSKA-ELR  KTNKPIMEKR  RRARINHCLN
                                   MKSLTAVC    QTGA------  -SGMPALNAS  GRIQRHPTHR  GDGEN---A  EMKMYLSKLK
CTT         FLQLLVLFPH  SVLSLLRSPP  PVLRIMKVAS  GSAAAAAGPS  CSLKA-----  GRTAGEVVLG  LSEQSVAISR  CAGTRLPALL  DEQQVNVLLY  DMNGCYSRLK
MAIQGCPIER  PGRVHIKDAP  PGSRFILNRA  WCRAVSSAPC  GGSLPVSPPT  SSMKAFR--S  GESVRKN--S  LSDHSLGISR  SKT---PV--  -DDP-MSLLY  NMNDCYSKLK
                                   MKALS--P    VRGCYEAVCC  LSERSLAIAR  GRGKSPST--  -EEP-LSLLD  DMNHCYSRLK
                                   MKAVSPVRP   SGRKAPSGCG  GGELALRCLA  EHGHSLGGSA  AAAAAAAAAR  CKAAEAAA--  -DEPALCLQC  DMNDCYSRLR

GVKPNTSLEG  MTSSPMESTQ  QSKNDMLIPL  AEHDRGPEHQ  QDDEDNDDAD  IDLKKDISMQ  PGRRGRK---  ------PTTL  ATTDEWKKQR  KDSHKEVERR  RRENINTAIN
PGPDSATSLF  ELPDSVIPTP  KPKPKPKQYP  KVILPSNSTR  RVSPVTAKTS  SSAEGVVVAS  ESPVIAPHGS  SHSRSLSKRR  SSGALVDDDK  RESHKHAEQA  RRNRLAVPLH
SESHLHIRSP  KKQHRYTELN  QRYPETHPHS  NTGELPTNTA  DVPTEFTTRE  GPHQPIGNDH  YNPPPPFSVPE  IRIPDSDIPA  NIEDDPVKVR  KWKHVQMEKI  RRINTKEAFE
                                   MTNDIKEIQ   TIQPGLSEIK  EIKGELANVK  KRKRRSKKIN  KLTDGQ---I  RINHVSSERK  RRELERAIFD
QNESANPPVQ  SPMQYSYSQG  QPFSYPQHKN  QSFSASPIDP  SMSYVYRAPE  SFSSINANVP  YGRNEYLRRV  TSLVPNQPEY  TGPYTRNPEL  RTSHKLAERK  RRKEIKELFD

VAADASRAPV  YGSRATSFMA  WTRSSQQSSC  ----SDDAAP  AAVVPAIEEP  QRLLKKVVAG  -----GGAWE  ----SCGGAT  GAAQEMSGTG  TKNHVMSERK  RREKLNEMFL
VAADASRAPV  YGSRATSFMA  WTRSSQQSSC  ----SDDAAP  -AVVPAIEEP  QRLLKKVVAG  -----GGAWE  ----SCGGAT  GAAQEMS--A  TKNHVMSERK  RREKLNEMFL
LPVDGSSAPA  DGSRATSFVV  WTRSSH--SC  ----SGEAA-  ---VPVIEEP  QKLLKKALAG  -----GGAWA  NTNCGGGGTT  VTAQE---NG  AKNHVMSERK  RREKLNEMFL
HYQGVLSNLL  KSSHQLVLGP  YFRNGNRESS  FVSWNKDGSS  GTHVPRSGTS  QRFLKKVLFE  VARMHENSRL  DAGKQKGNSD  CLAKPTADEI  DRNHVLSERK  RREKINERFM
```

Sequence alignment of 75 HLH protein sequences   **141**

```
Main section                           LOOP              ···HELIX 2······    LEUCINE ZIPPER·····
  bHLHZ proteins    ALRDQIP--- ---------- ELENNEKA-P KVVILKKATA YILSV--QAE EQKLISEEDL LRKRREQLKH KLEQLRNSCA
                    TLRDHVP--- ---------- ELVKNEKA-A KVVILKKATE YVHSL--QAE EHQLLLEKEK LQARQQQLLK KIEHARTC
                    ALRDQVP--- ---------- TLASCSKA-P KVVILSKALE YLQAL--VGA EKRMATEKRQ LRCRQQQLQK RIAYLSGY
                    ALRDQIP--- ---------- EVANNEKA-P KVVLSL--QSD EHKLIAEKEQ LRRRREQLKH NLEQLRNSRA
                    NLRDLVP--- ---------- ELVHNEKA-A KVVILKKATE YIHTL--QTD ESKLLVEREK LYERKQQLLE KIKQSAVC
                    SLRDSVPSL- -------QG EK------AS RAQILDKATE YIQYMRRKNH THQQDIDDLK --RQNALLE QQVRALEKAR
                    KLKGLVP-L- --------G PESSR---HT TLSLLTKAKL HIKKLEDCDR KAVH-Q--ID QLQREQRHLK RQLEK-----
                    RLKVLIP-L- --------G PDCTR---HT TLGLLNKAKA HIKKLEEAER KSQH-Q--LE NLEREQRFLK WRLEQ-----
                    SLKTLIPHT- --------DG E------KLS KAAILQQTAE YIFSLE---- ---------- ---------- --QEKTRLLQ
                    QLSKIIPDC- --------SM ESTKS--GQS KGGILSKACD YIQELRQSNH RLSEELQGLD QLQLDNDVLR QQVEDLKN--
                    QLSKIIPDC- --------NA DNSKT--GAS KGGILSKACD YIRELRQTNQ RMQETFKEAE RLQMDNELLR QQIEELKN--
                    ELGTLIPKS- --------SD PEMRW----N KGTILKASVD YIRKLQKEQQ RSKDLESRQR SLEQANRSLQ LRIQELELQA
                    ELGMLIPKA- --------ND LDVRW----N KGTILKASVD YIRRMQKDLQ KSRELENHSR RLEMTNKQLW LRIQELEIQA
                    ELGTLIPKS- --------ND PDIRW----N KGTILKASVD YIKWLQKEQQ RARELEHRQK KLEHANRQLM LRIQELEMQA
                    ELGTLIPKS- --------ND PDMRW----N KGTILKASVD YIRKLQREQQ RAKDLENRQK KLEHANRHLL LRVQELEMQA
                    ELKDLVVGT- --------EA -K------LN KSAVLRKAID YIRFLQHSNQ KLKQENLSLR TAVHKSKSLK DLVSACGSGG

  bHLH proteins     ELGRMCQ--- ---------- LHLNSEKPQT KLLILHQAVA VILNLEQQVR ERNLNPKAAC LKRREEKVS GVVG------
                    ELGRMVQ--- ---------- LHLKSDKPQT KLLILHQAVA VILSLEQQVR ERNLNPKAAC LKRREEKVS --SE------
                    ELGRMCQ--- ---------- LHLKSEKPQT KLLILHQAVA VILSLEQQVR ERNLNPKAAC LKRREEKVS AVSA------
                    ELGRMCM--- ---------- THLKSDKPQT KLGILNMAVE VIMTLEQQVR ERNLNPKAAC LKRREEKAE DGPKLSAQHH
                    ELAKLL---- ---------P LPAAITSQLD KASVIRLTTS YLKMRQVFPD GLG----EAW GS----SPAM QRGATIKEL-
                    NLRKVVP--- ---------- -CYSKTQKLS KIETLRLAKN YIWALSEILR SGKSPDLVSF VQTLCKGLSQ PTTNLVAGCL
                    ELRKLLP--- ---------- -TLPPDKKLS KIEILRLAIC YISYLNHVLD V
                    ELRKLLP--- ---------- -TLPPDKKLS KIEILRLAIC YISYLNHVLD V
                    QLRNVIP--- ---------- -SFNNDKKLS KYETLQMAQI YINALSELLQ TPNVGEQPPP PTASCKNDHH HLRTASSYEG
                    NLRKVVP--- ---------- -CYSKTQKLS KIETLRLAKN YIWALSEILR IGKRPDLLTF VQNLCKGLSQ PTTNLVAGCL
                    NLRQHIPQTV VNSLSNG--- -GRGSSKKLS KVDTLRIAVE YIRGLQDMLD DGTASSTRHI YNSA------ -DESSNDGSS
                    RLRQHIPQSI ITDLT---KG GGRGPHKKIS KVDTLRIAVE YIRSLQDLVD DLNGGSNIGA NNAVTQLQLC LDESSSHSSS
                    QLRQHIPAAV IADLSNGRRG IGPGANKKLS KVSTLKMAVE YIRRLQKVLH E------EAW NDQQKQKQLH LQ--------
                    LLREKIPEEV SEAFEA--QG AGRGASKKLS KVETLRMAVE YIRSLEKLLG FDFPPLNSQG NSSGSGDDSF MFIKDEFDCL
                    RL-RQYL--- ---------- PCLGNDRQLS KHETLQMAQT YISALGDLLR
                    TLREHVPNG- ---------- ---AANKKMS KVETLRSAVE YIRALQQLLD EHDAVSAAFQ AGVLSPTISP N---------
                    ALRQHVPHG- ---------- ---GANKKLS KVETLRSAVE YIRALQRLLA EHDAVRAALS GGLLTPATRP SDVCTQPSAS
                    TLKRC----- ---------- TSSNPNQRLP KVEILRNAIR YIEGLQALLR DQDAAPPGAA AFYAPGPLPP GRGGEHYSGD
                    ALKRS----- ---------- TLLNPNQRLP KVEILRSAIQ YIERLQALLS SLNQEER--- ----DLRYRG GGGPQ------
                    TLKRS----- ---------- TTTNPNQRLP KVEILRNAIR YIESLQELLR EQ------VE NYYS----LP GQSC------
                    ALKRR----- ---------- TVANPNQRLP KVEILRSAIS YIERLQDLLH RLDQQEKMQE LGVDPPFSYRP KQENL-----
                    ELRKLLP--- ---------- -THPPDRKLS KNEVLRLAMK YIGFLVRLLR DQTAVLTSGP SAPGSRKPPA RRGVEGSARF
                    ELRKLLP--- ---------- -THPPDRKLS KNEVLRLAMK YIGFLVRLLR DQTAVLTSGP SAPGSRKPPA RRGVEGSARF
                    ELRKLIP--- ---------- -THPPDRKLS KNEILRLAMK YINFLAKLLN DQEEEGTQRA KTGKDPVVGA GGGGGGGGGG
                    KLRKLIP--- ---------- -THPPDRKLS KNEVLRLAMK YINFLVKVLG EQSLQQT--- ---------- --------GV
                    ELSDMVP-T- ---------C SALAR--KPD KLTILRMAVS HMKSLRGTGN TSTD-GSYKP SFLTDQELKH LILEAADGFL
                    RLASLL---- ---------P FPQDVINKLD KLSVLRLSVS YLRAKSFFDV ALKSTPADRN GGQDQCRAQI RDWQDLQE--
                    SLQQIIP--- ---------- -TLPSD-KLS KIQTLKLATR YIDFLCRMLS SSDISLLKAL EAQGSPSAYG SASSLLSAAA
                    TLRHCVPEAI KGE------- DAANTNEKLT KITTLRLAMK YITMLTDSIR DPSYESEFIG ECLEESANRE ARVDLEANEE
                    ALRTLIP--- ---------- -TEPVDRKLS KIETLRLASS YIAHLANVLL LGDSADDGQP C--------- ------FRAA
                    ALRTLIP--- ---------- -TEPADRKLS KIETLRLASS YISHLGNVLL VGEACGDGQP CHSG------ --------PAFFHS
                    ELGRMCQ--- ---------- LHLKSEKPQT KLLILHQAVA VILSLEQQVR ERNLNPKAAC LKRREEKVS AVSA------
                    ELAKML---- ---------P LPAAITSQLD KASIIRLTIS YLKLRDFSGH GDPPWTREAS SSSKLKSAAI RRSPAVDLFE
                    ELRAVIPYA- ---------- -HSPSVRKLS KIATLLLAKN YILMQAQALE EMRRLVAYLN QGQAISAASL PSSAAAAAAA
                    ELRECIP--- ---------- -NVPADTKLS KIKTLRATS YIAYLMDVLA KDAQAGDPEA FKAELKKTDG GRESKRKREL
                    ELRECIP--- ---------- -NVPADTKLS KIKTLRATS YIAYLMDLLP KDDQNGEAEA FKAEIKKTD- VKEEKRKKEL

  HLH proteins (no  QLKTLILDA- --------LK KDSSRHSKLE KADILEMTVK HLRNLQ---- ---------- ---------- --RAQMTAAL
  functional DNA-   QLKGLVLPL- --------LG AETSRYSKLE KADILEMTVR FLRE-Q---- ---------- ---------- --PASVCST-
  binding domain    QLRSLLERH- --------YS HQ-IRKRKLE KADILELSVK YVRSLQ---- ---------- ---------- --NSLQGLWL
                    QLKLLLEQE- --------FA RHQP-NSKLE KADILEMAVS YLK------- ---------- ---------- --HSKAFAAA
                    TLKTLVAEF- --------QG DDAI--LRMD KAEMLEAALV FMRK-Q---- ---------- ---------- --VVKQQAPV
                    ELKDLMAEC- --------VA QTGD--AKFE KADILEVTVQ HLRK-L---- ---------- ---------- --KESKKHVP
                    NLKTLVAEL- --------RG DDGI--LRMD KAEMLESAVI FMRQ-Q---- ---------- ---------- --KTPKKVAQ
                    ELKTLILDA- --------TK KDPARHSKLE KADILEKTVK HLQELQ---- ---------- ---------- --RQQAAMQQ
                    ELKSLILEA- --------MK KDPARHTKLE KADILEMTVK HLQSVQ---- ---------- ---------- --RQQLNMAI
                    DLVPFMP--- ---------- ----KNRKLT KLEIIQHVID YICDLQ---T ELETHPEMGN FDAAAALTAV NGLHEDEDSD
                    ELVPTLP--- ---------- ----QNRKVS KVEILQHVID YIRDLQ---L ELNSESEV-- ---------- ----GTTGGR
                    ELVPSIP--- ---------- ----QNKKVT KMEILQHVID YILDLQ---I ALDSHPTIV- ---------- -SLHHQRPGQ
                    ELVPGVP--- ---------- ----RGTQLS QVEILQHVID YILDLQ---V VLAEPA---- ---------- -------PGP
                    RLVPTIP--- ---------- ----PNKKVS KVEILQHVID YILDLQ---L ALETHPALLR QPPPPA---- PPLHPAGACP

  Yeast proteins    VLSDLLPVR- --------ES S KAAILARAAE YIQKLKETDE ------ANIE KWTLQKLLSE QNASQLASAN
                    ELASLIPAEW ---------- KQQNVSAAPS KATTVEAACR YIRHLQQNGS T
                    RLIKSVR--- --------T PPKENGKRIP KHILLTCVMN DIKSIRSANE ALQHILDDS
                    ELVAVVPDL- ---------Q PQESR----S ELIIYLKSLS YLSWLYERNE K--------- --LRKQIIAK HEAKTGSSSS
                    DLKD--A--- ---------- LPLDKSTKSS KNGLLTRAIQ YI----EQLK SEQV-ALEAY VKSLEENMQS NKEVTKGT

  Plant proteins    VLKSLLP--- ---------- ----SIHRVN KASILAETIA YLKELQRRVQ ELESSREPAS RPSETTTR-- ---LITRPSR
                    VLKSLLP--- ---------- ----SIHRVN KASILAETIA YLKELQRRVQ ELESSREPAS RPSETTTR-- ---LITRPSR
                    VLKSLVP--- ---------- ----SIHKVD KASILAETIA YLKELQRRVQ ELESRRQGGS ---------- ----------
                    ILASLVP--- ---------- ----SGGKVD KVSILDHTID YLRGLERKVD ELESNKMVKG RGRESTTKTK LHDAIERTSD
```

```
SSAQLQ----  -------TNY  PSSDNSLYTN  AKGSTISAFD  GGSDSSSESE  PEEP---QSR  KKLRMEAS
L----GIERI  RMDSIGSTVS  SERSDSDR--  ----EEIDVD  --------V   ESTDYLTGDL  DW-SSSSVSD  SDERGSMQ-S  LGSDEGY---  ---SSTSIKR  IKLQDSHKAC
LQGPQEMERI  RMDSIGSTIS  SDRSDSER--  ----EEIEVD  --------V   ESTEFSHGEV  DNISTTSISD  IDDHSSLP-S  IGSDEGY---  ---SSASVK-  ----------
QNTQ--LKRF  IQELSGSSPK  RRRAEDKDEG  IGSP-DIWED  EKAEDLRREM  IELRQQLDKE  RSVRMMLEEQ  VRSLEAHMYP  EKLKVIAQQV  QLQQQQEQVR  LLHQEKLERE
KNLLLRAQLR  HHGLEVVIKN  DSN
ENALLRAQLQ  QHNLEMVGEG  TRQ
QIHGLPVPGT  PGLLSLATTS  TSDSLKPEQL  DIEEEGRPGA  RTFHVGGGPA  QNAPHQQPPA  PPSDALLDLH  FPSDHLGDLG  DPFHLGLEDI  LMEEEEGVVG  GLSGGALSPL
RVHGLPTTSP  SG---MNMAE  LAQQVVKQEL  PSEEG--PGE  ALMLGAEVPD  PEPLPALPPQ  APLPLPTQPP  SPFHHL-DFS  HSL-----SF  GGREDEGPPG  YPDRN
RAHGLPILAS  -----LGTAD  FGTHITKQQT  HSEKNSVGCC  QQL----TPS  QG-----TSP  EFYEQAVAFS  DPLSHFTDLS  --F-----SA  ALKEEQRLDG  MLLSDTICPF
RAHGLSLIPS  TG---LCSPD  LVNRIIKQEP  VLE----NCS  QEL----VQH  QADLTCTTTL  DLTDGTITFT  NNLGTMPESS  PAY-----SI  PRKMGSNLED  ILMDDALSPV
NTDVLMEGVK  TEVEDTLTPP  PSDAGSPFQS  SPLSLGSRGS  GSGGGSGSDSE  PDSPVFEDSK  AKPEQRPSLH  SRGMLDRSRL  ALCTLVFLCL  SCNPLASLLG  ARGLPSPSDT

-DPQMVLSAP  HPGLSEAHNP  AGHM
-PPPLSLAGP  HPGMGDASNH  MGQM
-EPPTTLPGT  HPGLSETTNP  MGHM
MIPQPQQVGG  TPGSSYHSQP  AQLVPPSSQT  ISTMTISLPV  NQANNGLPPH  LQQQQQQQSQ  LGHAQLPQ
---GSHLLQT  LDGFIFVVAP  DGKIMYISET  ASVHLGLSQV  ELTGNSIFEY  IHNYDQDEMN  AILSLHPHIN  QHPLAQTHTP  IGSPNGV---  ----QHPSAY  DHDRGSHTI-
QLNPRTFLPE  QNPDMPPHLP  TA-SASFPVH  PYSYQSPGLP  SPP-YGTMDS  SHVFQVKPPP  HAYSATLEPF  FESPLTDCTS  PSFDGPLS-P  PLSINGNFSF  KHEPSAEFEK

GAGASAVAGA  QPAPGGGPRP  TPPGPCRTRF  SGPASSGGYS  VQLDALHFPA  FEDRALTAMM  AQKDLSPSLP  GGILQPVQED  NSKTSPRSHR  SDGEFSPHSH  YSDSDEAS
QLNARSFLMG  QGGEAAHHTR  SPYSTFYP--  --PYHSPELA  TPPGHGTLDN  SKSMK----P  YNYCSAYESF  YESTSPECAS  PQFEGPLSPP  PINYNGIFSL  KQEETLDYGK
YNDYNDS---  ----------  ----------  LDSSQ-----  ----------  ----------  --QFLTGATQ  SAQ-------  ----------  --------S   RS--------
SSTCSSSGHN  TYYQNRISVS  PVQQQQQQLQR  QQFNH-----  ----------  ----------  --QPLTALSL  NTNLVGTSVP  GGDAGCVSTS  KNQQTCHSPT  SS--------
----------  ----------  --QQHLHFQQ  QQ-QH-----  ----------  ----------  --QHLYAWHQ  ELQL------  ----------  ---QSPTGST  SS--------
DEHFDDSLSN  YEMDEQQTVQ  QTLSEDMLNP  PQASDLLPSL  TTLNGLQYIR  IPGTNTYQLL  TTDLLGDLSH  EQKLEETAAS  GQLSRSPVPQ  KVVRSPCSSP  VSPVASTELL

-YSNDLN---  --------SM  AGSPVSSYSS  DEGSYDPLSP  EEQELLDFTN  WF
PASASLSCTS  TSPDRLGCSE  PASPRSAYSS  EDSSCEGETY  PMGQMFDFSN  WLGGY
SDASSP----  ----RSNCSD  GMMDYSGPPS  GARRRNCYEG  AYYNEAPSEP  RPGKSAAVSS  LDYLSSIVER  I-STESPAAP  ALLLADVPSE  SPPRRQEAAA  PSEGESSGDP
----------  ------PGVP  --SECSSHSA  SCSPEWGSAL  EFSANPGDHL  LTADPTDAHN  LHSLTSIVDS  I----TVEDV  SVAFPDETMP  N
SEPTSP----  ----TSNCSD  GMPECNSPVW  S-RKSSTFDS  IYCPDV-SNV  YATDKNSLSS  LDCLSNIVDR  I-T--SSEQP  GLPLQDLASL  S---------  ---------P
----------  ------EGAD  FLRTCSSQWP  SVS-DHSRGL  VITAKEGGAS  I--DSSASSS  LRCLSSIVDS  I----SSEER  KLPCVEEVVE  K
GAEHRVEAAR  SQPVLPGDCD  GDPNGSVRPI  KLEQTSLSPE  VR
GAEHRVEAAR  SQPVLPGDCD  GDPNGSVRPI  KLEQTSLSPE  VR
APPDDLLQDV  LSPNSSCGSS  LDGAASPDSY  -TEEPAPKHT  ARSLHPAMLP  AADGAGPR
AAQGNIL--G  LFPQGPHLPG  LEDRTLLENY  QVPSPGPSHH  IP
FIVSCETGRV  VYVSDSVTPV  LNQPQSEWFG  STLYDQVHPD  DVDKLREQLS  TSENALTGRI  LDLKTGTVKK  EGQQSSMRMC  MGSRRSFICR  MRCGSSSVDP  VSVNR-----
---GEFLLQA  LNGFVLVVTA  DALVFYASST  IQDYLGFQQS  DVIHQSVYEL  IHTEDRAEFQ  RQLHWALNPD  SAQGVDEAHG  PPQAAVYYTP  DQLPPENASF  ----------
NGAEGDLKCL  RKANGAPIIP  PEKLSYLFGV  WRMEGDAQHQ  KA
AEVELPVPVA  KKPAKTKGSG  KKSSAASKRQ  SQKQAKIVPQ  IPPISSGESC  YATSSDWIAC  LLAYASLSSS  SNSHSSSSSP  GLELDSLVGL  NGISALDSLL  LDTSDGDSLS
GSAKGAVPAA  PTRR------  ----QPRSIC  TFCLSNQRKG  GGRRDLGGSC  LKVRGVAPLR  GPRR
GRAGSPLPPP  PPPPLARDG   GENTQPKQIC  TFCLSNQRKL  SKDRDRKTAI  RS
-EPPTPHPGS  HPGLSETTNP  MGHM
QHQGTHILQS  LDGFALAVAA  DGRFLYISET  VSIYLGLSQV  EMTGSSIFDY  IHQADHSEIA  DQLGLSLTSG  GGGGGGGSSS  SGGGGGGAGG  GMASPTSGAS  DDGSGTHGTN
AALHPALGAY  EQAAGYPFSA  GLPPAASCPE  KCALFNSVSS  SLCKQCTEKP
PQQPESFPPA  SGPGEKRIKG  RTGW-PQQVW  ALELNQ
---NEILKST  VSSNDKKTKG  RTGW-PQHVW  ALELKQ

STDPSVLGKY  RAGFSECMNE  VTRFLSTCEG  VNTEVRTRLL  GHLANCMTQI  NAM-------  -TYPGQAHPA  LQAPPPPPP-  ----------  -----SGPGG  -PQHAPFAPP
-EAPGSLDSY  LEGYRACLAR  LARVLPACSV  LEPAVSARLL  EHL-------  RQR-------  -TVSGGPPSL  TPASASAPA-  ----------  -----PSPPV  -PPPSSLGLW
VPSGV---DY  PSGFRGGLPG  SSQRLRPGED  DSGLRCPLLL  QRRAGSTTDS  ANPQTASVLS  PCLPAIWAPG  PPAGGSQSPQ  SPFFPPLGGLL  ESSTGILAPP  PASNCQAENP
AGPKSLHQDY  SEGYSWCLQE  AVQFLTLHAA  SDTQM--KLL  YHFQR-----  ----------  PPAPAAPVKE  TPTPGAAPQP  ARSSTKAAAS  VSTSRQSACG  LWRPW
S--PLPMDSF  KNGYMNAVSE  ISRVMACTPA  MSVDVGKTVM  THLGVEFQRM  LQ-------A  DQVQTSVTTS  T--P------  ---RPLSPAS  SGYHSDNEDS  QSAASPKPVE
AN---PEQSF  RAGYIRAANE  VSRALASLPR  VDVAFGTTLM  THLGMRLNQL  EQPMEQPQAV  NTPLSIVCGS  SSSSSTYSSA  SSCSSISPVS  SGYASDNESL  LQISSPGQV-
EEQSLPLDSF  KNGYMNAVNE  VSRVMASTPG  MSVDLGKSVM  THLGRVYKNL  QQFHEAQSAA  DFIQNSMDCS  SMDK------  ---APLSPAS  SGYHSDCDS-  -PPPTPQPMQ
AADPKIVNKF  KAGFVECAEE  VSRF----PG  IRPAQRRRLL  QHLSNCINGV  KTELHQQQRQ  QQQQSIHAQM  LPSPPSSPEQ  DSQQGAAAPY  LFGIQQTASG  YFLPNGMQVI
QSDPSVVQKF  KTGFVECAEE  VNRYVSQMDG  IDTGVRQRLS  AHLNQCANSL  EQIGSMSNFS  NGYRGGLFPA  TAVTAAPTPL  FPSLPQDLNN  NSRTESSAPA  -IQMGGLQLI
MEDA------  ---------D  AEAEAEVDPD  VLAQRLNAEQ  PAKVSSPAAR  LPLTDRQTPN  TLVAPAHPQQ  HQQQQQLQLQ  QQQLQSQQQL  SNSLATPQNA  EKDSRQS
GLPV------  ---------R  APLSTLNGEI  SALAAEEAACV  PA------DD  RILCR
NQAS------  ---------R  TRLTTLNTDI  SILSLQASEF  PSEL-MSNDS  KVLCG
PDGP------  ---------H  ----------  --LPIQTAEL  TPELVISKDK  RSFCH
VAPP------  ---------R  TPLTALNTD-  ----------  PAGAVNKQGD  SILCR

EKLQEELGNA  YKEIEYMKRV  LRKEGIEYED  MHTHKKQENE  RKSTRSDNPH  EA

SDPVQEQNGN  IRDLVPKELI  WELGDGQSGQ

GNNESVRKEV  CAG--SKRKS  PELGRDDVER  PPVLTMDAGT  SNVTVTVSDK  DVLLEVQCRW  EELLMTRVFD  AIKSLHLDVL  SVQASAPDGF  MGLKIRAQFA  GSGAVVPWMI
GNNESVRKEV  CAG--SKRKS  PELGRDDVER  PPVLTMDAGS  SNVTVTVSDK  DVLLEVQCRW  EELLMTRVFD  AIKSLHLDVL  SVQASAPDGF  MGLKIRAQFA  GSGAVVPWMI
---GCVSKKV  CVGSNSKRKS  PEFAGGAKEH  PWVLPMD-GT  SNVTVTVSDT  NVLLEVQCRW  EKLLMTRVFD  AIKSLHLDAL  SVQASAPDGF  MRLKIGAQFA  GSGAVVPGMI
NYGATRTSNV  KKPLTNKRKA  SDTDKIGAVN  SRGRLKDSLT  DNITVNITNK  DVLIVVTCSS  KEFVLLEVME  AVRRLSLDSE  TVQQSSNRDGM  ISITIKAKCK  GLKVASASVI
```

Main section

bHLHZ proteins

```
               LGL
               LSFTS
               QQQLRTQLLP PPAPTHHPTV IVPAPPPPPS HHINVVTMGP SSVINSVSTS RQNLDTIVQA IQHIEGTQEK QELEEEQRRA

               RAASDPLLSS VSLLSPRPAA AAAASAWKR- SPDQASPLPW TFPPRKGGPC RMRPRLFPHP PMRLPRYLGR GDVIR

               -G-TDPLLSA IS-----PAV SKASS-RSSL SSEDGDEL
               -GVTDPLLSS VS-----PGA SKTSSRRSSM SAEETEHAC
```

bHLH proteins

```
               TSVYHSPGRN VLGTESRDGP GWAQWLLPPV VWLLNGLLVL VSLVLLFVYG EPVTRPHSGP AVYFWRHRKQ ADLDLARGDF


               ---------- -------EIE KTFFLRMKCV LAKRNAGLTT SGFKVIHCSG ---------- ---------- -----YLKAR
               NYAFTMHYPA ATLAGPQSHG SIFSGATAPR CEIPIDNIMS FDSHSHHERV -MSAQLNAIF HD

               NYNYGMHYCA VPPRGPLGQG AMFR------ --LPTDSHFP YDLHLRSQSL TMQDELNAVF HN
               ---------- ---------Y HSASPTPSYS GSEISGG--- -----GYIKQ ELQEQ---DL KFD-SFDSF- ---SDEQPD-
               ---------- ---------F NSSMSFDSGT YEGVPQQIST HLDRLDHLDN ELHTHSQLQL KFEP-YEHFQ LDEEDCTPD-
               ---------- ---------C NSISSYCKPA TSTIPGATPP ---------N NFHT------ KLEASFEDYR NNSCSSGTE-
               LQTQTCATPL QQQVIKQEYV STNISSSSNA QTSPQQQQQV QNLGSSPILP AFYDQEPVSF YDNVVLPGFK KEFSDILQQD


               TQSPDAAPQC PAGANPNPIY QVL

               VASTDSQPRT PGASSSRLIY HVL



               LSFVRNRCRN GLGSVKDGEP HFVVVHCTGY IKAWPPAGVS LPDDDPEAGQ GSKFCLVAIG RLQVTSSPNC TDMSNVCQPT
               ---------- --------ME RCFRCRLRCL LDN------S SGFLAMNFQG RLKY----- ---------- ----------
               CLSPGYGSLL TGSGESLLPG CRGDLPMSGL EKSDVELSLR LLDQRFQGFL RLCQRSAPVG LY

               NPDVAASMTQ ASTSGYKGYD RSFCVRMKST LTKRGCHFKS SGYRASDATS NCNNGNNASN NAKNVKNPGS NYSVVLLLCK
```

HLH proteins (no functional DNA-binding domain

```
               PPLVPI---- -----PGGAA PPPGSAPCKL GSQAGEAAKV FGGFQVVPAP DGQFAFLIPN GAFAHSGPV- ----------
               RPW
               RPGFRVWRPW

               ETMWRPW
               ---WRPW
               QPLWRPW
               PTKLPNGSIA LVLPQSLPQQ QQQQLLQHQQ QQQQLAVAAA AAAAAAAQQQ PMLVSMPQRT ASTGSASS-- ----------
               PSRLPSGEFA LIMPNTGSAA PPPGPFAWPG SAAGVAAGTA SAALASIANP THLNDYTQSF RMSAFSKPVN TSVPANLPEN
```


Yeast proteins

Plant proteins

```
               SEALRKAIGK R-
               SEALRKAIGK R
               SQSLRKAIGK R-
               KQALQKVTMK S
```

```
                                                           439        c-Myc
                                                           464        N-Myc
                                                           364        L-Myc
                                                           422        v-Myc
                                                           429        S-Myc
                                                           160         Max
                                                           221        Mad1
                                                           220        Mxi4
VIVKPVRSCP EAPTSDTASD SEASDSDAMD QSREEPSGDG                 318         AP4
                                                           310        USF1
                                                           254        USF2
                                                           411        TFE3
                                                           514        TFEB
                                                           317        TFEC
                                                           419         Mi
AQAAQQLWLA LRALGRPLPT SHLDLACSLL WNLIRHLLQR                 638       SREBP1a

                                                           654         E12
                                                           622        1TF2
                                                           682         HEB
                                                           710         Da
IYPD--RGDG QGSLIQNLGL VAVGHSLPSS AITEIKLHQN                 254        Sim
                                                           355       NeuroD
                                                           133        Hen1
                                                           135        Hen2
                                                           351       MATH1
                                                           337       MATH2
---------- -DEELLDYIS SWQEQ                                 257        L-Sc
---------- -DEEILDYIS LWQEQ                                 345       Scute
---------- -DEDILDYIS LWQDDL                                201       Achaete
QPNNTTAGCL SDESMIDAID WWEAHAPKSN GACTNLSV                   486       Asense
                                                           312       Atonal
                                                           233       Mash1
                                                           260       Mash2
                                                           319       Myod
                                                           224      Myogenin
                                                           255       Myf5
                                                           242       MRF4
                                                           278       Ly11
                                                           245       Ly12
                                                           331       Tal1
                                                           108       Tal2
EFISRHNIEG IFTFVDHRCV ATVGYQPQEL LGKNIVEFCH                 401       Arnt1
LHGQNKKGKD GALLPPQLAL FAIATPLQPP SILEIRTKNF                 279        AhR
                                                           490       Twist
                                                           361      Delilah
                                                           199     bHLH-EC2
                                                           207     Scleraxis
                                                           490      GbHLH1.4
LRPQYTFSHS RKSQPPLLGM VALAIALPPP SVHEIRLECD                 369        Trh
                                                           367       BETA3
                                                           216       Thing1
                                                           217       Thing2

----IPVYTS NSGTSVGPNA VSPSSGSSLT ADSMWRPWRN                 281        Hes1
                                                           157        Hes2
                                                           175        Hes3
                                                           166        Hes5
                                                           178      E(spl)M5
                                                           186      E(spl)M7
                                                           179      E(spl)M8
--HSSAGYES APGSSSSCSY APSSPANSSY EPMDIKPSVI                 309       Hairy
LIHTLPGQTQ LPVKNSTSPP LSPISSISSH CEESRAASPT                 335        Dpn
                                                           199        Emc
                                                           176        Id1
                                                           186        Id2
                                                           119        Id3
                                                           161        Id4

                                                           351        Cbf1
                                                           312        Pho4
                                                           304       Ino2p
                                                           151       Ino4p
                                                           414        Esc1

                                                           610        R-Lc
                                                           612        R-S
                                                           562      B-Peru
                                                           644        Del
```

$\underline{N\text{-terminal section}}$

```
c-Myc       1
N-Myc       1
L-Myc       1
v-Myc       1
S-Myc       1
USF1        1
USF2        1
TFEB        1
TFEC        1
Mi          1
SREBP1a     1

E12         1  MNQPQRMAP VGTDKELSDL LDFSMMFPLP VTNGKGRPAS LAGAQFGGSG LEDRPSSGSW GSGDQSSSSF DPSRTFSEGT
ITF2        1                                                        EFGG VEDRSSSGSW GNGGHPSP-- --SRNYGDGT
HEB         1  MNPQQQRMAA IGTDKELSDL LDFSAMFSPP VNSGKTRPTT LGSSQFSGSG IDERGGTTSW GTSGQPSPSY DSSRGFTDSP
Da          1                                                                               MATSDDEP
MATH1       1
Atonal      1
Tal1        1
Twist       1
GbHLH1.4    1
BETA3       1

Cbf1        1
Pho4        1
Ino2p       1
Escl        1

R-Lc        1
R-S         1
B-Peru      1
Del         1
```

$\underline{C\text{-terminal section}}$

```
AP4       319  ELP
SREBP1a   639  LWVGRWLAGR AGGLQQDCAL RVDASASARD AALVYHKLHQ LHTMGKHTGG HLTATNLALS ALNLAECAGD AVSVATLAEI

Sim       255  MFMFRAKLDM KLIFFDARVS QLTGYEPQDL IEK-TLYQYI HAADIMAMRC SHQILLYKGQ VTTKYYRFLT KGGGWVWVQS
Arnt1     402  PEDQQLLRDS FQQVVKLKGQ VLSVMFRFRS KNQEWLWMRT SSFTFQNPYS DEIEYIICTN TNVKNSSQEP RPTLSNTIQR
AhR       280  IFRTKHKLDF TPIGCDAKGQ LILGYTEVEL CTRGSGYQFI HAADMLHCAE SHIRMIKTGE SGMTVFRLLA KNSRWRWVQS
Trh       370  MFVTRVNFDL RVAHCEPRVS DLLDYSPEDL VNK-SLYSLC HAEDANRLRK SHSDLIEKGQ VLTGYYRLMN KSGGYTWLQT

Hairy     310  QRVPMEQQPL SLVIKKQIKE EEQPWRPW
Dpn       336  VDVLSKHSFA GVFSTPPPTS AETSFNTSGS LNLSAGSHDS SGCSRPLAHL QQQQVSSTSG IAKRDREAEA ESSDCSLDEP
```

```
HFTE------  --SHSSLSSS  TFLGPGLGGK  SGERGAYASF  GRDAGVGGLT  QAGFLSGELA  LNSPGPLSPS  GMKGTSQYYP  SYSGSSRRRA  ADGSL---DT  QPKKVRKVPP
PY-DHMTSRD  LGSHDNLSP-  PFVNSRIQSK  T-ERGSYSSY  GRESNLQGCH  QQSLLGGDMD  MGNPGTL-SP  T-KPGSQYYQ  YSSNNPRRRP  LHSSAM--EV  QTKKVRKVPP
HYSDHLNDSR  LGAHEGLSPT  PFMNSNLMGK  TSERGSFSLY  SRDTGLPGC-  QSSLLRQDLG  LGSPAQLSSS  G-KPGTAYYS  FSATSSRRRP  LHDSAALDPL  QAKKVRKVPP
MHLYEVFQNC  FNKIANKQPT  GTVGADRGGG  GGYHSPYGSL  GVENGMYPSD  FNS-MHDTVN  GGNNRYANAS  TVDQYFDSAA  AGSGGAWCQP  QMSSANSYMG  QSAYQNSGPL


YVAAALRVKT  SLPRALHFLT  RFFLSSARQA  CLAQSGSVPP  AMQWLCHPVG  HRFFVDGDWS  VLSTPWESLY  SLAGNPVDPL  AQVTQLFREH  LLERALNCVT  QPNPSPGSAD

YATLVHNSRS  SREVFIVSVN  YVLSEREVKD  LVLN----EI  QTGVVKRE--  ------PISP  AAQAAQAAQ-  ----------  ----------  ----------  ----------
PQLGPTANLP  LEMGSGQLAP  RQQQQQTELD  MVPGRDGLAS  YNHSQVVQPV  TTTGPEHSKP  LEKSDGLFAQ  DRDPRFSEIY  HNINADQSKG  ISSSTVPATQ  QLFSQGNTFP
NARLIY--RN  GRPDYIIVTQ  RPLTDEEGRE  H-LQKRSTSL  PFMFATGEAV  LYEISSPFSP  IMDP------  ------LPIR  TKSNTSRKDW  APQSTPSKDS  FHPSSLMSAL
CATVVCSTKN  ADEQNIICVN  YVISNRENEN  MILDCCQLEP  SPDSIKHEEG  LGNDKSSGSP  GGDASGEGNS  HLSAGDMKLN  SPKTDSEGHS  HRGRGRSAAA  SHGSSMNSLT

SSKKFLAGAI  EKSSSAWRPW
```

N-terminal section

```
         MPLNVS FTNRNYDLDY DSVQPYFYC- DEEENFY--Q QQQQSELQPP APSEDIW---
       M PSCSTSTMPG MICKNPDLEF DSLQPCFY-- PDEDDFYFGG P------DST PPGEDIW---
             MDY DSYQHYFYDY DCGEDFY--- -------RST APSEDIW---
      QA AAAAMPLSAS LPSKNYDYDY DSVQPYFYFE EEEENFYLAA QQRGSELQPP APSEDIW---
       M LSCTTSTMPG MICKNSDLEF DSLKPCFY-- PEDDDIYFGG R------NST PPGEDIW---


GLPSSVYPPS -SGEDYGRDA TAYPSAKTPS STYPAPFYVA DGSLHPSAEL WSPPG--QAG FG---PMLGG GSSPLPLPPG
GLPSSVYAPS ASTADYNRDS PGYPSSKPAT STFPSSFFMQ DG-HHSSDPW SSSSGMNQPG YA---GMLGN S-SHIP----
GLPSSVYAPS PNSDDFNRES PSYPSPKPPT SMFASTFFMQ DGTHNSSDLW SSSNGMSQPG FG---GILGT STSHMS----
SGHSIDQQQQ QVHQADGLGM GGGGGGGVGA DGMHCP--VT TGLPPISSFR PTSGGIGGPG AGQQAPVNVN VNPPAVFNSP


MFASTFFMQ DGTHNSSDLW SSSNGMSQPG YG---GMLGG SSSHMS----


MAL SASRVQQAEE LLQRPAERQL MRSQLAAAAR SINWSYALFW SISDTQ-PGV
MAV SASRVQQAEE LLQRPAERQL MRSQLAAAAR SINWSYALFW SISDTQ-PGV
MAL SASPAQ--EE LLQ-PAGRPL -RKQLAAAAR SINWSYALFW SISSTQRPRV
MATG IQNQKIVPEN LRKQLAIAVR SIQWSYAIFW SNSVAQ-PGV
```

C-terminal section

```
GDKEFSDALG YLQLLNSCSD AAGAPAYSFS ISSSMATTTG VDPVAKWWAS LTAVVIHWLR RDEEAAERLC PLVEHLPRVL

---------- ---------- --AAQAAQAA QAAQAAQAAQ AAQAAHVAQA V---QAQVVV VPQQSVVVQP QCAGATGQP-
PTPRPAENFR NSGLAPPVTI VQPSASAGQM LAQISRHSNP TQGATPTWTP TTRSGFSAQQ VATQATAKTR TSQFGVGSFQ
IQQDESIYLC PPSSPAPLDS HFLMGSVSKC GSWQDSFAAA GSEAALKHEQ IGHAQDVNLA LSGGPSELFP DNKNNDLYNI
MIKDSPTPLG VEIDSGVLPT TVATPVPAAT PPVQSTKRKR KTKASQHAED ----QGQEQV ISEQPLPKLP TMEQRDQQPR
```

```
-----KKFEL LPTPPLSPSR RSGLCSPSYV AVTPFSLRGD NDGGGGSFST   ADQLEMVTEL LGGDMVNQSF ICDPDDETFI KN---IIIQD CMWSGFSAAA KL---VSEKL
-----KKFEL LPTPPLSPSR --GFAEHSSE PPS------ -------WV             TEMLL-ENEL WGSPA-EEDA FGLGGLGGLT PN--PVILQD CMWSGFSARE KLERAVSEKL
-----KKFEL VPSPPTSPPW GLGPGAGDPA PG------- ----------           ----IGPPEP WPGGCTGDEA ESRGHSKGWG RNYASIIRRD CMWSGFSARE RLERAVSDRL
-----KKFEL LPMPPLSPSR RSSLAAASCF P-------- -------ST            ADQLEMVTEL LGGDMVNQSF ICDPDDESFV KS---IIIQD CMWSGFSAAA KLEKVVSEKL
-----KKFEL LPTPRLSPGR --ALAEDSLE PAN------ -------WA            TEMLLPEADL WSNPAEEEDI FGLKGLSGSS SN--PVVLQD CMWSGFSSRE KPETVVSEKL

                       EFRGG VTAGARAPAR GSVTAEAAAR AGRGSGRGAD GGREGRTGRA SLVARGRSRP GAGGGHSLRA RHPNLRQVAG

                                                                        M DEPPFSEAAL EQALGEPCDL DAALLTDIED MLQLINNQDS DFPGLFDPPY

SGPVGSSGSS STFGGLHQHE RMGYQLH--- GAEVNGGLPS ASSF--SSAP   GATYGGVSSH TPPVSGADSL LGSRGTTAGS S---GDALGK ALASIYSPDH SSNNFSSSPS
-------QS SSYCSLHPHE RLSYPSH--S SADINSSLPP MSTFHRSGT-             -NHYST-SSC TPPANGTDSI MANRGSGAAG SSQTGDALGK ALASIYSSDH TNNSFSSNPS
-------QS SSYGNLHSHD RLSYPPHSVS PTDINTSLPP MSSFHRGSTS             SSPYVA-ASH TPPINGSDSI LGTRG-NAAG SSQTGDALGK ALASIYSPDH TSSSFPSNPS
QAHNHNHTVQ AQHSALSTAG PLGHHSLNHT PHAHSHTLPL PHALPHGHTL   PHPHHSQQ-N SPAVQSSDAF SGAGASVKVA GAGNSSAAAL RQQMYMPADQ SISSFGSNPS

         M SSSEIYRYYY KTSEDLQGFK TAAAEPYFNP MAAYNPGVTH   ------YQFN GNTLASSSNY LSANGFIS-- ---------- -----FEQAS SDGWISSSP-

        MM SARSVSPKVL LDISYKPTLP NIMELQNNVI KLIQVEQQAY MHSGYQLQHQ QQHLHSHQHH QQHHQQQHAQ YAPLPSEYAA
--------QS GSYGSLHTHD RLSYPPHSVS PTDINASLPP MSSFHRGSTS   SSPYVA-ASH TPPVNGSENI LGNRG-NGAG GSQTGDALGK ALASIYSPDH TSSSFPSNPS

                      MSSYALPSMQ PTPTSSIPLR QMSQPTTSAP SNSASSTPYS PQQVPLTHNS YPLSTPSSFQ HGQTRLPPIN CLAEPFNRPQ PWHSNSAAPA
LTWTDGFYNG EVKTRKISNS VELTSDQLVM QRSDQLRELY EALLSGEGDR   RAAPARPAGS LSPEDLGDTE WYYVVSMTYA FRPGQGLPGR SFASDEHVWL CNAHLAGSKA
LTWTDGFYNG EVKTRKISNS VELTSDQLVM QRSDQLRELY EALLSGEGDR   RAAPARPAGS LSPEDLGDTE WYYVVSMTYA FRPGQGLPGR SFASDEHVWL CNAHLAGSKA
LTWTDGFYNG EVKTRKISHS VELTADQLLM QRSEQLRELY EALRSGECDR   RG--ARPVGS LSPEDLGDTE WYYVICMTYA FLPGQGLPGR SSASNEHVWL CNAHLAGSKD
LEWGDGFYNG DIKTRKTVQS VELNQDQLGL QRSDQLRELY ESLSLGETNT   QA--KRPTAA LSPEDLTDAE WFFLVCMSFI FNIGQGLPGR TLARNQAVWL CNAHRADTKV

QESERPLPRA ALHSFKAARA LLGCAKAESG PASLTICEKA SGYLQDSLAT   TPASSSIDKA VQLFLCDLLL VVRTSLWRQQ QPPAPAPAAQ GASSRPQASA LELRGFQRDL
-----VGPGT PVSLALSASP KLDPYFEPEL PLQPAVTP-- -VPPTNNSSS           SSNNNNGVWH HHHVQQQQQS GSMDHDSLSY TQLYPP---- --LNDLVVSS SSSV------
TPSSFSSMSL PGAPTASPGA AAYPSLTNRG SNFAPETGQT AGQFQTRTAE   GVGVWPQWQG QQPHHRSSSS EQHVQQPPAQ QPGQPEVFQE MLSMLGDQSN SYNNEEFPDL
MRNLGIDFED IRSMQNEEFF RTDSTAAGEV DFKDIDITDE ILTYVQDSLN   NSTLMNSACQ QQPVTQHLSC MLQERLQLEQ QQQLQQPPPQ ALEPQQQLCQ MVCPQQDLGP
SRLPSIVDEQ PSSAADSAVK DLEQAMSKHL TPTGVGPGVF YGDQQTGPLP   ADSLLKQQQQ QQQLDPNEKS STIQWIGTPY QQPPAPMPAT TPTGVGPGVF YGDQQTGPLP
```

N-terminal section

```
ASYQAARKDS  GSP--NPARG  HSVCST----  -------SSL  YLQDLSAAAS  ECIDPSVVFP  YPLNDSSS--  ----PKSCAS  QDSSAFSPSS
QHGRGPPTAG  STAQSPGAGA  ASPAGRGHGG  AAGAGRAGAA  LPAELAHPAA  ECVDPAVVFP  FPVNKREPAP  VPAAPASAPA  AGPAVASGAG
A--------  --------P   GAPRGNPPKA  SAAPDCTPSL  ----------  EAGNPAPAAP  CPL-------  ----------  ----------
ATYQASRQEG  GPA--AASRP  GPPPSGPPPP  PAGPAASAGL  YLHDLGAAAA  DCIDPSVVFP  YPLSERAP--  ----RAAPPG  ANPAAL----
PGGCGSLAVG  AGTLVPGAAA  ATSAGHARSG  TAGVGRRKAA  WLTELSHLDS  ECVDSAVI--  FPANKRESMP  VATIPASAGA  A---------
                                                                                  MKGQQKTAET  EEGTVQIQEG

AGARAADRLT  FRAREPAPAA  TMASRIGLRM  QLMREQAQQE  EQRERMQQQA  VMHYMQQQQQ  QQQQQLGGPP  TPAINTPVHF  QSPPPVPGEV

                                                                                              MLEMLEYSH
AGSGAGGTDP  ASPDTSSPGS  LSPPPATLSS  SLEAFLSGPQ  AAPSPLSPPQ  PAPTPLKMYP  SMPAFSPGPG  IKEESVPLSI  LQTPTPQPLP

TPVGSPQGL-  ----------  --AGTSQWPR  AGAPGALSPS  YDGGLHGL--  ----------  ------- --  --QSKIED--  -HLDEAIHVL
TPVGSPPSLS  ----------  --AGTAVWSR  NGGQASSSPN  YEGPLHSL--  ----------  -------     --QSRIEDRL  ERLDDAIHVL
TPVGSPSPL-  ----------  --TGTSQWPR  PGGQAPSSPS  YENSLHSL--  ----------  ----------  --QSRMEDRL  DRLDDAIHVL
TPVNSPPPLT  QSVVGGGGEP  SVSGGSGWGH  SVLNGGPSSS  YASEMVPV--  ----------  -SSLHTMASV  FQGVRMEE--  -RLDDALNVL

----------  ----------  ----ASHRSE  SPEYVDLNTM  YNGGCNNMAQ  NQQYGMI---  ----------  -----MEQSV  VSTAPAIPV-

YGITELEDTD  YNIPSNEVLS  TSSNQSAQSA  SLELNNNNTS  SNTNSSGNNP  SGFDGQASSG  SSWNEHGKRA  RSSGDYDCQT  GGSLVMQPEH
TPVGSPSPL-  ----------  --TGASQWSR  SGGQAPSSPN  YENSLHSLKN  RVEQQLHEHL  QDAMSFLKDV  CEQSRMEDRL  DRLDDAIHVL
                                                                      MAMERGLHL   GAAAASEDDL  FLHKSLGAST

                                                          MN  SLANNNKLST  EDEEIHSARK  RGYNEEQNYS
                                              M  GRTTSEGIHG  FVDDLEPKSS  ILDKVGDFIT  VNTKRHDGRE  DFNEQNDELN
                                                 MQQATGN    ELLGILDLDN  DIDFETAYQM  LSSNFDDQMS
SSSPTSATLS  ----------  -TAAHPVHTN  AAQVAGSSSS  YVYSVPP---  ----------  ----------  ------TNST  TSQASAKHSA

FPRALLAKSA  SIQSILCIPV  MGGVLELGTT  DTVPEAPDLV  SRATAAFWEP  QC------PS  --SSPSGRAN  ETGEAAADDG  TFAFEELDH-
FPRALLAKSA  SIQSILCIPV  MGGVLELGTT  DTVPEAPDLV  SRATAAFWEP  QCPTYSEEPS  --SSPSGRAN  ETGEAAADDG  TFAFEELDH-
FPRALLAKSA  SIQTIVCIPL  MGGVLELGTT  DKVPEDPDLV  SRATVAFWEP  QCPTYSKEPS  --SNPS--AY  ETGEAAY---  IVVLEDLDH-
FSRSLLAKSA  SIQTVVCFPY  SEGVVELGAT  ELVPEDLNLI  QHIKTSFLDS  P-ATVPKIPN  YVSNSITNNN  DLICEALEHA  NIPENDLDQL
```

C-terminal section

```
SSLRRLAQSF  RPAMRRVFLH  EATARLMAGA  SPTRTHQLLD  RSLRRRAGPG  GKGGAVAELE  PRPTRREHAE  ALLLASCYLP  PGFLSAPGQR
----------  -----GGGTA  SSAGGGSS--  ------ASAS  SSGVYSTEMQ  YPDTTTGNLY  YNNNNHYYYD  YDATVDVATS  MIR-------
TMFPPPFSE-  ----------
KHTQINGTF-  -----ASWNP  TPPVSFNCPQ  QELKHYQLFS  SLQGTAQEFP  YKPEVDSVPY  TQNFAPCN--  -QPLLPEHSK  SVQLDFPGRD
ALLRQLYANR  ESVIRATARQ  TPPGSESSYE  NQYLQLHSAA  SGGHPGGQKT  SADAFTNLVS  TYGGYHSSID  YHNAMTPPSS  VSPRDSNQPG
```

```
DSLLSSTESS PQGSPEPLVL HEETPPTTSS                                                              250   c-Myc
IAAPAGAPGV APPRPGGRQT SGGDHKALST                                                              254   N-Myc
---------- ----------  --GEPKTQAC                                                             156   L-Myc
---------- ---------L GVDTPPTTSS                                                              233   v-Myc
---------- ---------I SLGDHQGLSS                                                              226   S-Myc
AVATGEDPTS VAIASIQSAA TFPDPNVKYV                                                               50   USF1
                      EFHSWRRHV                                                                 9   USF2
LKVQSYLENP TSYHLQQSQH QKVREYLSET                                                              195   TFEB
                      MT                                                                        2   TFEC
YQVQTHLENP TKYHIQQAQR HQVKQYLSTT                                                               39   Mi
GALLPQSFPA PAPPQFSSTP VLGYPSPPGG                                                              171   SREBP1a

RSH------- AVGTA----- --GDMHTLL-                                                              419   E12
RNH------- AVGPSTAMPG GHGDMHGIIG                                                              378   ITF2
RNH------- AVGPSTSLPA GHSDIHSLLG                                                              437   HEB
RNHCEPEMLA GVNQSLASID NIDALTSFVP                                                              409   Da
           MSRLLH AEEWAEVKEL                                                                   16   MATH1
---------- ---------- ----------                                                             124   Atonal
MTERPPSEA ARSDPQLEGR DAAEASMAPP                                                                29   Tal1
KKLIHQQQQ QQQHQQQIYV DYLPTTVDEV                                                               202   Twist
RNH------- AVGPSTSLSG GHGDIHSLLG                                                              242   GbHLH1.4
AKRLEAAFRS TPPGMDLSLA PPPRERPASS                                                               59   BETA3

EARKKQRDQG LLSQESNDGN IDSALLSEGA                                                               62   Cbf1
SQENHNSSEN GNENENEQDS LALDDLDRAF                                                               81   Pho4
AHIHENTFSA TSPPLLTHEL GIIPNVATVQ                                                               67   Ino2p
VPHRSSQF-- ---QSTTLTP STTDSSSTDV                                                              165   Esc1

---------- -NNGMDDIEA ---MTAAGG-                                                              258   R-Lc
---------- -NNGM-DIEA ---MTAAGG-                                                              263   R-S
---------- -NA--MDMET ---VTAAAGR                                                              253   B-Peru
LNCPDTNICS PDNSLDDFAD NLLIDESNLA                                                              270   Del


VGMLAEAART LEKLGDRRLL HDCQQMLMRL GGGTTVTSS-                                                    321   AP4

---PFSANSN SCSSSSESER -QLSTGNASI VNETSPSQTT YSDLSHNFEL SYFSDNSSQQ HQHQQQQQHL MEQQHLQYQY ATW   1147   SREBP1a

FEPSLHPTTS NLDFVS---C LQVPENQSHG INSQSAMVSP QAYYAG--AM SMYQCQPGPQ RTPVDQTQYS SEIPGSQAFL SKVQSRGIFN ETYSS   673   Sim
KAAPVLASNG GYDYAPDPLR GQYATSSGDV VPATLPLKPQ ASYTATMHPS GSTTTEGGVT YSNLDQPQYF APHSSFHLYH KGSPASGWYS TPS     789   Arnt1
                                                                                             815   AhR
                                                                                             925   Trh

                                                                                             337   Hairy
                                                                                             435   Dpn
```